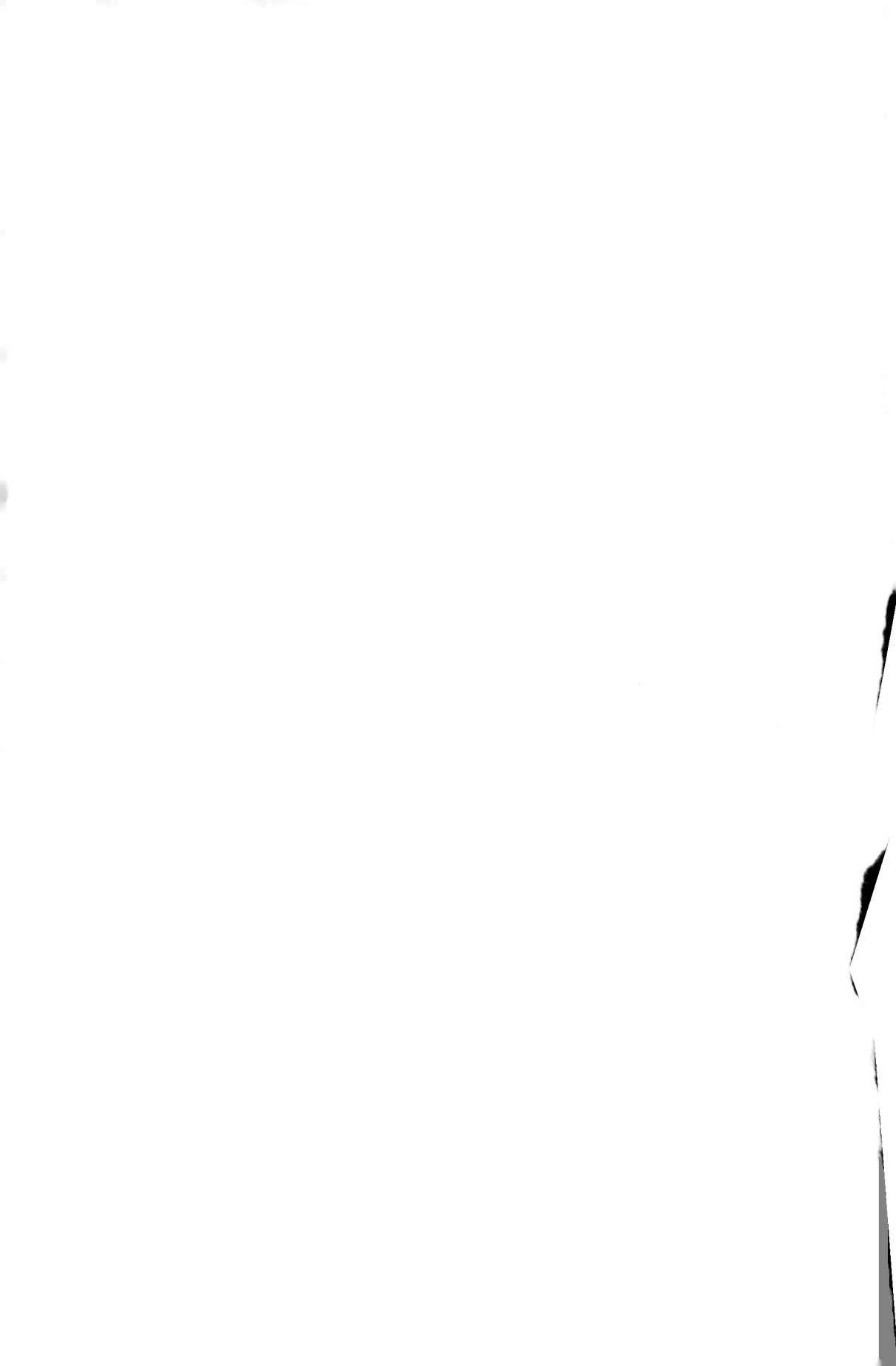

Acute Respiratory Distress Syndrome (ARDS): Personalized Therapies and Beyond

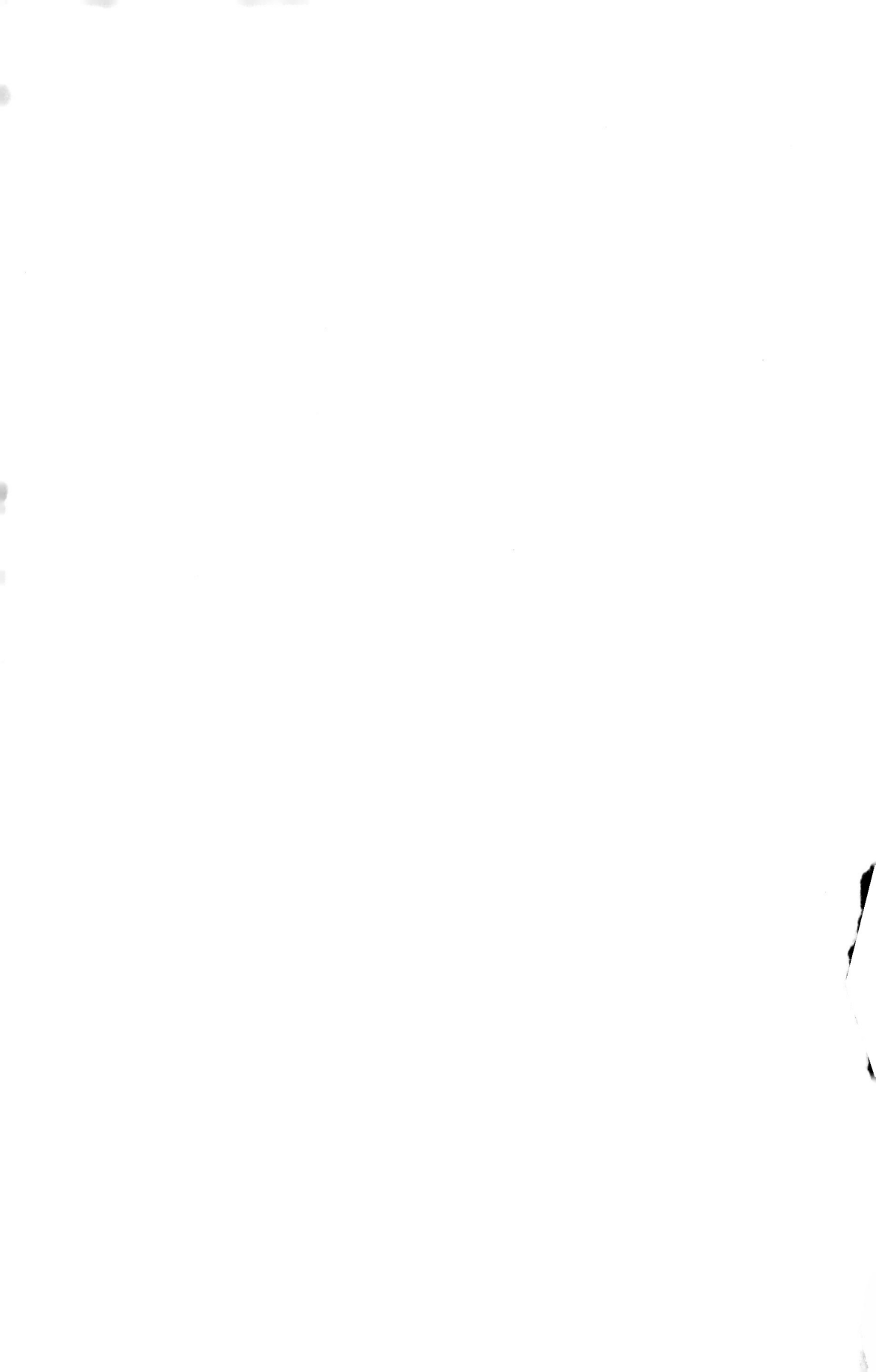

Acute Respiratory Distress Syndrome (ARDS): Personalized Therapies and Beyond

Topic Editors

Denise Battaglini
Paolo Pelosi

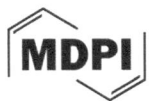

Basel • Beijing • Wuhan • Barcelona • Belgrade • Novi Sad • Cluj • Manchester

Topic Editors
Denise Battaglini
University of Genoa
Genoa
Italy

Paolo Pelosi
University of Genoa
Genoa
Italy

Editorial Office
MDPI AG
Grosspeteranlage 5
4052 Basel, Switzerland

This is a reprint of the Topic, published open access by the journals *Journal of Clinical Medicine* (ISSN 2077-0383), *Diagnostics* (ISSN 2075-4418) and *Advances in Respiratory Medicine* (ISSN 2543-6031), freely accessible at: https://www.mdpi.com/topics/4HGSMU0Y3W.

For citation purposes, cite each article independently as indicated on the article page online and as indicated below:

Lastname, A.A.; Lastname, B.B. Article Title. *Journal Name* **Year**, *Volume Number*, Page Range.

ISBN 978-3-7258-2837-1 (Hbk)
ISBN 978-3-7258-2838-8 (PDF)
https://doi.org/10.3390/books978-3-7258-2838-8

© 2024 by the authors. Articles in this book are Open Access and distributed under the Creative Commons Attribution (CC BY) license. The book as a whole is distributed by MDPI under the terms and conditions of the Creative Commons Attribution-NonCommercial-NoDerivs (CC BY-NC-ND) license (https://creativecommons.org/licenses/by-nc-nd/4.0/).

Contents

Mark R. Lutz, Jacob Charlamb, Joshua R. Kenna, Abigail Smith, Stephen J. Glatt, Joaquin D. Araos, et al.
Inconsistent Methods Used to Set Airway Pressure Release Ventilation in Acute Respiratory Distress Syndrome: A Systematic Review and Meta-Regression Analysis
Reprinted from: *J. Clin. Med.* **2024**, *13*, 2690, https://doi.org/10.3390/jcm13092690 1

Ida Giorgia Iavarone, Lou'i Al-Husinat, Jorge Luis Vélez-Páez, Chiara Robba, Pedro Leme Silva, Patricia R. M. Rocco and Denise Battaglini
Management of Neuromuscular Blocking Agents in Critically Ill Patients with Lung Diseases
Reprinted from: *J. Clin. Med.* **2024**, *13*, 1182, https://doi.org/10.3390/jcm13041182 16

Davide Chiumello, Silvia Coppola, Giulia Catozzi, Fiammetta Danzo, Pierachille Santus and Dejan Radovanovic
Lung Imaging and Artificial Intelligence in ARDS
Reprinted from: *J. Clin. Med.* **2024**, *13*, 305, https://doi.org/10.3390/jcm13020305 33

Shin-Hwar Wu, Chew-Teng Kor, Shu-Hua Chi and Chun-Yu Li
Categorizing Acute Respiratory Distress Syndrome with Different Severities by Oxygen Saturation Index
Reprinted from: *Diagnostics* **2024**, *14*, 37, https://doi.org/10.3390/diagnostics14010037 53

Martina Piluso, Clarissa Ferrari, Silvia Pagani, Pierfranco Usai, Stefania Raschi, Luca Parachini, et al.
COVID-19 Acute Respiratory Distress Syndrome: Treatment with Helmet CPAP in Respiratory Intermediate Care Unit by Pulmonologists in the Three Italian Pandemic Waves
Reprinted from: *Adv. Respir. Med.* **2023**, *91*, 30, https://doi.org/10.3390/arm91050030 65

Athiwat Tripipitsiriwat, Orawan Suppapueng, David M. P. van Meenen, Frederique Paulus, Markus W. Hollmann, Chaisith Sivakorn and Marcus J. Schultz
Epidemiology, Ventilation Management and Outcomes of COPD Patients Receiving Invasive Ventilation for COVID-19—Insights from PRoVENT-COVID
Reprinted from: *J. Clin. Med.* **2023**, *12*, 5783, https://doi.org/10.3390/jcm12185783 79

Stany Sandrio, Manfred Thiel and Joerg Krebs
The Outcome Relevance of Pre-ECMO Liver Impairment in Adults with Acute Respiratory Distress Syndrome
Reprinted from: *J. Clin. Med.* **2023**, *12*, 4860, https://doi.org/10.3390/jcm12144860 90

Laura Textoris, Ines Gragueb-Chatti, Florence Daviet, Sabine Valera, Céline Sanz, Laurent Papazian, et al.
Response to Prone Position in COVID-19 and Non-COVID-19 Patients with Severe ARDS Supported by vvECMO
Reprinted from: *J. Clin. Med.* **2023**, *12*, 3918, https://doi.org/10.3390/jcm12123918 108

Konrad Peukert, Andrea Sauer, Benjamin Seeliger, Caroline Feuerborn, Mario Fox, Susanne Schulz, et al.
Increased Alveolar Epithelial Damage Markers and Inflammasome-Regulated Cytokines Are Associated with Pulmonary Superinfection in ARDS
Reprinted from: *J. Clin. Med.* **2023**, *12*, 3649, https://doi.org/10.3390/jcm12113649 120

Xiaojun Pan, Jiao Liu, Sheng Zhang, Sisi Huang, Limin Chen, Xuan Shen and Dechang Chen
Application of Neuromuscular Blockers in Patients with ARDS in ICU: A Retrospective Study Based on the MIMIC-III Database
Reprinted from: *J. Clin. Med.* **2023**, *12*, 1878, https://doi.org/10.3390/jcm12051878 . . . . **130**

Jorge Luis Vélez-Páez, Paolo Pelosi, Denise Battaglini and Ivan Best
Biological Markers to Predict Outcome in Mechanically Ventilated Patients with Severe COVID-19 Living at High Altitude
Reprinted from: *J. Clin. Med.* **2023**, *12*, 644, https://doi.org/10.3390/jcm12020644 . . . . **142**

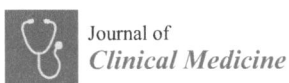

Systematic Review

Inconsistent Methods Used to Set Airway Pressure Release Ventilation in Acute Respiratory Distress Syndrome: A Systematic Review and Meta-Regression Analysis

Mark R. Lutz [1,†], Jacob Charlamb [1,†], Joshua R. Kenna [1,†], Abigail Smith [2], Stephen J. Glatt [3,4,5], Joaquin D. Araos [6], Penny L. Andrews [7], Nader M. Habashi [7], Gary F. Nieman [1,*,‡] and Auyon J. Ghosh [8,‡]

1. Department of Surgery, SUNY Upstate Medical University, Syracuse, NY 13210, USA; charlaja@upstate.edu (J.C.); kennajo@upstate.edu (J.R.K.)
2. Health Sciences Library, SUNY Upstate Medical University, Syracuse, NY 13210, USA; smithab@upstate.edu
3. Department of Psychiatry and Behavioral Sciences, SUNY Upstate Medical University, Syracuse, NY 13210, USA
4. Department of Neuroscience and Physiology, SUNY Upstate Medical University, Syracuse, NY 13210, USA
5. Department of Public Health and Preventive Medicine, SUNY Upstate Medical University, Syracuse, NY 13210, USA
6. Department of Clinical Sciences, College of Veterinary Medicine, Cornell University, Ithaca, NY 14853, USA; jda246@cornell.edu
7. Department of Critical Care, R Adams Cowley Shock Trauma Center, Baltimore, MD 21201, USA
8. Division of Pulmonary, Critical Care, and Sleep Medicine, SUNY Upstate Medical University, Syracuse, NY 13210, USA; ghosha@upstate.edu
* Correspondence: niemang@upstate.edu; Tel.: +1-315-464-4508
† These authors contributed equally to this work.
‡ These authors jointly supervised this study and are co-senior authors.

Abstract: Background: Airway pressure release ventilation (APRV) is a protective mechanical ventilation mode for patients with acute respiratory distress syndrome (ARDS) that theoretically may reduce ventilator-induced lung injury (VILI) and ARDS-related mortality. However, there is no standard method to set and adjust the APRV mode shown to be optimal. Therefore, we performed a meta-regression analysis to evaluate how the four individual APRV settings impacted the outcome in these patients. **Methods:** Studies investigating the use of the APRV mode for ARDS patients were searched from electronic databases. We tested individual settings, including (1) high airway pressure (P_{High}); (2) low airway pressure (P_{Low}); (3) time at high airway pressure (T_{High}); and (4) time at low pressure (T_{Low}) for association with PaO_2/FiO_2 ratio and ICU length of stay. **Results:** There was no significant difference in PaO_2/FiO_2 ratio between the groups in any of the four settings (P_{High} difference −12.0 [95% CI −100.4, 86.4]; P_{Low} difference 54.3 [95% CI −52.6, 161.1]; T_{Low} difference −27.19 [95% CI −127.0, 72.6]; T_{High} difference −51.4 [95% CI −170.3, 67.5]). There was high heterogeneity across all parameters (P_{hHgh} I^2 = 99.46%, P_{Low} I^2 = 99.16%, T_{Low} I^2 = 99.31%, T_{High} I^2 = 99.29%). **Conclusions:** None of the four individual APRV settings independently were associated with differences in outcome. A holistic approach, analyzing all settings in combination, may improve APRV efficacy since it is known that small differences in ventilator settings can significantly alter mortality. Future clinical trials should set and adjust APRV based on the best current scientific evidence available.

Keywords: ARDS; VILI; APRV

1. Introduction

Acute respiratory distress syndrome (ARDS) is a heterogeneous disorder that arises from a variety of pulmonary and extrapulmonary insults and is uniformly associated with high mortality [1,2]. Current treatment is supportive, including mechanical ventilation, prone positioning, and extracorporeal membrane oxygenation [3]. Despite several advances in the role of mechanical ventilation in the mitigation of lung injury, incorrectly adjusted ventilator settings can lead to unintended ventilator-induced lung injury (VILI), which has been shown to increase mortality in ARDS [4].

Repetitive alveolar collapse and expansion (RACE) is the primary cause of atelectrauma, which, along with volutrauma, comprise the two main mechanical mechanisms of VILI [4,5]. Low tidal volume ventilation (LTVV) has been shown to reduce mortality in ARDS, ostensibly by limiting volutrauma in the remaining normal tissue. However, even after the application of LTVV, mortality from ARDS remains unacceptably high [6–8]. Therefore, there is a need for novel protective modes of ventilation that can ameliorate both volutrauma and atelectrauma [NO_PRINTED_FORM].

Airway pressure release ventilation (APRV) is a form of mechanical ventilation that has been shown to have a superior physiologic profile compared to conventional LTVV in pre-clinical studies [9]. Specifically, a time-controlled adaptive ventilation protocol for setting the APRV mode, which is personalized based on changes in respiratory system compliance (C_{RS}), has several important plausible mechanisms to reduce the propagation of lung injury [10]. These mechanisms include: (i) a brief expiratory time personalized to lung pathophysiology (C_{RS}) that stabilizes lung tissue via pressure and time, and (ii) the extended inspiratory time that leads to the recruitment of small volumes of lung tissue with each breath. In the first mechanism, the lung does not have time to fully depressurize, generating a time-controlled PEEP. In the second mechanism, lung tissue is gradually "ratcheted" open over time, while the brief expiratory time prevents the newly opened lung tissue from re-collapsing. These elements of the physiologic rationale for APRV stem, in part, from the literature supporting the use of higher vs. lower positive end-expiratory pressure (PEEP) strategies [11,12]. Accordingly, recent practice guidelines, supported by the American Thoracic Society (ATS), suggest using higher PEEP in moderate to severe ARDS [13]. Given the inverse ratio nature of APRV, PEEP tends to be lower, but the resulting increase in mean airway pressure approximates the goal of higher PEEP in normal ratio ventilation strategies. However, clinical trials have demonstrated mixed results, with a recent meta-analysis comparing APRV, using multiple protocols to set the mode, to LTVV, finding that APRV was associated with overall improved outcomes, albeit with relatively poor study quality [14].

One of the factors that contribute to the variability in APRV vs. LTVV clinical trials may be the lack of an optimal or even standardized protocol for initiating and adjusting APRV settings on a mechanical ventilator. We therefore sought to examine the effect of the four main APRV settings on outcomes in ARDS. The objectives of our study were to (i) identify if there were studies that used similar methods to set APRV and, if so, (ii) whether there is a method of setting APRV that was associated with an improvement in ARDS-related outcomes. We analyzed the four settings used to adjust APRV, including the highest level of pressure applied to the respiratory system (P_{high}), the lowest level of pressure applied to the respiratory system (P_{low}), and the time spent at each pressure setting (T_{high} and T_{low}, respectively). We hypothesized that personalizing the four settings to lung pathophysiology (C_{RS}) would be associated with reduced mortality and length of stay and improved oxygenation.

2. Methods

2.1. Search Strategy

This systematic review and meta-regression is reported according to the Preferred Reporting for Items for Systematic Reviews and Meta-analyses (PRISMA) guidelines. A health sciences librarian with experience in systematic reviews and literature searching developed the search strategies in consultation with the research team. Systematic search queries related to ARDS and APRV using a combination of keywords and controlled vocabulary (where available) were conducted in PubMed, Embase, Scopus, Web of Science Core Collection, and CENTRAL. The included databases are standard among medical systematic reviews and meta-analyses, and we chose not to include other, specialty-specific databases that are not representative of critical care to avoid additional publication biases. All databases and registers were searched from inception to 12 October 2023. There were no search restrictions on language, publication status, or outcomes. The details of all the search strategies, including specific terms and Boolean operators, can be found in Supplementary Materials File S1. The search identified 2131 records. Duplicates were removed using EndNote 20 (Endnote, Clarivate, available at www.endnote.com, accessd on 1 January 2023). The remaining 1755 records were uploaded into Covidence (Covidence, Veritas Health Innovation, Melbourne, Australia; available at ww.covidence.org) for title and abstract screening.

2.2. Study Inclusion Criteria and Outcomes Measured

We included all experimental studies that used APRV as a mode of ventilation within their study. All patients were adults (age $\geq$18 years) who underwent mechanical ventilation. We excluded case reports, literature reviews, and conference proceedings as they generally lacked the data specificity necessary for our intended analyses. There were no search restrictions on language, publication status, or outcomes. All studies were conducted on humans.

We chose to categorize ventilator settings into groups based on how each setting impacts lung physiology and their alignment with the preponderance of the basic science literature that has been shown to be lung-protective [10,15]. Specifically, we compared P_{high} set by plateau pressure vs. P_{high} not set by plateau pressure, P_{low} set to 0 vs. P_{low} not set to 0, T_{low} set to 50–75% of peak expiratory flow rate vs. T_{low} not set to 50–75% of peak expiratory flow rate, and T_{high} set based on $PaCO_2$ vs. T_{high} set arbitrarily.

The primary outcomes of this study were mortality (percentage of patients surviving in the APRV group), P/F ratio (PaO_2/FiO_2), number of ventilator-free days, static lung compliance, and intensive care unit length of stay (LOS).

2.3. Data Extraction and Quality Assessment

All procedures were independently reviewed by three authors (JC, JK, ML) in accordance with the prespecified inclusion criteria. The general information extracted included study and subject characteristics (age, gender, etiology, study design, aim of study, inclusion and exclusion criteria, method of recruitment, ventilator mode, population size, and population characteristics), specific APRV settings, including the time at high pressure, the time at low pressure, the high pressure, and the low pressure (T_{high}, T_{low}, P_{high}, P_{low}), and outcome results. Data were recorded as either percentage or mean and standard deviation. The Cochrane Risk of Bias tool was used for the quality assessments. Any disagreements regarding data collection, data extraction, and quality assessment were resolved by consensus.

2.4. Statistical Analysis

Data extracted from the individual studies are presented as published (e.g., means and standard deviations) where available; when standard deviation (SD) was unavailable, we estimated the standard deviation (SD) from the range using a previously published method [16]. Between-study heterogeneity was assessed using the Cochran Q-test and I-squared test. We performed mixed-effects meta-regression to assess the association of APRV setting strategy and clinical outcomes of interest, using the maximum likelihood (ML) estimator for mixed-effect modeling. We chose to perform a meta-regression analysis as opposed to a traditional meta-analysis given the limitations of the meta-analysis framework. Specifically, a meta-analysis does not allow for a comparison of outcomes within a single arm (i.e., P_{low} set to 0 vs. not set to 0) as opposed to a comparison of outcomes between an intervention and a control (i.e., P_{low} set to 0 vs. LTVV). To maximize statistical power, we compared strategies in individual ventilator setting parameters (i.e., P_{high}, P_{low}, T_{low}, T_{high}) instead of groups of settings, because, given there is no standardized protocol and a limited number of studies available, there were several combinations of ventilator settings presented as APRV in individual studies. We similarly chose not to perform sub-group analyses due to the small number of studies across parameter combinations, which could limit the validity and interpretability of any tests of interaction between subgroups. We defined statistical significance as a 2-sided alpha < 0.5. Statistical analysis was performed using the *metafor* R package in R (version 4.3.2, The R Foundation for Statistical Computation, Vienna, Austria).

3. Results
3.1. Study Selection and Characteristics

We identified 2,131 records from a systematic search of the included databases (PubMed $n = 1248$, Embase $n = 370$, Scopus $n = 192$, Web of Science $n = 321$, CENTRAL $n = 43$). In total, 419 duplicative records were excluded. After screening 1755 titles and abstracts, 1432 records were excluded for irrelevance. After full-text assessment, 20 studies were included in our data extraction and subsequent analysis (Figure 1). The majority of studies excluded at full-text assessment ($n = 303$) were for incorrect study design (i.e., the study was not a RCT or cohort study), incorrect publication type (i.e., conference proceeding, and/or incomplete data). The remaining excluded studies were for languages other than English, incorrect outcomes (i.e., did not include any of the outcomes of interest), incorrect patient population or pediatric population, incorrect intervention, incorrect clinical setting, or repeat study.

We included 9 cohort studies, 10 randomized controlled trials, and one cross-over study (Table 1) [17–36]. The average number of participants from randomized controlled trials was 37 while the average number of participants from cohort studies was 22. The included studies were published between 1994 and 2022. Six of the included studies were conducted in the United States. The other studies were performed in Australia, China, Egypt, Finland, Germany, India, Japan, Mexico, and Turkey. The sample sizes ranged from 6 to 71, for a total of 538 study participants.

Table 1. Characteristics from included studies.

Study	Design	Sample Size of APRV Group	T_{low} (%)	P_{low} Set to 0	T_{high} Adjusted for PCO_2	P_{high} Set Based on P_{plat}	Outcomes
Momtaz 2022 [36]	RCT	-	75	No	No	Yes	1
Li 2023 [17]	Cohort study	12	50–75	Yes	Yes	Yes	1,2
Varpula 2004 [18]	RCT	30	Arbitrary	No	No	No	1, 2, 3
Kaplan 2001 [19]	Cohort study	12	Arbitrary	-	No	-	2
Ibrahim 2022 [20]	RCT	30	Arbitrary	Yes	No	No	1, 4, 5
Wrigge 2001 [21]	Cohort study	14	Arbitrary	No	No	No	2
Lim 2016 [22]	Cohort study	50	Arbitrary	No	No	No	1, 2, 5
Li 2016 [23]	RCT	26	Arbitrary	Yes	No	No	1, 2, 3, 4, 5
Zhou 2017 [24]	RCT	71	50–75	No	Yes	Yes	1, 2, 3, 5
Marik 2009 [25]	Cohort study	22	Arbitrary	No	No	Yes	1, 2
Kucuk 2022 [26]	RCT	32	Arbitrary	Yes	No	Yes	1, 2, 3, 5
Daoud 2013 [27]	Cohort study	6	50–75	Yes	No	Yes	2
Yoshida 2009 [28]	Cohort study	9	50–75	Yes	No	No	2
Manjunath 2021 [29]	RCT	30	Arbitrary	Yes	No	No	2, 4, 5
Sydow 1994 [30]	Cross-over study	18	Arbitrary	No	No	No	1
Liu 2009 [31]	Cohort study	19	Arbitrary	Yes	No	No	1, 2, 5
Dart 2005 [32]	Cohort study	46	Arbitrary	Yes	Yes	No	1, 2, 3
Hirshberg 2018 [34]	RCT	35	50–75	Yes	Yes	No	1, 2, 3, 5
Maxwell 2010 [33]	Cohort study	31	Arbitrary	Yes	No	Yes	1, 5
Ibarra-Estrada 2022 [35]	RCT	45	50–75	Yes	No	Yes	1, 2, 3, 5

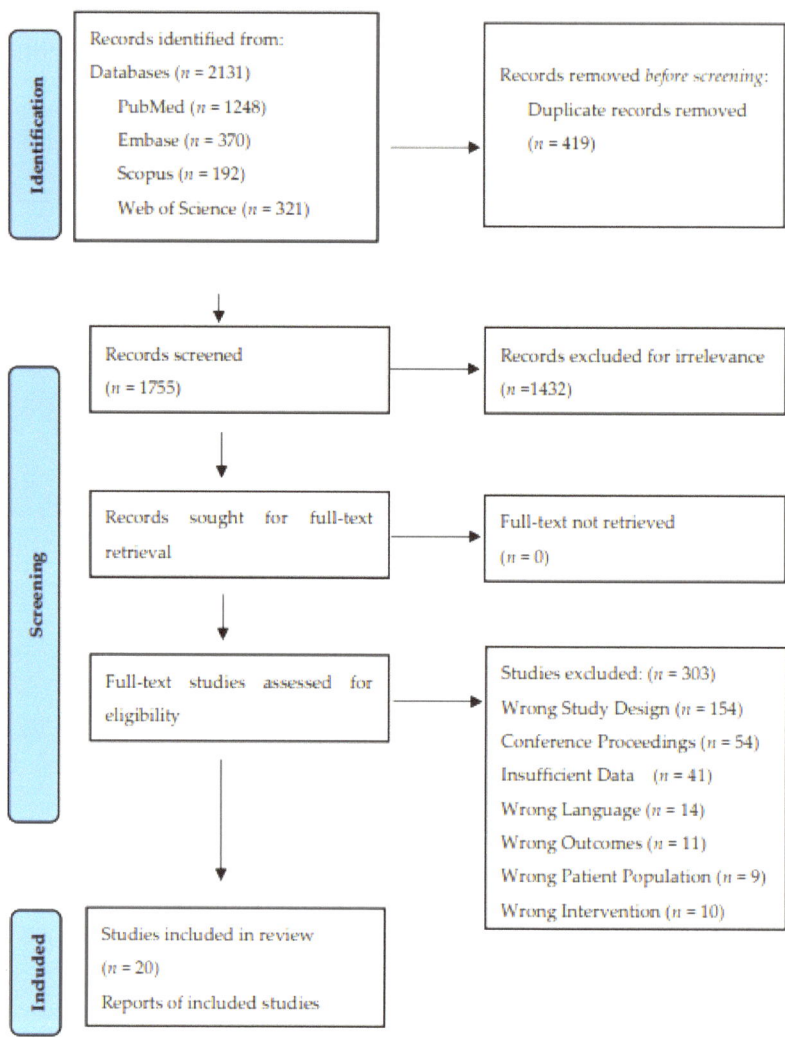

Figure 1. PRISMA flowchart.

3.2. Bias and Study Quality Assessment

Table 2 documents the quality assessment of the included studies as determined through the Cochrane Risk of Bias tool. While most of the studies employed adequate random sequence generation and allocation concealment, the overwhelming majority of studies lacked blinding of both participants and personnel as well as an outcome assessment. We found that there was a very heterogeneous assessment of outcomes across the included studies. Most studies had complete outcome data for PaO_2/FiO_2 (P/F) ratio and intensive care unit (ICU) length of stay (LOS). However, the majority of studies did not include complete data for mortality, ventilator-free days, and static lung compliance. Therefore, we were only able to perform meta-regression analyses for the P/F ratio and ICU LOS. There was limited evidence of selective reporting, and we detected a low risk of other bias.

Table 2. Quality assessment of included studies.

Study ID	Sequence Generation (Selection Bias)	Allocation Concealment (Selection Bias)	Blinding of Participants and Personnel (Performance Bias)	Blinding of Outcome Assessment (Detection Bias)	Incomplete Outcome Data (Attrition Bias)	Selective Reporting (Reporting Bias)	Other Sources of Bias
Momtaz 2022 [36]	Low	Low	Low	Low	Low	Low	Low
Li 2023 [17]	Low	Unsure	Low	Low	Low	Low	Low
Varpula 2004 [18]	Low	Low	High	Unsure	High	Low	Low
Kaplan 2001 [19]	Unsure	High	High	High	High	Unsure	Low
Ibrahim 2022 [20]	Low	Low	High	High	Low	Low	Low
Wrigge 2001 [21]	Unsure	Unsure	High	High	High	Unsure	Low
Lim 2016 [22]	Low	Low	Unsure	Unsure	Low	High	Low
Li 2016 [23]	Low	Low	Unsure	Unsure	Unsure	Low	Low
Zhou 2017 [24]	Unsure	Low	High	Unsure	Low	Low	Low
Marik 2009 [25]	Unsure	High	High	High	High	High	Low
Küçük 2022 [26]	Low	Low	High	High	Low	Low	Low
Daoud 2013 [27]	High	High	Low	High	Low	Low	Low
Yoshida 2009 [28]	High	High	High	High	High	Unsure	Low
Manjunath 2021 [29]	Unsure	Low	High	High	High	Low	Low
Sydow 1994 [30]	Low	Unsure	Unsure	Unsure	Low	Unsure	Low
Liu 2009 [31]	Low	High	Unsure	Unsure	Low	Low	Low
Dart 2005 [32]	Unsure	Low	Low	Low	Low	Low	Low
Hirshberg 2018 [34]	Low	Low	Low	High	Low	Unsure	Low
Maxwell 2010 [33]	Low	Low	High	Unsure	Low	Unsure	Low
Ibarra-Estrada 2022 [35]	Low	Low	High	High	Low	Low	Low

7

3.3. Meta-Regression Analyses

We performed mixed model meta-regression analyses with each ventilator setting individually as the categorical independent variable and outcome measure of interest as the dependent variable with a study-level random intercept to account for between-study heterogeneity. In total, 15 studies had complete data (i.e., both mean and SD) for the P/F ratio. There was no significant difference in P/F ratio between groups defined on the basis of any of the four settings (P_{high} difference −12.0 [95% CI −100.4, 86.39]; P_{low} difference 54.3 [95% CI −52.6, 161.1]; T_{low} difference −27.19 [95% CI −127.0, 72.6]; T_{high} difference −51.4 [95% CI −170.3, 67.5]). The forest plots are shown in Figure 2. There was high heterogeneity across all parameters (P_{high} I^2 = 99.46%, P_{low} I^2 = 99.16%, T_{low} I^2 = 99.31%, T_{high} I^2 = 99.29%).

There were 9 studies with complete data for ICU LOS. Similarly, there was no significant difference in ICU LOS between the groups in any of the four settings (P_{high} difference 2.8 days [95% CI −4.8, 10.3], P_{low} difference −2.0 days [95% CI −11.7, 7.7], T_{low} difference −1.8 days [95% CI −9.4, 5.7], T_{high} difference 3.5 days [95% CI −3.5, 10.4]). The forest plots are shown in Figure 3. As with the P/F ratio analysis, there was high heterogeneity across all four ventilator setting parameters (P_{high} I^2 = 99.63%, P_{low} I^2 = 99.67%, T_{low} I^2 = 99.63%, T_{high} I^2 = 99.59%).

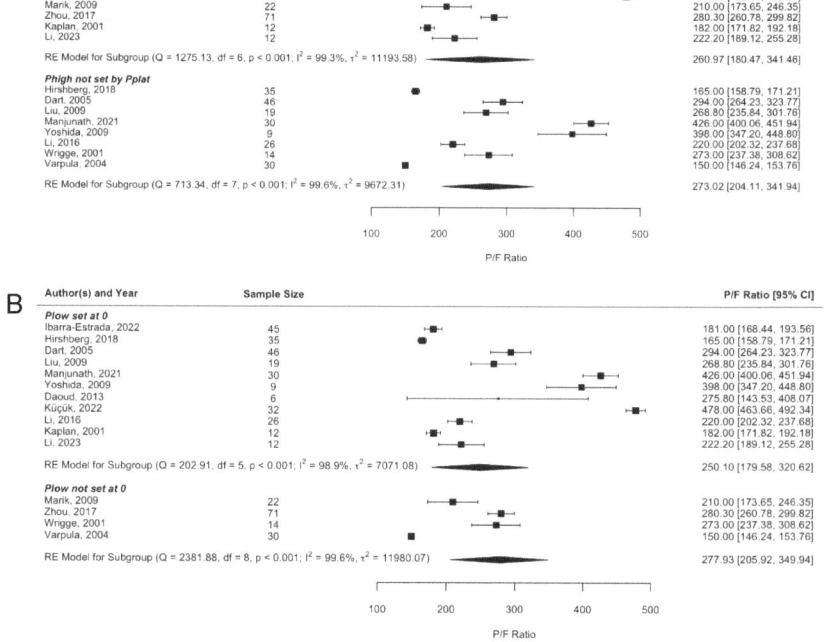

Figure 2. *Cont.*

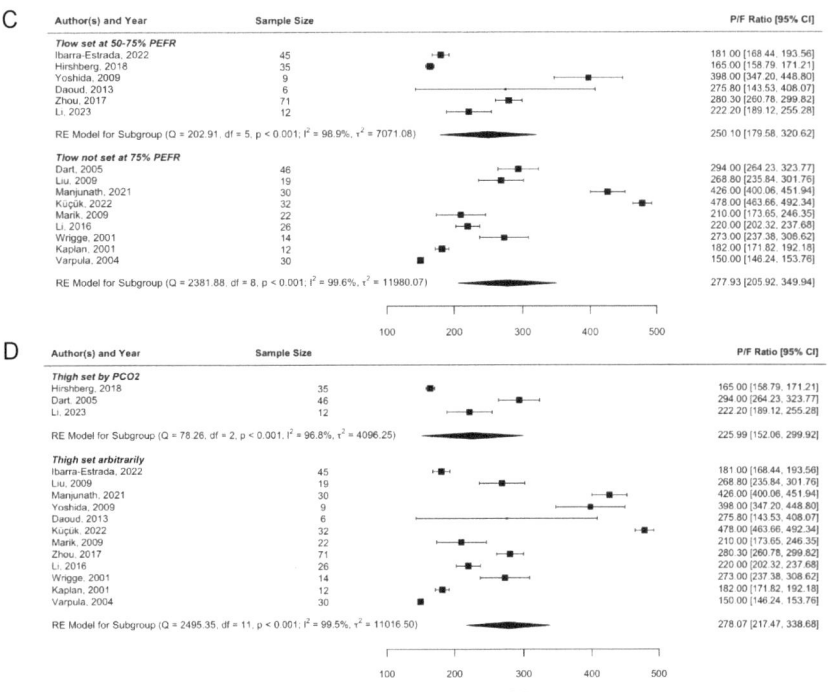

Figure 2. P/F ratio forest plots. Forest plots of P/F ratio analysis by APRV setting. (**A**) P_{high} forest plot. (**B**) P_{low} forest plot. (**C**) T_{low} forest plot. (**D**) T_{high} forest plot [17–36].

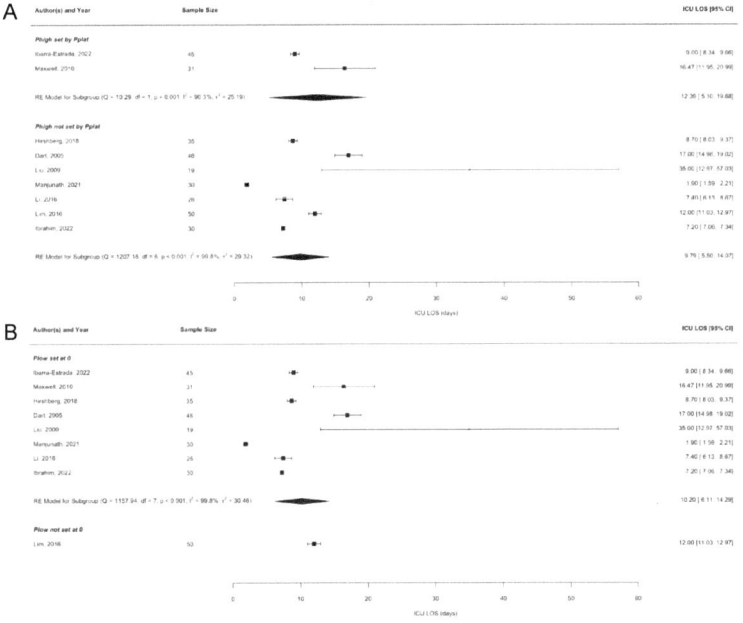

Figure 3. *Cont.*

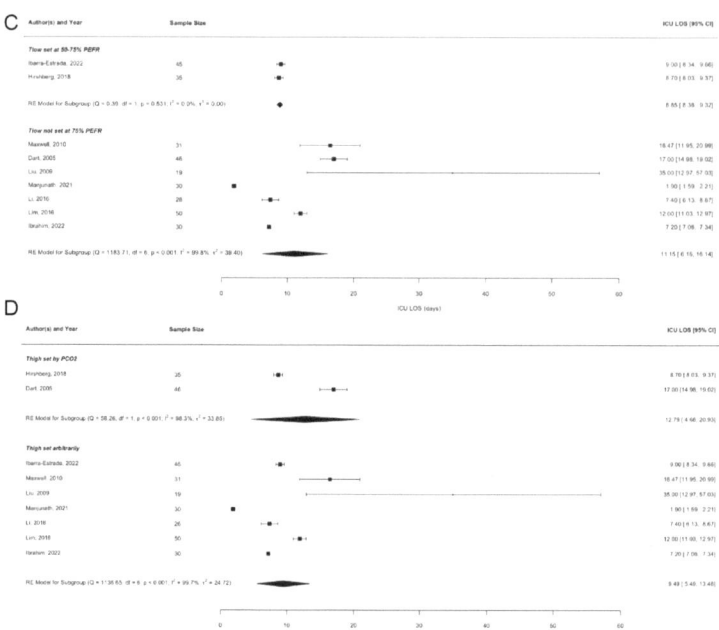

Figure 3. ICU LOS forest plots. Forest plots of ICU LOS analysis by APRV setting. (**A**) P_{high} forest plot. (**B**) P_{low} forest plot. (**C**) T_{low} forest plot. (**D**) T_{high} forest plot [17–36].

4. Discussion

In our systematic review and meta-regression analysis, we found no difference in oxygenation or ICU LOS between strategies in setting individual APRV-related ventilator parameters. In addition, we also demonstrate significant variability in the setting and adjustment of APRV in patients with ARDS. Taken together, these findings suggest that the most effective combination of APRV settings has not been established, and the design of existing trials comparing APRV to LTVV may be suboptimal.

The variability in APRV settings among the included studies was one of the most striking findings of our study. Among the 20 studies included in our analyses, 11 of the 16 possible combinations of the 4 ventilator settings were represented, with only 2 combinations represented by more than 2 studies each. Given the inconsistency in APRV protocols used across the studies and the limited number of studies in each combination, comparisons of APRV to LTVV are limited by study heterogeneity, and comparisons of APRV protocols are limited by the low number of studies with matching ventilator setting configurations. We attempted to address some of the between-study variability by pursuing a meta-regression analysis of single APRV arms instead of the traditional meta-analysis comparing APRV to LTVV. Given the relatively even distribution of studies within each parameter, aside from T_{low}, we were similarly able to employ meta-regression analysis to circumvent some of these issues.

We categorized APRV settings based on extensive physiologic data from studying the four APRV setting categories in animal models of ARDS. Although ARDS pathophysiology is highly complex, the dynamic change in alveolar mechanics predisposes the lung to a secondary VILI. In this setting, the lung becomes time- and pressure-dependent, such that it takes more time to open lung tissue and less time to re-collapse at any given airway pressure [37]. Thus, a longer inspiratory time (T_{High}) and a very brief expiratory time (T_{Low}) may rapidly stabilize and then gradually recruit collapsed lung tissue, eliminating both atelectrauma and volutrauma.

Arguably, the most important APRV setting is the T_{Low}. If the T_{Low} is set to be sufficiently brief, it will not allow sufficient time for the alveoli to collapse, even with very rapid collapse time constants. Preventing alveolar collapse during expiration has two important lung-protective benefits: (1) progressive lung collapse moving the lung into the "VILI Vortex" would be prevented, and (2) atelectrauma, a primary VILI mechanism, would be minimized [4,38]. The slope of the expiratory flow curve ($Slope_{EF}$) has been shown to be a measure of C_{RS} and can be used to personalize the T_{Low} based on changes in lung pathophysiology [39]. Importantly, the expiratory flow curve is a breath-by-breath assessment of C_{RS} only when the P_{low} is set to 0 cmH_2O. We have previously demonstrated that if the expiratory flow is terminated (T_{EF}) at 75% of the peak expiratory flow (P_{EF}) (P_{EF} L/min x 75% = T_{EF} L/min), alveolar collapse and dynamic heterogeneity is prevented, whereas increasing the T_{Low} (P_{EF} x 10%, 25%, or 50%) does not. We have further shown that using this method to set T_{Low} is highly lung-protective both in a clinically relevant large animal model and in clinical case series [40–42]. Despite the volume of data supporting its use, only one study included in our present analysis used P_{EF} 75% to set the T_{Low} [36].

In addition, we have previously demonstrated that, when using P_{EF} 75% to set T_{Low}, alveoli are stabilized even when P_{Low} was set at 0 cmH_2O [43]. Interestingly, the majority of studies included in the present analysis set P_{Low} to 0 cmH_2O (Table 1). Using this method, T_{Low} is sufficiently brief such that the lung does not have time to fully depressurize. Therefore, alveolar stability is maintained by a combination of time and pressure. While P_{Low} is set at 0 cmH_2O, the end-expiratory pressure remains approximately half of the P_{High} value [44]. On the other hand, P_{Low} set above 0 cmH_2O has two negative effects: (i) the added resistance slows the expiratory flow, and the $Slope_{EF}$ is no longer an accurate assessment of C_{RS}, and (ii) the reduced rate of expiration may cause an increase in $PaCO_2$.

APRV can be adjusted to increase $PaCO_2$ removal using two basic methods that increase minute ventilation. The T_{Low} could be increased to augment tidal volume (V_T), but from a physiologic perspective, this is problematic. It is well known that a large V_T can cause VILI, and lengthening the T_{Low} can cause alveolar instability (atelectrauma) and alveolar duct overdistension (volutrauma) [8,43,45]. Alternatively, reducing the length of the T_{High} to increase respiratory rate can increase $PaCO_2$ removal. While decreasing T_{High} is likely more lung protective than increasing T_{Low}, which would increase V_T and compromise alveolar stability, the shorter inspiratory time may slow progressive lung recruitment. Only three of the studies analyzed in this meta-analysis changed T_{High} to eliminate $PaCO_2$ (Table 1).

One of the main limiting factors of existing clinical trials comparing APRV to LTVV has been sample size. Assuming an effect size comparable to the ARMA trial (approximately 10% reduction in mortality), $\alpha = 0.05$, and 80% power, the estimated sample size needed would be over 700 individuals. Among the studies included in our analysis, the largest sample size was 71 individuals, with a total of 538 individuals across all included studies, which only makes up just above 60% of the estimated sample size of an adequately powered clinical trial. Any future trial will thus need to address these considerations to study APRV in the clinical setting appropriately.

The primary limitation of our analysis was the substantial heterogeneity in the included studies. The I^2 for all the analyses was over 99%, suggesting that almost all the observed variation was due to between-study, as opposed to within-study, differences. As mentioned above, at least some and perhaps a large proportion of the heterogeneity is clearly due to the multiple combinations of parameters across the studies. However, rather than showing that all APRV protocols are the same, our study demonstrates that the optimal strategy has not yet been demonstrated. There are also likely many other unknown sources of variability due to the diverse etiologies and clinical presentations of ARDS. For example, the study by Ibarra-Estrada et al. included only individuals with ARDS secondary to the novel coronavirus disease 2019 (COVID-19). While there are several clinical and biologic similarities between COVID-19 ARDS and non-COVID-19 ARDS, there are notable pathophysiologic differences, including the severity of endothelial injury, microangiopathy, and thrombosis [46]. In addition, there is a growing body of literature delineating two molecular phenotypes that have distinct biological profiles and mortality trajectories. Post hoc analyses have not demonstrated the interaction between randomized treatment and phenotype, but future studies that are designed with these heterogeneous groups in mind are necessary to better understand the role of APRV and other management strategies in ARDS [47].

Our results further highlight heterogeneity in clinical trial design as an important barrier to scientific advancement in the practice of critical care. In particular, the lack of standardization in protocols for mechanical ventilation limits the generalizability of any given clinical trial and the comparability of clinical trials in meta-analysis. For example, despite a consistent signal toward reduced mortality and improved oxygenation with higher PEEP, the authors of the recent ATS practice guideline offered only a conditional recommendation for the use of higher PEEP due to heterogeneity noted in the meta-analyses [13]. Future trials designed to evaluate APRV as a ventilation strategy for ARDS should include a clear justification for the method of setting each individual parameter, rather than comparing ventilator modes in name only.

Despite the number of criticisms of the existing APRV trials, we acknowledge that the ideal clinical trial design is complex. There may be several viable approaches, but a multi-arm parallel-group design is likely the most familiar and straightforward method for studying the multiple parameters required for APRV [48]. In this scenario, each arm would consist of a given combination of settings for the duration of the study period. Alternatively, a stepped wedge with or without cluster randomization could achieve similar results.

The principal source of bias for the included studies was the lack of blinding for participants and personnel, which was unfortunately unavoidable due to the nature of the intervention. In addition, several of the outcomes of interest, including, notably, mortality, had missing data, precluding inclusion in our analysis. However, there was sufficient data to analyze both the P/F ratio and ICU LOS, an important physiologic outcome and an important patient-centered outcome, respectively.

In conclusion, we found no differences in outcomes in individual APRV parameter strategies. Specifically, 68% of the included studies set the expiratory time (T_{low}) arbitrarily and without scientific rationale. Setting the expiratory time to a specific physiologic parameter, such as C_{RS}, may be the most important of the four settings since, if sufficiently short, it may eliminate recruitment/derecruitment-induced atelectrama. Only one study set expiratory time to 75% of P_{EF}; thus, we could not further assess this method in subgroup analysis. While our analysis had several strengths, including the inclusion of a wide breadth of studies and meta-regression study design, the main limitation was the profound heterogeneity between included studies. With mortality related to ARDS remaining unacceptably high, further investigation into novel ventilation strategies is imminently necessary. Understanding the physiologic impact of each setting, both individually and in combination, is critical to optimizing the lung-protective impact of APRV. Our findings suggest that future studies are needed to establish the optimal combination of APRV settings to improve ARDS-related patient outcomes.

Supplementary Materials: The following supporting information can be downloaded at: https://www.mdpi.com/article/10.3390/jcm13092690/s1, File S1: Search Strategy Details

Author Contributions: Concept and design, M.R.L., J.C., J.R.K., G.F.N., and A.J.G.; Data Collection, M.R.L., J.C., J.R.K., and A.S.; Data Analysis, M.R.L., J.C., J.R.K., S.J.G., and A.J.G.; Manuscript Writing, M.R.L., J.C., J.R.K., S.J.G., J.D.A., P.L.A., N.M.H., G.F.N., and A.J.G. All authors have read and agreed to the published version of the manuscript.

Funding: A.J.G. is supported by U.S. National Institutes of Health K08HL168205. J.A. is supported by U.S. National Institutes of Health R21EB034562. S.J.G. is supported by U.S. National Institutes of Health R01AG064955. N.M.H. is supported by U.S. Department of Defense W81XWH-20-1-0696. G.F.N. is supported by U.S. Department of Defense W81XWH-20-1-0696 and U.S. National Institutes of Health R01HL142702.

Institutional Review Board Statement: Not applicable.

Informed Consent Statement: Not applicable.

Data Availability Statement: The original data presented in the study are openly available in PubMed, Embase, Scopus, Web of Science Core Collection, and CENTRAL.

Conflicts of Interest: G.F.N. has received honoraria and/or travel reimbursement at event(s) sponsored by Dräger Medical Systems, Inc., outside of the published work. G.F.N. has lectured for Intensive Care On-line Network, Inc. (ICON). N.M.H. has an Unrestricted Educational Grant from Dräger Medical Systems, Inc. N.M.H. is the founder of ICON. N.M.H. holds patents on a method of initiating, managing, and/or weaning airway pressure release ventilation, as well as controlling a ventilator in accordance with the same.

References

1. Matthay, M.A.; Zemans, R.L.; Zimmerman, G.A.; Arabi, Y.M.; Beitler, J.R.; Mercat, A.; Herridge, M.; Randolph, A.G.; Calfee, C.S. Acute respiratory distress syndrome. *Nat. Rev. Dis. Primers* **2019**, *5*, 18. [CrossRef]
2. Bellani, G.; Laffey, J.G.; Pham, T.; Fan, E.; Brochard, L.; Esteban, A.; Gattinoni, L.; Van Haren, F.; Larsson, A.; McAuley, D.F.; et al. Epidemiology, Patterns of Care, and Mortality for Patients with Acute Respiratory Distress Syndrome in Intensive Care Units in 50 Countries. *JAMA* **2016**, *315*, 788–800. [CrossRef] [PubMed]
3. Fan, E.; Brodie, D.; Slutsky, A.S. Acute Respiratory Distress Syndrome: Advances in Diagnosis and Treatment. *JAMA* **2018**, *319*, 698–710. [CrossRef]
4. Slutsky, A.S.; Ranieri, V.M. Ventilator-induced lung injury. *N. Engl. J. Med.* **2013**, *369*, 2126–2136. [CrossRef] [PubMed]
5. Seah, A.S.; Grant, K.A.; Aliyeva, M.; Allen, G.B.; Bates, J.H. Quantifying the roles of tidal volume and PEEP in the pathogenesis of ventilator-induced lung injury. *Ann. Biomed. Eng.* **2011**, *39*, 1505–1516. [CrossRef] [PubMed]
6. Pham, T.; Serpa Neto, A.; Pelosi, P.; Laffey, J.G.; De Haro, C.; Lorente, J.A.; Bellani, G.; Fan, E.; Brochard, L.J.; Pesenti, A.; et al. Outcomes of Patients Presenting with Mild Acute Respiratory Distress Syndrome: Insights from the LUNG SAFE Study. *Anesthesiology* **2019**, *130*, 263–283. [CrossRef]
7. Writing Group for the Alveolar Recruitment for Acute Respiratory Distress Syndrome Trial Investigators; Cavalcanti, A.B.; Suzumura, E.A.; Laranjeira, L.N.; Paisani, D.M.; Damiani, L.P.; Guimarães, H.P.; Romano, E.R.; de Moraes Regenga, M.; Taniguchi, L.N.; et al. Effect of Lung Recruitment and Titrated Positive End-Expiratory Pressure (PEEP) vs. Low PEEP on Mortality in Patients with Acute Respiratory Distress Syndrome: A Randomized Clinical Trial. *JAMA* **2017**, *318*, 1335–1345. [CrossRef] [PubMed]
8. Acute Respiratory Distress Syndrome Network; Brower, R.G.; Matthay, M.A.; Morris, A.; Schoenfeld, D.; Thompson, B.T.; Wheeler, A. Ventilation with lower tidal volumes as compared with traditional tidal volumes for acute lung injury and the acute respiratory distress syndrome. *N. Engl. J. Med.* **2000**, *342*, 1301–1308. [CrossRef]
9. Jain, S.V.; Kollisch-Singule, M.; Sadowitz, B.; Dombert, L.; Satalin, J.; Andrews, P.; Gatto, L.A.; Nieman, G.F.; Habashi, N.M. The 30-year evolution of airway pressure release ventilation (APRV). *Intensive Care Med. Exp.* **2016**, *4*, 11. [CrossRef]
10. Cressoni, M.; Chiurazzi, C.; Gotti, M.; Amini, M.; Brioni, M.; Algieri, I.; Cammaroto, A.; Rovati, C.; Massari, D.; di Castiglione, C.B.; et al. Lung inhomogeneities and time course of ventilator-induced mechanical injuries. *Anesthesiology* **2015**, *123*, 618–627. [CrossRef]
11. Briel, M.; Meade, M.; Mercat, A.; Brower, R.G.; Talmor, D.; Walter, S.D.; Slutsky, A.S.; Pullenayegum, E.; Zhou, Q.; Cook, D.; et al. Higher vs Lower Positive End-Expiratory Pressure in Patients with Acute Lung Injury and Acute Respiratory Distress Syndrome. *JAMA* **2010**, *303*, 865. [CrossRef] [PubMed]
12. Dianti, J.; Tisminetzky, M.; Ferreyro, B.L.; Englesakis, M.; Del Sorbo, L.; Sud, S.; Talmor, D.; Ball, L.; Meade, M.; Hodgson, C.; et al. Association of Positive End-Expiratory Pressure and Lung Recruitment Selection Strategies with Mortality in Acute Respiratory Distress Syndrome: A Systematic Review and Network Meta-analysis. *Am. J. Respir. Crit. Care Med.* **2022**, *205*, 1300–1310. [CrossRef] [PubMed]
13. Qadir, N.; Sahetya, S.; Munshi, L.; Summers, C.; Abrams, D.; Beitler, J.; Bellani, G.; Brower, R.G.; Burry, L.; Chen, J.-T.; et al. An Update on Management of Adult Patients with Acute Respiratory Distress Syndrome: An Official American Thoracic Society Clinical Practice Guideline. *Am. J. Respir. Crit. Care Med.* **2024**, *209*, 24–36. [CrossRef] [PubMed]
14. ZZhong, X.; Wu, Q.; Yang, H.; Dong, W.; Wang, B.; Zhang, Z.; Liang, G. Airway pressure release ventilation versus low tidal volume ventilation for patients with acute respiratory distress syndrome/acute lung injury: A meta-analysis of randomized clinical trials. *Ann. Transl. Med.* **2020**, *8*, 1641. [CrossRef]
15. Camporota, L.; Rose, L.; Andrews, P.L.; Nieman, G.F.; Habashi, N.M. Airway pressure release ventilation for lung protection in acute respiratory distress syndrome: An alternative way to recruit the lungs. *Curr. Opin. Crit. Care* **2024**, *30*, 76–84. [CrossRef] [PubMed]
16. Wan, X.; Wang, W.; Liu, J.; Tong, T. Estimating the sample mean and standard deviation from the sample size, median, range and/or interquartile range. *BMC Med. Res. Methodol.* **2014**, *14*, 135. [CrossRef]

17. Li, R.; Wu, Y.; Zhang, H.; Wang, A.; Zhao, X.; Yuan, S.; Yang, L.; Zou, X.; Shang, Y.; Zhao, Z. Effects of airway pressure release ventilation on lung physiology assessed by electrical impedance tomography in patients with early moderate-to-severe ARDS. *Crit. Care* **2023**, *27*, 178. [CrossRef] [PubMed]
18. Varpula, T.; Valta, P.; Niemi, R.; Takkunen, O.; Hynynen, M.; Pettilä, V. Airway pressure release ventilation as a primary ventilatory mode in acute respiratory distress syndrome. *Acta Anaesthesiol. Scand.* **2004**, *48*, 722–731. [CrossRef] [PubMed]
19. Kaplan, L.J.; Bailey, H.; Formosa, V. Airway pressure release ventilation increases cardiac performance in patients with acute lung injury/adult respiratory distress syndrome. *Crit. Care* **2001**, *5*, 221. [CrossRef]
20. Ibrahim, R.; Mohamed, Y.; Abd El-kader, M.; Azouz, A. Airway pressure release ventilation versus pressure-controlled ventilation in acute hypoxemic respiratory failure. *Egypt. J. Chest Dis. Tuberc.* **2022**, *71*, 74.
21. Wrigge, H.; Zinserling, J.; Hering, R.; Schwalfenberg, N.; Stüber, F.; von Spiegel, T.; Schroeder, S.; Hedenstierna, G.; Putensen, C. Cardiorespiratory Effects of Automatic Tube Compensation during Airway Pressure Release Ventilation in Patients with Acute Lung Injury. *Anesthesiology* **2001**, *95*, 382–389. [CrossRef]
22. Lim, J.; Litton, E.; Robinson, H.; Das Gupta, M. Characteristics and outcomes of patients treated with airway pressure release ventilation for acute respiratory distress syndrome: A retrospective observational study. *J. Crit. Care* **2016**, *34*, 154–159. [CrossRef] [PubMed]
23. Li, J.-Q.; Li, N.; Han, G.-J.; Pan, C.-G.; Zhang, Y.-H.; Shi, X.-Z.; Xu, J.-Y.; Lu, B.; Li, M.-Q. Clinical research about airway pressure release ventilation for moderate to severe acute respiratory distress syndrome. *Eur. Rev. Med. Pharmacol. Sci.* **2016**, *20*, 2634–2641.
24. Zhou, Y.; Jin, X.; Lv, Y.; Wang, P.; Yang, Y.; Liang, G.; Wang, B.; Kang, Y. Early application of airway pressure release ventilation may reduce the duration of mechanical ventilation in acute respiratory distress syndrome. *Intensive Care Med.* **2017**, *43*, 1648–1659. [CrossRef]
25. Marik, P.E.; Delgado, E.M.; Baram, M.; Gradwell, G.; Romeo, S.; Dutill, B. Effect of Airway Pressure Release Ventilation (APRV) with Pressure Support. (PS) on Indices of Oxygenation and Ventilation in Patients with Severe ARDS: A Cohort Study. *Crit Care Shock* **2009**, *12*, 43–48.
26. Küçük, M.P.; Öztürk, Ç.E.; İlkaya, N.K.; Küçük, A.O.; Ergül, D.F.; Ülger, F. The effect of preemptive airway pressure release ventilation on patients with high risk for acute respiratory distress syndrome: A randomized controlled trial. *Braz. J. Anesthesiol. (Engl. Ed.)* **2022**, *72*, 29–36. [CrossRef] [PubMed]
27. Daoud, E.G.; Chatburn, R.L. Comparing surrogates of oxygenation and ventilation between airway pressure release ventilation and biphasic airway pressure in a mechanical model of adult respiratory distress syndrome. *Respir. Investig.* **2014**, *52*, 236–241. [CrossRef] [PubMed]
28. Yoshida, T.; Rinka, H.; Kaji, A.; Yoshimoto, A.; Arimoto, H.; Miyaichi, T.; Kan, M. The Impact of Spontaneous Ventilation on Distribution of Lung Aeration in Patients with Acute Respiratory Distress Syndrome: Airway Pressure Release Ventilation Versus Pressure Support Ventilation. *Anesth. Analg.* **2009**, *109*, 1892–1900. [CrossRef] [PubMed]
29. Manjunath, V.; Reddy, B.; Prasad, S. Is airway pressure release ventilation, a better primary mode of post-operative ventilation for adult patients undergoing open heart surgery? A prospective randomised study. *Ann. Card. Anaesth.* **2021**, *24*, 288.
30. Sydow, M.; Burchardi, H.; Ephraim, E.; Zielmann, S.; Crozier, T.A. Long-term effects of two different ventilatory modes on oxygenation in acute lung injury. Comparison of airway pressure release ventilation and volume-controlled inverse ratio ventilation. *Am. J. Respir. Crit. Care Med.* **1994**, *149*, 1550–1556. [CrossRef]
31. Liu, L.; Tanigawa, K.; Ota, K.; Tamura, T.; Yamaga, S.; Kida, Y.; Kondo, T.; Ishida, M.; Otani, T.; Sadamori, T.; et al. Practical use of airway pressure release ventilation for severe ARDS—A preliminary report in comparison with a conventional ventilatory support. *Hiroshima J. Med. Sci.* **2009**, *58*, 83–88. [PubMed]
32. Dart, B.W.; Maxwell, R.A.; Richart, C.M.; Brooks, D.K.; Ciraulo, D.L.; Barker, D.E.; Burns, R.P. Preliminary Experience with Airway Pressure Release Ventilation in a Trauma/Surgical Intensive Care Unit. *J. Trauma Inj. Infect. Crit. Care* **2005**, *59*, 71–76. [CrossRef] [PubMed]
33. MMaxwell, R.A.; Green, J.M.; Waldrop, J.; Dart, B.W.; Smith, P.W.; Brooks, D.; Lewis, P.L.; Barker, D.E. A Randomized Prospective Trial of Airway Pressure Release Ventilation and Low Tidal Volume Ventilation in Adult Trauma Patients with Acute Respiratory Failure. *J. Trauma Inj. Infect. Crit. Care* **2010**, *69*, 501–511. [CrossRef] [PubMed]
34. Hirshberg, E.L.; Lanspa, M.J.; Peterson, J.; Carpenter, L.; Wilson, E.L.; Brown, S.M.; Dean, N.C.; Orme, J.; Grissom, C.K. Randomized Feasibility Trial of a Low Tidal Volume-Airway Pressure Release Ventilation Protocol Compared with Traditional Airway Pressure Release Ventilation and Volume Control Ventilation Protocols. *Crit. Care Med.* **2018**, *46*, 1943–1952. [CrossRef] [PubMed]
35. Ibarra-Estrada, M.; García-Salas, Y.; Mireles-Cabodevila, E.; López-Pulgarín, J.A.; Chávez-Peña, Q.; García-Salcido, R.; Mijangos-Méndez, J.C.; Aguirre-Avalos, G. Use of Airway Pressure Release Ventilation in Patients with Acute Respiratory Failure Due to COVID-19: Results of a Single-Center Randomized Controlled Trial*. *Crit. Care Med.* **2022**, *50*, 586–594. [PubMed]
36. Momtaz, O.M.; Ahmed El Hefeny, R.; Fawzy, R.M.; Fathy, A.; Khateeb, E. Study of Airway pressure release ventilation versus low tidal volume ventilation in hospital outcome of acute respiratory distress syndrome. *Neuroquantology* **2022**, *20*, 3436–3445.
37. Nieman, G.F.; Kaczka, D.W.; Andrews, P.L.; Ghosh, A.; Al-Khalisy, H.; Camporota, L.; Satalin, J.; Herrmann, J.; Habashi, N.M. First Stabilize and then Gradually Recruit: A Paradigm Shift in Protective Mechanical Ventilation for Acute Lung Injury. *J. Clin. Med.* **2023**, *12*, 4633. [CrossRef]

38. Marini, J.J.; Gattinoni, L. Time Course of Evolving Ventilator-Induced Lung Injury: The "Shrinking Baby Lung". *Crit. Care Med.* **2020**, *48*, 1203–1209. [CrossRef]
39. Habashi, N.M. Other approaches to open-lung ventilation: Airway pressure release ventilation. *Crit. Care Med.* **2005**, *33*, S228–S240. [CrossRef]
40. Roy, S.; Habashi, N.; Sadowitz, B.; Andrews, P.; Ge, L.; Wang, G.; Roy, P.; Ghosh, A.; Kuhn, M.; Satalin, J.; et al. Early airway pressure release ventilation prevents ards—A novel preventive approach to lung injury. *Shock* **2013**, *39*, 28–38. [CrossRef]
41. Rola, P.; Daxon, B. Airway Pressure Release Ventilation with Time-Controlled Adaptive Ventilation (TCAV^{TM}) in COVID-19: A Community Hospital's Experience. *Front. Physiol.* **2022**, *13*, 787231. [CrossRef] [PubMed]
42. Janssen, M.; Meeder, J.H.; Seghers, L.; den Uil, C.A. Time controlled adaptive ventilation^{TM} as conservative treatment of destroyed lung: An alternative to lung transplantation. *BMC Pulm. Med.* **2021**, *21*, 176. [CrossRef]
43. Kollisch-Singule, M.; Jain, S.; Andrews, P.; Smith, B.J.; Hamlington-Smith, K.L.; Roy, S.; DiStefano, D.; Nuss, E.; Satalin, J.; Meng, Q.; et al. Effect of Airway Pressure Release Ventilation on Dynamic Alveolar Heterogeneity. *JAMA Surg.* **2016**, *151*, 64. [CrossRef] [PubMed]
44. Kollisch-Singule, M.; Emr, B.; Jain, S.V.; Andrews, P.; Satalin, J.; Liu, J.; Porcellio, E.; Van Kenyon, V.; Wang, G.; Marx, W.; et al. The effects of airway pressure release ventilation on respiratory mechanics in extrapulmonary lung injury. *Intensive Care Med. Exp.* **2015**, *3*, 35. [CrossRef] [PubMed]
45. Kollisch-Singule, M.; Emr, B.; Smith, B.; Ruiz, C.; Roy, S.; Meng, Q.; Jain, S.; Satalin, J.; Snyder, K.; Ghosh, A.; et al. Airway pressure release ventilation reduces conducting airway micro-strain in lung injury. *J. Am. Coll. Surg.* **2014**, *219*, 968–976. [CrossRef] [PubMed]
46. Ackermann, M.; Verleden, S.E.; Kuehnel, M.; Haverich, A.; Welte, T.; Laenger, F.; Vanstapel, A.; Werlein, C.; Stark, H.; Tzankov, A.; et al. Pulmonary Vascular Endothelialitis, Thrombosis, and Angiogenesis in COVID-19. *N. Engl. J. Med.* **2020**, *383*, 120–128. [CrossRef] [PubMed]
47. Sinha, P.; Neyton, L.; Sarma, A.; Wu, N.; Jones, C.; Zhuo, H.; Liu, K.D.; Sanchez Guerrero, E.; Ghale, R.; Love, C.; et al. Molecular Phenotypes of Acute Respiratory Distress Syndrome in the ROSE Trial Have Differential Outcomes and Gene Expression Patterns That Differ at Baseline and Longitudinally over Time. *Am. J. Respir. Crit. Care Med.* **2024**, *209*, 816–828. [CrossRef]
48. Juszczak, E.; Altman, D.G.; Hopewell, S.; Schulz, K. Reporting of Multi-Arm Parallel-Group Randomized Trials. *JAMA* **2019**, *321*, 1610. [CrossRef]

Disclaimer/Publisher's Note: The statements, opinions and data contained in all publications are solely those of the individual author(s) and contributor(s) and not of MDPI and/or the editor(s). MDPI and/or the editor(s) disclaim responsibility for any injury to people or property resulting from any ideas, methods, instructions or products referred to in the content.

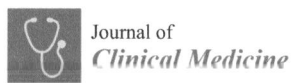 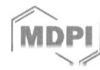

Review

Management of Neuromuscular Blocking Agents in Critically Ill Patients with Lung Diseases

Ida Giorgia Iavarone [1,2], Lou'i Al-Husinat [3], Jorge Luis Vélez-Páez [4,5], Chiara Robba [1,2,4], Pedro Leme Silva [6], Patricia R. M. Rocco [6] and Denise Battaglini [1,*]

1. Anesthesia and Intensive Care, IRCCS Ospedale Policlinico San Martino, 16132 Genova, Italy; idagiorgia.iavarone@gmail.com (I.G.I.); kiarobba@gmail.com (C.R.)
2. Department of Surgical Sciences and Integrated Diagnostics, University of Genova, 16132 Genova, Italy
3. Department of Clinical Sciences, Faculty of Medicine, Yarmouk University, Irbid 21163, Jordan; loui.husinat@yu.edu.jo
4. Facultad de Ciencias Médicas, Universidad Central de Ecuador, Quito 170129, Ecuador; jorgeluisvelez13@hotmail.com
5. Unidad de Terapia Intensiva, Hospital Pablo Arturo Suárez, Centro de Investigación Clínica, Quito 170129, Ecuador
6. Laboratory of Pulmonary Investigation, Carlos Chagas Filho Institute of Biophysics, Federal University of Rio de Janeiro, Rio de Janeiro 21941, Brazil; pedroleme@biof.ufrj.br (P.L.S.); prmrocco@gmail.com (P.R.M.R.)
* Correspondence: battaglini.denise@gmail.com

Abstract: The use of neuromuscular blocking agents (NMBAs) is common in the intensive care unit (ICU). NMBAs have been used in critically ill patients with lung diseases to optimize mechanical ventilation, prevent spontaneous respiratory efforts, reduce the work of breathing and oxygen consumption, and avoid patient–ventilator asynchrony. In patients with acute respiratory distress syndrome (ARDS), NMBAs reduce the risk of barotrauma and improve oxygenation. Nevertheless, current guidelines and evidence are contrasting regarding the routine use of NMBAs. In status asthmaticus and acute exacerbation of chronic obstructive pulmonary disease, NMBAs are used in specific conditions to ameliorate patient–ventilator synchronism and oxygenation, although their routine use is controversial. Indeed, the use of NMBAs has decreased over the last decade due to potential adverse effects, such as immobilization, venous thrombosis, patient awareness during paralysis, development of critical illness myopathy, autonomic interactions, ICU-acquired weakness, and residual paralysis after cessation of NMBAs use. The aim of this review is to highlight current knowledge and synthesize the evidence for the effects of NMBAs for critically ill patients with lung diseases, focusing on patient–ventilator asynchrony, ARDS, status asthmaticus, and chronic obstructive pulmonary disease.

Keywords: neuromuscular blocking agents; intensive care unit; acute respiratory distress syndrome; status asthmaticus; chronic obstructive pulmonary disease

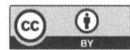

1. Introduction

Neuromuscular blocking agents (NMBAs) represent a landmark in modern anesthesia, acting on the neuromuscular junction by blocking the transmission of nervous impulses in the motor endplate of striated muscles, resulting in skeletal muscle paralysis [1].

The use of NMBAs is common in the intensive care unit (ICU), especially in cases of acute distress respiratory syndrome (ARDS). It is used in 25–45% of cases, with different practices associated with geographic differences [2]. NMBAs are used in pulmonary critical care patients, such as those with ARDS, to optimize mechanical ventilation (MV), prevent spontaneous respiratory efforts, reduce the work of breathing and oxygen consumption, reduce the risk of barotrauma, and avoid patient–ventilator asynchrony [3,4]. NMBAs have many other beneficial effects on lung function, improving alveolar recruitment, and they can reduce the concentration of interleukins and tumor necrosis factor-alpha, leading to anti-inflammatory effects [5].

Patients with severe ARDS, status asthmaticus, and chronic obstructive pulmonary disease (COPD) often need MV support, which is frequently insufficiently controlled with sedative and analgesic drugs [2,6,7]. NMBAs seem to have beneficial effects on airway pressures. In a small trial conducted on mechanically ventilated children with severe acute hypoxemic respiratory failure, NMBAs decreased the mean airway pressure ($p = 0.039$) and the oxygenation index (OI) ($p = 0.039$) in all patients [8]. In a recent trial conducted on 30 patients with moderate-to-severe ARDS, neuromuscular blockade treatment did not affect the transpulmonary driving pressure (expressed as inspiratory lung pressure minus expiratory lung pressure and defined as a surrogate of the stress applied to the lungs) at 48 h [9]. NMBAs also seem to play a role in gas exchange. In their study, Gainnier et al. [10] reported a higher PaO_2/FiO_2 ratio at 48, 96, and 120 h in patients randomized to the NMBA group ($p = 0.021$).

Thus, when deep sedation fails or is not tolerated, NMBAs could be administered to harmonize the respiratory function [4].

Although these beneficial effects, especially in patients with ARDS, the impact of NMBAs on mortality remains controversial [11]. The routine use of NMBAs in ICUs has decreased in the last decade due to potential harmful effects resulting from immobilization such as venous thrombosis, development of critical illness myopathy, ICU-acquired weakness (ICUAW), autonomic interactions, awareness during paralysis, and residual paralysis after cessation of NMBAs [4,12]. However, the real benefits and complications of NMBAs in critically ill patients with lung diseases have not been completely elucidated.

The aim of this review is to highlight current knowledge and synthesize the evidence concerning the effects of NMBAs in critically ill patients with lung diseases, particularly in cases of patient–ventilator asynchrony, ARDS, status asthmaticus, and COPD.

2. Methods

We searched PubMed, MEDLINE, Embase, and Scopus for observational studies, randomized controlled trials, meta-analyses, and current guidelines evaluating the administration of NMBAs in critically ill patients with lung diseases (ARDS or status asthmaticus or COPD).

3. Classification of NMBAs, Pharmacokinetics and Pharmacodynamics

Neuromuscular blockade acts at the neuromuscular junction. When an electric impulse is released in the motor neuron, acetylcholine (ACh) is accumulated in vesicles of the presynaptic membrane acting on the nicotinic receptors on the postsynaptic membrane and causing muscle contraction [13]. Pharmacokinetics and pharmacodynamics of the most commonly used NMBAs are reported in Table 1.

Besides the neuromuscular blockading action, NMBAs have an anti-inflammatory effect [14]. Particularly in patients with ARDS, NMBAs decreased the pro-inflammatory response [15], as well as the levels of biomarkers associated with epithelial and endothelial lung injury [16].

Recently, a new series of neuromuscular complexes called the chlorofumarates (gantacurium, CW002, and CW011) are being developed with a promising pharmacodynamic profile; however, availability for clinical use remains undefined. Other studies are required to establish the role of these drugs in clinical practice [17].

Table 1. Pharmacokinetics and pharmacodynamics of the most commonly used NMBAs.

Agent	Duration	ED95 (mg/kg)	Onset Time (min)	Duration (min)	Dosing	Metabolism
			Depolarizing *			
Succinylcholine	Ultra-short	0.3	1–1.5	5–10	1 mg/kg bolus NA	Plasma cholinesterase

Table 1. Cont.

Agent	Duration	ED95 (mg/kg)	Onset Time (min)	Duration (min)	Dosing	Metabolism
Non-Depolarizing **						
Aminosteroids						
Rocuronium	Intermediate-duration agent	0.3	1.5–3	20–35	0.6–1.2 mg/kg bolus 8–12 mcg/kg/min infusion	Hepatic, no active metabolites
Vecuronium	Intermediate-duration agent	0.05	3–4	20–45	0.08–0.1 mg/kg bolus 0.8–1.7 mcg/kg/min infusion	Hepatic, bile, urinary metabolites
Pancuronium	Long-duration agent	0.07	2–4	60–100	0.05–1 mg/kg bolus 0.8–1.7 mcg/kg/min infusion	Renal elimination
Benzylisoquinolines						
Cisatracurium	Intermediate-duration agent	0.05	5–7	30–60	0.1–0.2 mg/kg bolus 1–3 mcg/kg/min	Hoffmann reaction, renal elimination
Atracurium	Intermediate-duration agent	0.2–0.25	3–4	20–35	0.4–0.5 mg/kg bolus 5–10 mcg/kg/min	Hoffmann reaction, plasmatic esterase
Mivacurium	Short-duration agent	0.08	3–4	15–20	0.15–0.25 mg/kg bolus 9–10 mcg/kg/min infusion	Plasmatic esterase
Doxacurium	Long-duration agent	0.025	5–10	40–120	0.03–0.06 mg/kg NA	Renal elimination
Chlorofumarate diesters						
Gantacurium	Ultra-short duration agent	0.19	1.7	6–8	0.2–0.5 mg/kg NA	Addition of cysteine and ester hydrolysis

* Depolarizing NMBA causes depolarization of the postsynaptic membrane, resulting in resistance to the activity of acetylcholine [18]. ** Non-depolarizing NMBAs compete with acetylcholine for the binding site on the alpha subunit of the nicotinic receptors, preventing its action and establishing a neuromuscular blockade [19]. NA, not available.

4. General Advantages and Disadvantages of Using NMBAs in Critically Ill Patients with Lung Diseases

NMBAs can ameliorate the management of ventilation [20], limiting recruitment, inspiratory effort, and expiratory alveolar collapse [9]. Some studies demonstrated improved oxygenation using NMBAs, possibly related to the effects on reducing the work of breathing [12,21]. In a randomized controlled trial on patients with ARDS receiving conventional therapy plus placebo or NMBAs, treatment with cysatracurium exerted anti-inflammatory effects by reducing the concentration of interleukins and tumor necrosis factor-alpha in serum and bronchoalveolar lavage [5].

Intra-abdominal hypertension (IAH), defined as an intra-abdominal pressure (IAP) above 12 mmHg, is one of the possible conditions in which the use of NMBAs can improve lung function. It is estimated that around 20% of patients present with IAH on admission to the ICU and almost 50% will develop IAH within the first week in the ICU [21,22]. IAH often progresses with an upper shift of the diaphragm and decreased lung volume and chest wall compliance, resulting in increased airway pressures [23] and decreased oxygenation [24]. Although abdominal contractions can falsely increase IAP values, to date, no recommendation on increasing sedation or using NMBAs to accurately measure IAP has been defined [24]. A recent guideline for the management of IAH and abdominal compartment syndrome in critically ill patients highlighted the possibility of considering the use of NMBAs for persistent IAH [25].

When paralyzing the patient, it is always important to consider the possibility of the development of complications associated with the administration of NMBAs, such as corneal abrasions [4] and venous thrombosis [26], and complications associated with prolonged immobilization such as ICUAW and myopathy. The relationship between ICUAW and NMBAs is controversial [4]. Although a recent meta-analysis did not show an association between NMBAs and neuromuscular dysfunction acquired in critical illness (odds ratio (OR), 1.21; 95% confidence interval (CI), 0.67–2.19), merged data from all the included studies suggested a modest association (OR, 1.25; 95% CI, 1.06–1.48; I = 16%) between NMBA use and ICUAW [27]. Many other studies have confirmed the association [28,29] or the potential risk [30] of the development of ICUAW with the use of NMBAs, but with a weak study design and high risk of bias because of the multi-factorial causes of ICUAW and heterogeneous outcomes [31]. In this uncertainty, the association between the use of NMBAs and critical weakness does not seem to be reasonable. Thus, recent SCCM guidelines did not relate the use of NMBAs with the risk of ICUAW, rather associating it with prolonged immobility and muscle disuse [32]. In addition, NMBAs impaired airway protective reflexes [33] and increased the risk of upper airway obstruction and pneumonia. Moreover, these patients needed deep sedation due to prolonged treatment with NMBAs [34].

Critically ill patients often have multi-organ-system disorders and receive treatments for longer periods; thus, the elimination of NMBAs and metabolites can be delayed, resulting in greater accumulation [4,35] and adverse events, difficulty in weaning from the ventilator [36], and the risk of venous thrombosis [26].

5. Patient–Ventilator Asynchrony

Patient–ventilator asynchrony is frequently observed during MV and is associated with worse outcomes and higher mortality [37].

Ventilatory under-assistance or over-assistance translates to different types of asynchronies [38]. Under-assistance could lead to an increased load on respiratory muscles, air hunger, and lung injury caused by excessive tidal volumes (V_T). Over-assistance could yield decreased inspiratory drive, which may result in reverse triggering, thus worsening lung injury. In addition, asynchronies may increase intrathoracic pressure, thus modifying cardiac output and hemodynamic status [39].

Yoshida et al. [40] demonstrated that an increase in distending pressure, caused by spontaneous effort in mechanically ventilated patients, could worsen a pre-existing lung injury through a pendelluft effect from non-dependent lung areas toward dependent areas because the diaphragm contraction is poorly transmitted across the pleural surface in an injured lung. Therefore, management of patient–ventilator asynchrony with neuromuscular blockade may be considered to minimize the lung and diaphragm injury associated with spontaneous breathing [41], especially in patients with ARDS [42].

The use of NMBAs in the critical care setting is frequently guided by personal experience and local practice, more than validated guidelines and recommendations [32]. NMBAs minimize the risk of ventilator-induced lung injury (VILI). However, the use of NMBAs requires adequate sedation to prevent VILI and may lead to extended time on MV, longer ICU stays, and increased risk of ventilator-associated pneumonia (VAP) [43,44]. NMBAs should be administered with adequate sedation. Nevertheless, the sedation level is a factor that could affect the incidence of asynchrony. Observational studies showed an association between deep sedation and a higher incidence of patient–ventilator asynchronies [37,45].

A multi-center study showed a lower incidence of asynchronies with lighter sedation with dexmedetomidine compared with deeper sedation with propofol [46]. So, increasing sedation does not always represent an effective strategy to reduce asynchrony. When asynchrony is related to double triggering, deeper sedation associated with neuromuscular blockade could be taken into consideration. In contrast, in the case of reverse triggering, muscle effort could result in inflation so that a reduced sedation and NMBA strategy could be considered [47].

6. Acute Respiratory Distress Syndrome

To date, pharmacologic therapies have shown no beneficial effects in patients with ARDS, but supportive treatments such as MV can improve ARDS outcomes [48]. NMBAs have been largely used in patients with ARDS over the years [49], given that they can minimize VILI in the presence of increased respiratory drive or patient ventilatory asynchrony [50]. Lighter sedation and an early active breathing strategy are increasingly used for patients with ARDS to reduce muscle wasting [3,51–53]. Therefore, the use of NMBAs in this population is controversial.

Many trials focusing on the use of NMBAs have been conducted on patients with ARDS (Table 2), but no consensus has been reached, and specific recommendations are currently being formulated.

Table 2. Randomized trials and metanalysis focusing on the use of NMBAs in patients with ARDS.

Authors/Year	Type of Study/Population	Subtypes of Drugs	Objective	Outcome
Gainnier et al. [10] 2004	Multi-center, prospective, controlled, randomized trial: 56 patients with $PaO_2/FiO_2 < 150$ with PEEP ≥ 5 cm H_2O randomized in control ($n = 28$) and NMBA ($n = 28$) groups	not specified	Evaluate the effects of a 48 h NMBAs infusion on gas exchange over a 120 h time period in patients with ARDS	NMBAs were administered for 48 h; oxygenation (PaO_2/FiO_2 ratio) was better in NMBA compared to control group
Papazian et al. (ACURASYS trial) [54] 2010	Multi-center, prospective, controlled, randomized trial: 340 patients with severe ARDS randomized in placebo ($n = 162$) and NMBA ($n = 178$) groups	cisatracurium	Evaluate clinical outcomes after 48 h of therapy with NMBAs in patients with early, severe ARDS	Early administration of NMBAs for 48 h decreased 90-day mortality (31.6% with NMBAs vs. 40.7% in the placebo group) and risk of barotrauma in patients with moderate to severe ARDS
Forel et al. [14] 2006	Multi-center, prospective, controlled, and randomized trial: 36 patients with $PaO_2/FiO_2 < 200$ at a PEEP ≥ 5 cm H_2O randomized in placebo ($n = 18$) and NMBA ($n = 18$) groups	cisatracurium	Evaluate the effects of NMBAs on pulmonary and systemic inflammation in patients with ARDS ventilated with a lung-protective strategy	At 48 h after randomization, pulmonary concentrations of IL-1β ($p = 0.005$), IL-6 ($p = 0.038$), and IL-8 ($p = 0.017$) and serum concentration of IL-6 ($p = 0.05$) and IL-8 ($p = 0.003$) were lower in the NMBA group as compared with the control group; improvement in PaO_2/FiO_2 ratio was observed and reinforced in the NMBA group ($p < 0.001$)
The National Heart, Lung, and Blood Institute PETAL Clinical Trials Network (ROSE trial) [52] 2019	Multi-center, prospective, controlled, randomized trial: 1006 patients with moderate-to-severe ARDS $PaO_2/FiO_2 < 150$ with PEEP ≥ 8 cm H_2O, randomized in intervention ($n = 501$) and control ($n = 505$) groups	cisatracurium	Evaluate mortality at 90 days in patients with moderate-to-severe ARDS randomly divided into two groups: the intervention group, treated with 48 h infusion of NMBA with concomitant deep sedation, or the control group (no NMBA)	Mortality rate at 90 days did not differ between groups (42.5% in the control group vs. 42.8% in the intervention group

Table 2. *Cont.*

Authors/Year	Type of Study/Population	Subtypes of Drugs	Objective	Outcome
Lyu et al. [55] 2014	Prospective study: 96 patients randomized into severe ARDS ($n = 48$) and moderate ARDS ($n = 48$) groups according to the Berlin definition of ARDS; patients were than randomly divided into treatment ($n = 24$) and control ($n = 24$) groups	vecuronium	Observe the clinical effects of early use of NMBA in patients with severe sepsis and ARDS	Sepsis scores improved after treatment with NMBAs in severe ARDS group compared with control group (APACHEII score: 16.58 ± 2.41 vs. 19.79 ± 3.52, $t = 3.679$, $p = 0.010$; SOFA score: 12.04 ± 2.17 vs. 14.75 ± 3.26, $t = 3.385$, $p = 0.010$; PaO$_2$/FiO$_2$: 159.31 ± 22.57 mmHg vs. 131.81 ± 34.93 mmHg, $t = 3.239$, $p = 0.020$; ScvO$_2$: 0.673 ± 0.068 vs. 0.572 ± 0.142, $t = 3.137$, $p = 0.030$; Lac: 3.10 ± 1.01 mmol/L vs. 4.39 ± 1.72 mmol/L, $t = 3.161$, $p = 0.030$), while the value of CRP showed no significant difference (180.91 ± 37.14 mg/L vs. 174.66 ± 38.46 mg/L, $t = 0.572$, $p = 0.570$); 21-day mortality in treatment group was significantly lower than that in the control group [20.8% (5/24) vs. 50.0% (12/24), $\chi(2) = 4.463$, $p = 0.035$].
Guervilly et al. [9] 2017	Randomized controlled trial: 30 patients with moderate to severe ARDS; 6 of them were defined as severe ARDS and treated with 7ysatracurium; 24 patients were classified as moderate ARDS; 13/24 treated with 7ysatracurium; 11/24 not treated with NMBA	cisatracurium	Investigate whether NMBA exert beneficial effects in ARDS by reason of their action on respiratory mechanics, particularly transpulmonary pressures (P$_L$)	NMBA infusion was associated with an improvement in oxygenation (higher PaO$_2$/FiO$_2$) in moderate and severe ARDS, accompanied by a decrease in both P$_{plat}$ and total PEEP; the mean inspiratory and expiratory P$_L$ were higher in the moderate ARDS group receiving NMBA than in the control group; no change driving pressure or ΔP$_L$ related to NMBA administration

Table 2. *Cont.*

Authors/Year	Type of Study/Population	Subtypes of Drugs	Objective	Outcome
		Meta-analyses		
Alhazzani et al. [56] 2013	Metanalysis: three trials (431 patients)	cisatracurium	Evaluate mortality effect and risk of ICU-acquired weakness in patients with ARDS treated with neuromuscular blockade	Short-term infusion of 7ysatracurium was associated with lower hospital mortality (RR, 0.72; 95% CI, 0.58 to 0.91); lower risk of barotrauma (RR, 0.43; 95% CI, 0.20 to 0.90); no effect on the duration of MV was reported (MD, 0.25 days; 95% CI, 5.48 to 5.99), or the risk of ICU-acquired weakness (RR, 1.08; 95% CI, 0.83 to 1.41)
Torbic et al. [5] 2021	Metanalysis: six studies (1558 subjects)	not specified	Evaluate differences in mortality comparing subjects with ARDS who received NMBA to those who received placebo or usual care	NMBAs were associated with a reduction in 21 to 28-day mortality (RR = 0.71 [95% CI 0.52–0.98], but not at 90-day mortality RR = 0.81 [95% CI 0.64–1.04])
Chang et al. [55] 2020	Metanalysis: seven trials (1598 patients)	not specified	Evaluate the effects of NMBA use in patients with moderate-to-severe ARDS	Improvement in oxygenation and reduction in barotrauma risk (RR 0.56, 95% CI 0.36 to 0.87); decreasing mortality at 28 days (RR 0.74, 95% CI 0.56 to 0.9) and 90 days (RR 0.77, 95% CI 0.60 to 0.99)
Hua et al. [56] 2020	Metanalysis: six RCTs (1557 patients)	not specified	Evaluate mortality effects of NMBAs on patients with ARDS; the analysis was performed by comparing placebo or NMBAs treatment	Improvement in oxygenation (PaO_2/FiO_2 ratio) at 48 h (MD 27.26 mmHg, 95% CI 1.67, 52.84, I^2 = 92%) and reduction in barotrauma risk (RR 0.55, 95% CI 0.35, 0.85); compared with placebo or usual treatment, NMBAs were associated with lower 21 to 28-day mortality (RR 0.72, 95% CI 0.53–0.97)

Table 2. *Cont.*

Authors/Year	Type of Study/Population	Subtypes of Drugs	Objective	Outcome
Ho et al. [3] 2020	Metanalysis: five RCTs (1461 patients)	cisatracurium	Evaluate NMBAs benefits for Patients with ARDS	The 8ysatracurium group had the same risk of death at 28 days (RR, 0.90; 95% CI, 0.78–1.03; I^2 = 50%, p = 0.12) and 90 days (RR, 0.81; 95% CI, 0.62–1.06; I^2 = 56%, p = 0.06) as the control group (no 8ysatracurium); no differences in MV duration and ventilator-free days; cisatracurium had a significantly lower risk of barotrauma than the control group with no difference in intensive care unit (ICU)-induced weakness; the PaO_2/FiO_2 ratio was higher in the 8ysatracurium group but not until 48 h

NMBA, neuromuscular blocking agent; ARDS, acute respiratory distress syndrome; CRP, C-reactive protein; IL, interleukin; PaO_2/FiO_2, arterial partial pressure of oxygen/ fraction of inspired oxygen ratio; PEEP, positive end-expiratory pressure; RR, relative risk; CI, confidence interval; ICU, intensive care unit; MV, mechanical ventilation, MD, mean difference; $ScvO_2$, central venous saturation of oxygen; RCT, randomized controlled trial.

Controversial results were shown concerning the mortality rate in two larger studies: the ACURASYS and ROSE trials [52,54].

The ACURASYS trial reported a reduction in mortality in patients with moderate to severe ARDS; in contrast, the ROSE trial did not find significant changes in mortality. The differences between these two trials may be attributed to certain factors. (1) Differences in the definition of ARDS: even though, in both studies, patients presented PaO2/FiO2 < 150 mmHg, in the baseline of the ROSE trial, positive end-expiratory pressure was higher ($\geq$8 cm H2O) [52]. (2) The enrollment of patients was later in the ACURASYS trial (16 h) compared with the ROSE trial [54] (8 h), resulting in different study populations and potential bias. (3) Pharmacologic treatments differed between the studies. (4) In the ROSE trial [52], a lighter sedation strategy was used in the control group, whereas in the ACURASYS trial [54], deep sedation was used in both the treatment and placebo groups. (5) Although both studies used protective lung ventilation strategies, in the ROSE trial, a lower FiO2 was applied, but PEEP was higher and tidal volume was lower in both study arms [52].

Some meta-analyses showed improvement in oxygenation and reduction in barotrauma risk in patients with ARDS treated with NMBAs [55–58]. These controversial results were also confirmed in a recent analysis of the administration of NMBAs in cases of ARDS [59]. In contrast, another recent meta-analysis of five trials endorsed by the European Society of Intensive Care Medicine (ESICM) found no significant effect on outcomes and 28-day mortality in patients with ARDS treated with NMBAs compared with patients with ARDS who were not treated [14,52]. These controversial results may be associated with high data heterogeneity. In addition, Plens et al., in a recent study, demonstrate that NMBA infusion during ARDS could reduce expiratory muscles activity and increase end expiratory lung volume leading to a benefit in MV [60].

During the COVID-19 pandemic, NMBAs were frequently administered in patients with ARDS to reduce spontaneous efforts and thus transpulmonary pressures [53]. To date, no randomized controlled trials using NMBAs in patients with COVID-19 ARDS have been published [53,54]. A recent study observed a reduction in the duration of MV and mortality in patients with COVID-19 ARDS treated with NMBAs [61]. However, in a study conducted on 1953 patients with COVID-19 and moderate/severe ARDS, early and short courses of NMBAs did not reduce 90-day mortality and ventilator-free days [62]. The 2017 ESICM clinical practice guideline did not investigate NMBAs in the treatment of ARDS because of resource constraints [63]. More recent guidelines concluded that there is no evidence to support the routine use of NMBAs in cases of ARDS [32]. The ESICM guidelines on ARDS, published in 2023 [53], recommend against the routine use of continuous infusions of NMBAs to reduce mortality in patients with moderate/severe ARDS with a strong recommendation and a moderate level of evidence. Furthermore, because of the lack of evidence, the routine use of continuous infusions of NMBAs in patients with ARDS due to COVID-19 was not recommended [53]. In contrast, an update of the American Thoracic Society guidelines suggests neuromuscular blockade in patients with early ($\leq$48 h from MV therapy) severe ARDS (PaO2/FiO2 $\leq$ 100) [64]. In short, clinical evidence suggests that NMBAs might be considered in selected cases with early and severe ARDS with deep sedation, invasive MV, and the need for prone positioning within 48 h [32,56]. The use of NMBAs must be individualized, and further studies are required [4]. Two new trials investigating the use of cisatracurium in cases of moderate/severe ARDS are ongoing: (1) a comparison between bolus and continuous infusion (NCT05153525); and (2) early NMBAs versus sedation alone (NCT04922814). Another trial, which titrated NMBAs in spontaneous breathing patients with severe ARDS (partial neuromuscular blockade in acute respiratory distress syndrome (PNEUMA)) supported with venovenous extracorporeal membrane oxygenation recently finished, but no results have been published.

7. Status Asthmaticus

Status asthmaticus is a severe, persistent asthma attack that does not respond to usual treatments; it is characterized by hypoxemia, hypercapnia, and secondary respiratory failure [65]. A retrospective review reported that 61.2% of patients hospitalized for status asthmaticus required intubation and MV [7]. In the case of deterioration of respiratory conditions, despite initial pharmacologic treatment, intubation and MV are required. In addition, when patient–ventilator asynchronies, hypoxemia, or dynamic hyperinflation occur, even with deep sedation, the risk of generating auto-PEEP or barotrauma is high, thus requiring NMBAs [66], which then improve oxygenation and hemodynamics.

In an analysis of 30 years of ICU admissions for status asthmaticus, the use of NMBAs in mechanically ventilated patients with status asthmaticus has increased in the last 10 years [7], but this therapy remains controversial.

In a retrospective large study, Adnet et al. [28] analyzed the morbidity of intubated asthmatic patients receiving long-term (>12 h) NMBAs and found that VAP, post-intubation myopathy, and duration of ICU stay were higher in the group of patients treated with NMBAs.

Peters et al. [7] reported similar findings and an equivalent overall rate of myopathy incidence in patients with status asthmaticus receiving NMBAs. In contrast, Kesler et al. [29] demonstrated that the risk of myopathy in status asthmaticus was not associated with the duration of NMBAs because patients who underwent a short period of neuromuscular blockade also developed weakness. Replacing NMBAs with a continuous deep sedation strategy did not seem to modify the incidence of muscle weakness in patients with status asthmaticus. A recent paper from Qiao et al. [67] evaluated the risk of rhabdomyolysis, a rare but potentially fatal complication, in patients with status asthmaticus treated with high doses of steroids or theophylline combined with NMBAs, thus enhancing the debate on the use of NMBAs in status asthmaticus.

Current knowledge and the 2016 guideline for sustained neuromuscular blockade in critically ill patients suggest against the routine administration of NMBAs to mechanically ventilated patients with status asthmaticus [32].

8. Chronic Obstructive Pulmonary Disease

COPD is a heterogeneous lung condition characterized by chronic respiratory symptoms (dyspnea, cough, expectoration, and/or exacerbations) due to abnormalities of the airways (bronchitis, bronchiolitis) and/or alveoli (emphysema) that cause persistent, often progressive, airflow obstruction [68]. COPD is characterized by expiratory flow limitation, resulting in air trapping and dynamic hyperinflation, leading to auto-PEEP, increased intrathoracic pressure, and breathing efforts, as well as the risk of barotrauma. Acute respiratory failure due to an exacerbation of COPD has been associated with severe respiratory acidosis, increased levels of dyspnea, muscle fatigue, compromised neurologic status, and hemodynamic instability [6], which may require MV, either invasive or non-invasive. Sedation and occasionally paralysis with NMBAs may be needed to decrease patient–ventilator asynchrony [68,69].

In the ICU, half of patients with COPD are considered difficult to wean from MV [70]. As already described for status asthmaticus [28,29,65,71], weaning failure has been attributed to muscle weakness caused by a combination of NMBAs and corticosteroids [72]. In addition, the continuous administration of NMBAs and high doses of sedatives contribute to muscle atrophy [73]; thus, it is recommended that they are used for as short a time as possible [72]. The occurrence of respiratory muscle dysfunction caused by NMBAs may further worsen the respiratory pump performance in patients with COPD [72].

9. Monitoring of Neuromuscular Blockade and Adequacy of Sedation

Neuromuscular monitoring is indispensable for optimal management of NMBAs [35]. A peripheral nerve stimulator was introduced in the 1950s and is useful for monitoring neuromuscular blockade. In 1970, Ali et al. [74] reported train-of-four (TOF) testing to measure the degree of neuromuscular blockade through the use of a peripheral nerve stimulator. The goal of TOF monitoring is to ensure that the minimum amount of NMBA is administered to adequately paralyze the patient. TOF stimulation releases four electrical pulses to a peripheral nerve. The pattern involves stimulating the ulnar nerve with a TOF supramaximal twitch stimuli with a frequency of 2 Hz, i.e., four stimuli each separated by 0.5 s. The TOF is then repeated every 10 s (train frequency of 0.1 Hz). As well as enabling the observer to compare T1 (first twitch of the TOF) to T0 (control), it also enables comparison of T4 (fourth twitch of the TOF) to T1. This is known as the TOF ratio. [75]. There is a lack of evidence in the current ICU guidelines [32] relating to monitoring neuromuscular blockade. In the postoperative setting, a residual neuromuscular blockade (TOF < 0.9) is still related to a high incidence of unfavorable outcomes such that quantitative monitoring is considered necessary in the intraoperative management of neuromuscular blockade [75], as recommended by the latest French guidelines [76] on muscle relaxants in 2020 and by new European Society of Anesthesia and Intensive Care and American Society of Anesthesiologists guidelines [75,77]. In accordance with these guidelines, the Italian intersociety consensus on perioperative anesthesia care in thoracic surgery recommends strict neuromuscular monitoring for correct administration of both NMBAs and reversal agents [78].

Titration of the level of a neuromuscular blockade based on the patient's condition (such as renal or hepatic failure) might be considered to avoid prolonged paralysis in the ICU [26]. Residual neuromuscular blockade in the ICU is unrecognized and underreported because monitoring is not commonly carried out in this setting. In a recent study, residual neuromuscular weakness was often considered unrecognized before extubation [79]. A case report described by Workum et al. [80] reported an unusual protracted effect of NMBAs, highlighting the complexity of neuromuscular blockade in the ICU. Thus, monitoring using TOF measurements in the ICU and choosing cisatracurium over rocuronium in critically ill patients should be considered [80].

A recent trial explored the efficacy of TOF monitoring to guide clinical neuromuscular blockade compared with clinical monitoring alone in patients with ARDS. They found no significant change in ICU mortality between the two groups [81]. New research is needed to better assess which is the best NMBA in each clinical situation and how to monitor neuromuscular blockade in the ICU context.

The use of deep sedation and analgesia is always required with NMBAs [32,82]. Patients undergoing MV are often in pain; thus, sedation is necessary to facilitate tolerance to the endotracheal tube, endotracheal suction, and prolonged immobility [83,84]. Strictly sedation monitoring in the ICU could be performed with the bi-spectral index of the electroencephalogram (BIS) or E-entropy, a non-invasive technique easily obtained at the bedside [85]. However, the BIS score is not always considered reliable because of variability in the patient response caused by forehead muscle tone and electrical and mechanical interference, particularly in ICU patients [82]. In this case, NMBAs could be useful to abolish muscle contractions. A small study, conducted by Messner et al. [86], considered the effect of complete muscle relaxation on BIS in fully awake and non-sedated individuals and reported a significant decrease in BIS levels when NMBAs were administered. Other studies showed similar results in sedated patients [87,88]. Even though the use of BIS is advantageous, its systematic use is not recommended in the ICU, [89], and more studies are required to better understand if this monitoring modality is valid for mechanically ventilated patients in the ICU [90].

In summary, the use of NMBAs in patients with lung diseases seems quite safe if the sedative state is adequately monitored [89]. Nevertheless, NMBAs use is still controversial, especially considering the lack of updated guidelines concerning sedation, reversal, and monitoring [31,75,76,90].

10. Conclusions

The appropriate use of NMBAs in critically ill patients with lung diseases is unclear, and proper indications for their use are still required, including appropriate timing and careful monitoring of the duration of administration to reduce side effects while allowing for the advantage of their benefits, such as improved oxygenation. The lack of well-designed prospective trials reflects the controversial results.

There is a lack of strong and updated recommendations for the use of NMBAs in the ICU setting. Precise monitoring of the neuromuscular blockade is considered a useful strategy by which to minimize residual weakness and other detrimental effects which are not so rare in the ICU. In this case, TOF might play a role, but its use in the ICU setting is still unclear. Although current knowledge is lacking concerning studies with long-term outcomes conducted on ICU patients, in accordance with the recent guidelines, the administration of NMBAs should be limited to avoid ventilator asynchrony with a personalized approach based on each individual clinical setting. Current knowledge suggests that the use of NMBAs in critically ill patients with lung diseases must be individualized, and further studies are required. Other indications will come from new ongoing clinical trials.

Author Contributions: Conceptualization: D.B., Methodology, D.B.; Data Curation, I.G.I.; Writing—Original Draft Preparation, I.G.I., P.R.M.R. and D.B.; Writing—Review and Editing, I.G.I., L.A.-H., J.L.V.-P., C.R., P.L.S., P.R.M.R. and D.B.; Supervision, D.B. All authors have read and agreed to the published version of the manuscript.

Funding: This research received no external funding. P.R.M.R. was supported by the Brazilian Council for Scientific and Technological Development (408124/2021-0) and the Rio de Janeiro State Research Foundation (E-26/010.001488/2019).

Institutional Review Board Statement: Not applicable.

Informed Consent Statement: Not applicable.

Data Availability Statement: Not applicable.

Conflicts of Interest: The authors declare no conflicts of interest.

References

1. Fierro, M.A.; Bartz, R.R. Management of Sedation and Paralysis. *Clin. Chest Med.* **2016**, *37*, 723–739. [CrossRef]
2. Bourenne, J.; Hraiech, S.; Roch, A.; Gainnier, M.; Papazian, L.; Forel, J.-M. Sedation and Neuromuscular Blocking Agents in Acute Respiratory Distress Syndrome. *Ann. Transl. Med.* **2017**, *5*, 291. [CrossRef] [PubMed]
3. Ho, A.T.N.; Patolia, S.; Guervilly, C. Neuromuscular Blockade in Acute Respiratory Distress Syndrome: A Systematic Review and Meta-Analysis of Randomized Controlled Trials. *J. Intensive Care* **2020**, *8*, 12. [CrossRef] [PubMed]
4. Renew, J.R.; Ratzlaff, R.; Hernandez-Torres, V.; Brull, S.J.; Prielipp, R.C. Neuromuscular Blockade Management in the Critically Ill Patient. *J. Intensive Care* **2020**, *8*, 37. [CrossRef] [PubMed]
5. Torbic, H.; Krishnan, S.; Harnegie, M.P.; Duggal, A. Neuromuscular Blocking Agents for ARDS: A Systematic Review and Meta-Analysis. *Respir. Care* **2021**, *66*, 120–128. [CrossRef] [PubMed]
6. O'Donnell, D.E. COPD Exacerbations · 3: Pathophysiology. *Thorax* **2006**, *61*, 354–361. [CrossRef] [PubMed]
7. Peters, J.I.; Stupka, J.E.; Singh, H.; Rossrucker, J.; Angel, L.F.; Melo, J.; Levine, S.M. Status Asthmaticus in the Medical Intensive Care Unit: A 30-Year Experience. *Respir. Med.* **2012**, *106*, 344–348. [CrossRef] [PubMed]
8. Wilsterman, M.E.F.; De Jager, P.; Blokpoel, R.; Frerichs, I.; Dijkstra, S.K.; Albers, M.J.I.J.; Burgerhof, J.G.M.; Markhorst, D.G.; Kneyber, M.C.J. Short-Term Effects of Neuromuscular Blockade on Global and Regional Lung Mechanics, Oxygenation and Ventilation in Pediatric Acute Hypoxemic Respiratory Failure. *Ann. Intensive Care* **2016**, *6*, 103. [CrossRef] [PubMed]
9. Guervilly, C.; Bisbal, M.; Forel, J.M.; Mechati, M.; Lehingue, S.; Bourenne, J.; Perrin, G.; Rambaud, R.; Adda, M.; Hraiech, S.; et al. Effects of Neuromuscular Blockers on Transpulmonary Pressures in Moderate to Severe Acute Respiratory Distress Syndrome. *Intensive Care Med.* **2017**, *43*, 408–418. [CrossRef]
10. Gainnier, M.; Roch, A.; Forel, J.-M.; Thirion, X.; Arnal, J.-M.; Donati, S.; Papazian, L. Effect of Neuromuscular Blocking Agents on Gas Exchange in Patients Presenting with Acute Respiratory Distress Syndrome*. *Crit. Care Med.* **2004**, *32*, 113–119. [CrossRef]
11. Savoie-White, F.H.; Tremblay, L.; Menier, C.A.; Duval, C.; Bergeron, F.; Tadrous, M.; Tougas, J.; Guertin, J.R.; Ugalde, P.A. The Use of Early Neuromuscular Blockage in Acute Respiratory Distress Syndrome: A Systematic Review and Meta-Analyses of Randomized Clinical Trials. *Heart Lung* **2023**, *57*, 186–197. [CrossRef] [PubMed]
12. Wang, W.; Xu, C.; Ma, X.; Zhang, X.; Xie, P. Intensive Care Unit-Acquired Weakness: A Review of Recent Progress With a Look Toward the Future. *Front. Med.* **2020**, *7*, 559789. [CrossRef]

13. Fagerlund, M.J.; Eriksson, L.I. Current Concepts in Neuromuscular Transmission. *Br. J. Anaesth.* **2009**, *103*, 108–114. [CrossRef] [PubMed]
14. Forel, J.-M.; Roch, A.; Marin, V.; Michelet, P.; Demory, D.; Blache, J.-L.; Perrin, G.; Gainnier, M.; Bongrand, P.; Papazian, L. Neuromuscular Blocking Agents Decrease Inflammatory Response in Patients Presenting with Acute Respiratory Distress Syndrome*. *Crit. Care Med.* **2006**, *34*, 2749–2757. [CrossRef] [PubMed]
15. Slutsky, A.S. Neuromuscular Blocking Agents in ARDS. *N. Engl. J. Med.* **2010**, *363*, 1176–1180. [CrossRef] [PubMed]
16. Sottile, P.D.; Albers, D.; Moss, M.M. Neuromuscular Blockade Is Associated with the Attenuation of Biomarkers of Epithelial and Endothelial Injury in Patients with Moderate-to-Severe Acute Respiratory Distress Syndrome. *Crit Care* **2018**, *22*, 63. [CrossRef] [PubMed]
17. Stäuble, C.G.; Blobner, M. The Future of Neuromuscular Blocking Agents. *Curr. Opin. Anaesthesiol.* **2020**, *33*, 490–498. [CrossRef] [PubMed]
18. Hager, H.H.; Burns, B. Succinylcholine Chloride. In *StatPearls*; StatPearls Publishing: Treasure Island, FL, USA, 2023. Available online: https://pubmed.ncbi.nlm.nih.gov/29763160/ (accessed on 15 November 2023).
19. Sparr, H.J.; Beaufort, T.M.; Fuchs-Buder, T. Newer Neuromuscular Blocking Agents: How Do They Compare with Established Agents? *Drugs* **2001**, *61*, 919–942. [CrossRef]
20. Hraiech, S.; Yoshida, T.; Annane, D.; Duggal, A.; Fanelli, V.; Gacouin, A.; Heunks, L.; Jaber, S.; Sottile, P.D.; Papazian, L. Myorelaxants in ARDS Patients. *Intensive Care Med.* **2020**, *46*, 2357–2372. [CrossRef]
21. Reintam Blaser, A.; Regli, A.; De Keulenaer, B.; Kimball, E.J.; Starkopf, L.; Davis, W.A.; Greiffenstein, P.; Starkopf, J. Incidence, Risk Factors, and Outcomes of Intra-Abdominal Hypertension in Critically Ill Patients—A Prospective Multicenter Study (IROI Study). *Crit. Care Med.* **2019**, *47*, 535–542. [CrossRef]
22. Malbrain, M.L.N.G.; Chiumello, D.; Cesana, B.M.; Reintam Blaser, A.; Starkopf, J.; Sugrue, M.; Pelosi, P.; Severgnini, P.; Hernandez, G.; Brienza, N.; et al. A Systematic Review and Individual Patient Data Meta-Analysis on Intra-Abdominal Hypertension in Critically Ill Patients: The Wake-up Project. World Initiative on Abdominal Hypertension Epidemiology, a Unifying Project (WAKE-Up!). *Minerva Anestesiol.* **2014**, *80*, 293–306.
23. Pelosi, P.; Quintel, M.; Malbrain, M.L.N.G. Effect of Intra-Abdominal Pressure on Respiratory Mechanics. *Acta Clin. Belg.* **2007**, *62* (Suppl. S1), 78–88. [CrossRef]
24. Regli, A.; Pelosi, P.; Malbrain, M.L.N.G. Ventilation in Patients with Intra-Abdominal Hypertension: What Every Critical Care Physician Needs to Know. *Ann. Intensive Care* **2019**, *9*, 52. [CrossRef]
25. De Laet, I.E.; Malbrain, M.L.N.G.; De Waele, J.J. A Clinician's Guide to Management of Intra-Abdominal Hypertension and Abdominal Compartment Syndrome in Critically Ill Patients. *Crit. Care* **2020**, *24*, 97. [CrossRef] [PubMed]
26. Deem, S.; Lee, C.M.; Curtis, J.R. Acquired Neuromuscular Disorders in the Intensive Care Unit. *Am. J. Respir. Crit. Care Med.* **2003**, *168*, 735–739. [CrossRef]
27. Price, D.R.; Mikkelsen, M.E.; Umscheid, C.A.; Armstrong, E.J. Neuromuscular Blocking Agents and Neuromuscular Dysfunction Acquired in Critical Illness: A Systematic Review and Meta-Analysis. *Crit. Care Med.* **2016**, *44*, 2070–2078. [CrossRef] [PubMed]
28. Adnet, F.; Dhissi, G.; Borron, S.W.; Galinski, M.; Rayeh, F.; Cupa, M.; Pourriat, J.; Lapostolle, F. Complication Profiles of Adult Asthmatics Requiring Paralysis during Mechanical Ventilation. *Intensive Care Med.* **2001**, *27*, 1729–1736. [CrossRef]
29. Kesler, S.M.; Sprenkle, M.D.; David, W.S.; Leatherman, J.W. Severe Weakness Complicating Status Asthmaticus despite Minimal Duration of Neuromuscular Paralysis. *Intensive Care Med.* **2009**, *35*, 157–160. [CrossRef]
30. Bellaver, P.; Schaeffer, A.F.; Leitao, C.B.; Rech, T.H.; Nedel, W.L. Association between Neuromuscular Blocking Agents and the Development of Intensive Care Unit-Acquired Weakness (ICU-AW): A Systematic Review with Meta-Analysis and Trial Sequential Analysis. *Anaesth. Crit. Care Pain Med.* **2023**, *42*, 101202. [CrossRef] [PubMed]
31. Puthucheary, Z.; Rawal, J.; Ratnayake, G.; Harridge, S.; Montgomery, H.; Hart, N. Neuromuscular Blockade and Skeletal Muscle Weakness in Critically Ill Patients: Time to Rethink the Evidence? *Am. J. Respir. Crit. Care Med.* **2012**, *185*, 911–917. [CrossRef]
32. Murray, M.J.; DeBlock, H.; Erstad, B.; Gray, A.; Jacobi, J.; Jordan, C.; McGee, W.; McManus, C.; Meade, M.; Nix, S.; et al. Clinical Practice Guidelines for Sustained Neuromuscular Blockade in the Adult Critically Ill Patient. *Crit. Care Med.* **2016**, *44*, 2079–2103. [CrossRef]
33. Cedborg, A.I.H.; Sundman, E.; Bodén, K.; Hedström, H.W.; Kuylenstierna, R.; Ekberg, O.; Eriksson, L.I. Pharyngeal Function and Breathing Pattern during Partial Neuromuscular Block in the Elderly. *Anesthesiology* **2014**, *120*, 312–325. [CrossRef]
34. Awadh Behbehani, N.; Al-Mane, F.; D'yachkova, Y.; Paré, P.; Fitz Gerald, J.M. Myopathy Following Mechanical Ventilation for Acute Severe Asthma. *Chest* **1999**, *115*, 1627–1631. [CrossRef] [PubMed]
35. Rodríguez-Blanco, J.; Rodríguez-Yanez, T.; Rodríguez-Blanco, J.D.; Almanza-Hurtado, A.J.; Martínez-Ávila, M.C.; Borré-Naranjo, D.; Acuña Caballero, M.C.; Dueñas-Castell, C. Neuromuscular Blocking Agents in the Intensive Care Unit. *J. Int. Med. Res.* **2022**, *50*, 030006052211281. [CrossRef]
36. Levy, B.D.; Kitch, B.; Fanta, C.H. Medical and Ventilatory Management of Status Asthmaticus. *Intensive Care Med.* **1998**, *24*, 105–117. [CrossRef] [PubMed]
37. Blanch, L.; Villagra, A.; Sales, B.; Montanya, J.; Lucangelo, U.; Luján, M.; García-Esquirol, O.; Chacón, E.; Estruga, A.; Oliva, J.C.; et al. Asynchronies during Mechanical Ventilation Are Associated with Mortality. *Intensive Care Med.* **2015**, *41*, 633–641. [CrossRef] [PubMed]

38. Pham, T.; Telias, I.; Piraino, T.; Yoshida, T.; Brochard, L.J. Asynchrony Consequences and Management. *Crit. Care Clin.* **2018**, *34*, 325–341. [CrossRef]
39. De Haro, C.; Ochagavia, A.; López-Aguilar, J.; Fernandez-Gonzalo, S.; Navarra-Ventura, G.; Magrans, R.; Montanyà, J.; Blanch, L. Patient-Ventilator Asynchronies during Mechanical Ventilation: Current Knowledge and Research Priorities. *ICMx* **2019**, *7*, 43. [CrossRef]
40. Yoshida, T.; Amato, M.B.P.; Kavanagh, B.P. Understanding Spontaneous vs. Ventilator Breaths: Impact and Monitoring. *Intensive Care Med.* **2018**, *44*, 2235–2238. [CrossRef]
41. Yoshida, T.; Fujino, Y.; Amato, M.B.P.; Kavanagh, B.P. FIFTY YEARS OF RESEARCH IN ARDS. Spontaneous Breathing during Mechanical Ventilation. Risks, Mechanisms, and Management. *Am. J. Respir. Crit. Care Med.* **2017**, *195*, 985–992. [CrossRef]
42. Yoshida, T.; Uchiyama, A.; Matsuura, N.; Mashimo, T.; Fujino, Y. The Comparison of Spontaneous Breathing and Muscle Paralysis in Two Different Severities of Experimental Lung Injury*. *Crit. Care Med.* **2013**, *41*, 536–545. [CrossRef] [PubMed]
43. Wei, X.; Wang, Z.; Liao, X.; Guo, W.; Qin, T.; Wang, S. Role of Neuromuscular Blocking Agents in Acute Respiratory Distress Syndrome: An Updated Meta-Analysis of Randomized Controlled Trials. *Front. Pharmacol.* **2020**, *10*, 1637. [CrossRef] [PubMed]
44. Balzer, F.; Weiß, B.; Kumpf, O.; Treskatsch, S.; Spies, C.; Wernecke, K.-D.; Krannich, A.; Kastrup, M. Early Deep Sedation Is Associated with Decreased In-Hospital and Two-Year Follow-Up Survival. *Crit. Care* **2015**, *19*, 197. [CrossRef]
45. Mellott, K.G.; Grap, M.J.; Munro, C.L.; Sessler, C.N.; Wetzel, P.A.; Nilsestuen, J.O.; Ketchum, J.M. Patient Ventilator Asynchrony in Critically Ill Adults: Frequency and Types. *Heart Lung* **2014**, *43*, 231–243. [CrossRef]
46. Conti, G.; Ranieri, V.M.; Costa, R.; Garratt, C.; Wighton, A.; Spinazzola, G.; Urbino, R.; Mascia, L.; Ferrone, G.; Pohjanjousi, P.; et al. Effects of Dexmedetomidine and Propofol on Patient-Ventilator Interaction in Difficult-to-Wean, Mechanically Ventilated Patients: A Prospective, Open-Label, Randomised, Multicentre Study. *Crit. Care* **2016**, *20*, 206. [CrossRef] [PubMed]
47. Holanda, M.A.; Vasconcelos, R.D.S.; Ferreira, J.C.; Pinheiro, B.V. Patient-Ventilator Asynchrony. *J. Bras. Pneumol.* **2018**, *44*, 321–333. [CrossRef] [PubMed]
48. Qadir, N.; Chang, S.Y. Pharmacologic Treatments for Acute Respiratory Distress Syndrome. *Crit. Care Clin.* **2021**, *37*, 877–893. [CrossRef] [PubMed]
49. Bellani, G.; Laffey, J.G.; Pham, T.; Fan, E.; Brochard, L.; Esteban, A.; Gattinoni, L.; van Haren, F.; Larsson, A.; McAuley, D.F.; et al. Epidemiology, Patterns of Care, and Mortality for Patients With Acute Respiratory Distress Syndrome in Intensive Care Units in 50 Countries. *JAMA* **2016**, *315*, 788–800. [CrossRef]
50. Tsolaki, V.; Zakynthinos, G.E.; Papadonta, M.-E.; Bardaka, F.; Fotakopoulos, G.; Pantazopoulos, I.; Makris, D.; Zakynthinos, E. Neuromuscular Blockade in the Pre- and COVID-19 ARDS Patients. *JPM* **2022**, *12*, 1538. [CrossRef]
51. Tarazan, N.; Alshehri, M.; Sharif, S.; Al Duhailib, Z.; Møller, M.H.; Belley-Cote, E.; Alshahrani, M.; Centofanti, J.; McIntyre, L.; Baw, B.; et al. Neuromuscular Blocking Agents in Acute Respiratory Distress Syndrome: Updated Systematic Review and Meta-Analysis of Randomized Trials. *ICMx* **2020**, *8*, 61. [CrossRef]
52. The National Heart, Lung, and Blood Institute PETAL Clinical Trials Network Early Neuromuscular Blockade in the Acute Respiratory Distress Syndrome. *N. Engl. J. Med.* **2019**, *380*, 1997–2008. [CrossRef]
53. Grasselli, G.; Calfee, C.S.; Camporota, L.; Poole, D.; Amato, M.B.P.; Antonelli, M.; Arabi, Y.M.; Baroncelli, F.; Beitler, J.R.; Bellani, G.; et al. ESICM Guidelines on Acute Respiratory Distress Syndrome: Definition, Phenotyping and Respiratory Support Strategies. *Intensive Care Med.* **2023**, *49*, 727–759. [CrossRef]
54. Papazian, L.; Forel, J.-M.; Gacouin, A.; Penot-Ragon, C.; Perrin, G.; Loundou, A.; Jaber, S.; Arnal, J.-M.; Perez, D.; Seghboyan, J.-M.; et al. Neuromuscular Blockers in Early Acute Respiratory Distress Syndrome. *N. Engl. J. Med.* **2010**, *363*, 1107–1116. [CrossRef]
55. Lyu, G.; Wang, X.; Jiang, W.; Cai, T.; Zhang, Y. Clinical study of early use of neuromuscular blocking agents in patients with severe sepsis and acute respiratory distress syndrome. *Zhonghua Wei Zhong Bing Ji Jiu Yi Xue* **2014**, *26*, 325–329. [CrossRef]
56. Alhazzani, W.; Alshahrani, M.; Jaeschke, R.; Forel, J.; Papazian, L.; Sevransky, J.; Meade, M.O. Neuromuscular Blocking Agents in Acute Respiratory Distress Syndrome: A Systematic Review and Meta-Analysis of Randomized Controlled Trials. *Crit. Care* **2013**, *17*, R43. [CrossRef] [PubMed]
57. Chang, W.; Sun, Q.; Peng, F.; Xie, J.; Qiu, H.; Yang, Y. Validation of Neuromuscular Blocking Agent Use in Acute Respiratory Distress Syndrome: A Meta-Analysis of Randomized Trials. *Crit. Care* **2020**, *24*, 54. [CrossRef]
58. Hua, Y.; Ou, X.; Li, Q.; Zhu, T. Neuromuscular Blockers in the Acute Respiratory Distress Syndrome: A Meta-Analysis. *PLoS ONE* **2020**, *15*, e0227664. [CrossRef] [PubMed]
59. Mefford, B.; Donaldson, J.C.; Bissell, B.D. To Block or Not: Updates in Neuromuscular Blockade in Acute Respiratory Distress Syndrome. *Ann. Pharmacother.* **2020**, *54*, 899–906. [CrossRef]
60. Plens, G.M.; Droghi, M.T.; Alcala, G.C.; Pereira, S.M.; Wawrzeniak, I.C.; Victorino, J.A.; Crivellari, C.; Grassi, A.; Rezoagli, E.; Foti, G.; et al. Expiratory Muscle Activity Counteracts PEEP and Is Associated with Fentanyl Dose in ARDS Patients. *Am. J. Respir. Crit. Care Med.* **2024**, rccm.202308-1376OC. [CrossRef] [PubMed]
61. Lee, B.Y.; Lee, S.-I.; Baek, M.S.; Baek, A.-R.; Na, Y.S.; Kim, J.H.; Seong, G.M.; Kim, W.-Y. Lower Driving Pressure and Neuromuscular Blocker Use Are Associated With Decreased Mortality in Patients With COVID-19 ARDS. *Respir. Care* **2022**, *67*, 216–226. [CrossRef]
62. Li Bassi, G.; Gibbons, K.; Suen, J.Y.; Dalton, H.J.; White, N.; Corley, A.; Shrapnel, S.; Hinton, S.; Forsyth, S.; Laffey, J.G.; et al. Early Short Course of Neuromuscular Blocking Agents in Patients with COVID-19 ARDS: A Propensity Score Analysis. *Crit. Care* **2022**, *26*, 141. [CrossRef]

63. Fan, E.; Del Sorbo, L.; Goligher, E.C.; Hodgson, C.L.; Munshi, L.; Walkey, A.J.; Adhikari, N.K.J.; Amato, M.B.P.; Branson, R.; Brower, R.G.; et al. An Official American Thoracic Society/European Society of Intensive Care Medicine/Society of Critical Care Medicine Clinical Practice Guideline: Mechanical Ventilation in Adult Patients with Acute Respiratory Distress Syndrome. *Am. J. Respir. Crit. Care Med.* **2017**, *195*, 1253–1263. [CrossRef]

64. Qadir, N.; Sahetya, S.; Munshi, L.; Summers, C.; Abrams, D.; Beitler, J.; Bellani, G.; Brower, R.G.; Burry, L.; Chen, J.-T.; et al. An Update on Management of Adult Patients with Acute Respiratory Distress Syndrome: An Official American Thoracic Society Clinical Practice Guideline. *Am. J. Respir. Crit. Care Med.* **2024**, *209*, 24–36. [CrossRef] [PubMed]

65. Chakraborty, R.K.; Basnet, S. Status Asthmaticus. In *StatPearls*; StatPearls Publishing: Treasure Island, FL, USA, 2022. Available online: https://www.ncbi.nlm.nih.gov/books/NBK526070 (accessed on 15 November 2023).

66. Goh, A.; Chan, P. Acute Myopathy after Status Asthmaticus: Steroids, Myorelaxants or Carbon Dioxide? *Respirology* **1999**, *4*, 97–99. [CrossRef]

67. Qiao, H.; Cheng, H.; Liu, L.; Yin, J. Potential Factors Involved in the Causation of Rhabdomyolysis Following Status Asthmaticus. *Allergy Asthma Clin. Immunol.* **2016**, *12*, 43. [CrossRef] [PubMed]

68. Venkatesan, P. GOLD COPD Report: 2023 Update. *Lancet Respir. Med.* **2023**, *11*, 18. [CrossRef]

69. Vassilakopoulos, T. Understanding Wasted/Ineffective Efforts in Mechanically Ventilated COPD Patients Using the Campbell Diagram. *Intensive Care Med.* **2008**, *34*, 1336–1339. [CrossRef] [PubMed]

70. Petrof, B.J.; Legaré, M.; Goldberg, P.; Milic-Emili, J.; Gottfried, S.B. Continuous Positive Airway Pressure Reduces Work of Breathing and Dyspnea during Weaning from Mechanical Ventilation in Severe Chronic Obstructive Pulmonary Disease. *Am. Rev. Respir. Dis.* **1990**, *141*, 281–289. [CrossRef]

71. Appleton, R.; Kinsella, J. Intensive Care Unit-Acquired Weakness. *Contin. Educ. Anaesth. Crit. Care Pain* **2012**, *12*, 62–66. [CrossRef]

72. Scaramuzzo, G.; Ottaviani, I.; Volta, C.A.; Spadaro, S. Mechanical Ventilation and COPD: From Pathophysiology to Ventilatory Management. *Minerva Med.* **2022**, *113*, 460–470. [CrossRef]

73. Goligher, E.C.; Dres, M.; Fan, E.; Rubenfeld, G.D.; Scales, D.C.; Herridge, M.S.; Vorona, S.; Sklar, M.C.; Rittayamai, N.; Lanys, A.; et al. Mechanical Ventilation–Induced Diaphragm Atrophy Strongly Impacts Clinical Outcomes. *Am. J. Respir. Crit. Care Med.* **2018**, *197*, 204–213. [CrossRef] [PubMed]

74. Ali, H.H.; Utting, J.E.; Gray, C. Stimulus Frequency in the Detection of Neuromuscular Block in Humans. *Br. J. Anaesth.* **1970**, *42*, 967–978. [CrossRef] [PubMed]

75. Thilen, S.R.; Weigel, W.A.; Todd, M.M.; Dutton, R.P.; Lien, C.A.; Grant, S.A.; Szokol, J.W.; Eriksson, L.I.; Yaster, M.; Grant, M.D.; et al. 2023 American Society of Anesthesiologists Practice Guidelines for Monitoring and Antagonism of Neuromuscular Blockade: A Report by the American Society of Anesthesiologists Task Force on Neuromuscular Blockade. *Anesthesiology* **2023**, *138*, 13–41. [CrossRef] [PubMed]

76. Brull, S.J.; Eriksson, L. The French Guidelines on Muscle Relaxants and Reversal in Anaesthesia: The Chain Is Finally Broken and the Soul Is Freed. *Anaesth. Crit. Care Pain Med.* **2020**, *39*, 31–33. [CrossRef] [PubMed]

77. Motamed, C. Sugammadex in Emergency Situations. *J. Pers. Med.* **2023**, *13*, 159. [CrossRef] [PubMed]

78. Piccioni, F.; Droghetti, A.; Bertani, A.; Coccia, C.; Corcione, A.; Corsico, A.G.; Crisci, R.; Curcio, C.; Del Naja, C.; Feltracco, P.; et al. Recommendations from the Italian Intersociety Consensus on Perioperative Anesthesa Care in Thoracic Surgery (PACTS) Part 2: Intraoperative and Postoperative Care. *Perioper. Med.* **2020**, *9*, 31. [CrossRef] [PubMed]

79. Calef, A.; Castelgrande, R.; Crawley, K.; Dorris, S.; Durham, J.; Lee, K.; Paras, J.; Piazza, K.; Race, A.; Rider, L.; et al. Reversing Neuromuscular Blockade without Nerve Stimulator Guidance in a Postsurgical ICU—An Observational Study. *J. Clin. Med.* **2023**, *12*, 3253. [CrossRef]

80. Workum, J.D.; Janssen, S.H.V.; Touw, H.R.W. Considerations in Neuromuscular Blockade in the ICU: A Case Report and Review of the Literature. *Case Rep. Crit. Care* **2020**, *2020*, 8780979. [CrossRef]

81. Rezaiguia-Delclaux, S.; Laverdure, F.; Genty, T.; Imbert, A.; Pilorge, C.; Amaru, P.; Sarfati, C.; Stéphan, F. Neuromuscular Blockade Monitoring in Acute Respiratory Distress Syndrome: Randomized Controlled Trial of Clinical Assessment Alone or with Peripheral Nerve Stimulation. *Anesth. Analg.* **2021**, *132*, 1051–1059. [CrossRef]

82. Tezcan, B.; Turan, S.; Clinic of Anaesthesiology and Reanimation, Department of Intensive Care, Turkiye Yuksek Ihtisas Training and Research Hospital, Ankara, Turkey; Ozgok, A.; Clinic of Anaesthesiology and Reanimation, Turkiye Yuksek Ihtisas Training and Research Hospital, Ankara, Turkey. Current Use of Neuromuscular Blocking Agents in Intensive Care Units. *Turk. J. Anaesthesiol. Reanim.* **2019**, *47*, 273–281. [CrossRef]

83. Puntillo, K.A.; Arai, S.; Cohen, N.H.; Gropper, M.A.; Neuhaus, J.; Paul, S.M.; Miaskowski, C. Symptoms Experienced by Intensive Care Unit Patients at High Risk of Dying*. *Crit. Care Med.* **2010**, *38*, 2155–2160. [CrossRef]

84. Desbiens, N.A.; Wu, A.W.; Broste, S.K.; Wenger, N.S.; Connors, A.F.; Lynn, J.; Yasui, Y.; Phillips, R.S.; Fulkerson, W. Pain and Satisfaction with Pain Control in Seriously Ill Hospitalized Adults: Findings from the SUPPORT Research Investigations. *Crit. Care Med.* **1996**, *24*, 1953–1961. [CrossRef]

85. Coleman, R.M.; Tousignant-Laflamme, Y.; Ouellet, P.; Parenteau-Goudreault, É.; Cogan, J.; Bourgault, P. The Use of the Bispectral Index in the Detection of Pain in Mechanically Ventilated Adults in the Intensive Care Unit: A Review of the Literature. *Pain Res. Manag.* **2015**, *20*, e33–e37. [CrossRef] [PubMed]

86. Messner, M.; Beese, U.; Romstöck, J.; Dinkel, M.; Tschaikowsky, A.K. The Bispectral Index Declines During Neuromuscular Block in Fully Awake Persons. *Anesth. Analg.* **2003**, *97*, 488–491. [CrossRef]

87. Inoue, S.; Kawaguchi, M.; Sasaoka, N.; Hirai, K.; Furuya, H. Effects of Neuromuscular Block on Systemic and Cerebral Hemodynamics and Bispectral Index during Moderate or Deep Sedation in Critically Ill Patients. *Intensive Care Med.* **2006**, *32*, 391–397. [CrossRef] [PubMed]
88. Vivien, B.; Di Maria, S.; Ouattara, A.; Langeron, O.; Coriat, P.; Riou, B. Overestimation of Bispectral Index in Sedated Intensive Care Unit Patients Revealed by Administration of Muscle Relaxant. *Anesthesiology* **2003**, *99*, 9–17. [CrossRef] [PubMed]
89. Shetty, R.M.; Bellini, A.; Wijayatilake, D.S.; Hamilton, M.A.; Jain, R.; Karanth, S.; Namachivayam, A. BIS Monitoring versus Clinical Assessment for Sedation in Mechanically Ventilated Adults in the Intensive Care Unit and Its Impact on Clinical Outcomes and Resource Utilization. *Cochrane Database Syst. Rev.* **2018**, *2019*, CD011240. [CrossRef]
90. Bilgili, B.; Montoya, J.C.; Layon, A.J.; Berger, A.L.; Kirchner, H.L.; Gupta, L.K.; Gloss, D.S. Utilizing Bi-Spectral Index (BIS) for the Monitoring of Sedated Adult ICU Patients: A Systematic Review. *Minerva Anestesiol* **2017**, *83*, 288–301. [CrossRef]

Disclaimer/Publisher's Note: The statements, opinions and data contained in all publications are solely those of the individual author(s) and contributor(s) and not of MDPI and/or the editor(s). MDPI and/or the editor(s) disclaim responsibility for any injury to people or property resulting from any ideas, methods, instructions or products referred to in the content.

Review

Lung Imaging and Artificial Intelligence in ARDS

Davide Chiumello [1,2,3,*], Silvia Coppola [2], Giulia Catozzi [1], Fiammetta Danzo [4,5], Pierachille Santus [4,5] and Dejan Radovanovic [4,5]

[1] Department of Health Sciences, University of Milan, 20122 Milan, Italy
[2] Department of Anesthesia and Intensive Care, ASST Santi Paolo e Carlo, San Paolo University Hospital Milan, 20142 Milan, Italy
[3] Coordinated Research Center on Respiratory Failure, University of Milan, 20122 Milan, Italy
[4] Division of Respiratory Diseases, Luigi Sacco University Hospital, ASST Fatebenefratelli-Sacco, 20157 Milan, Italy
[5] Department of Biomedical and Clinical Sciences, Università degli Studi di Milano, 20157 Milan, Italy
* Correspondence: davide.chiumello@unimi.it

Abstract: Artificial intelligence (AI) can make intelligent decisions in a manner akin to that of the human mind. AI has the potential to improve clinical workflow, diagnosis, and prognosis, especially in radiology. Acute respiratory distress syndrome (ARDS) is a very diverse illness that is characterized by interstitial opacities, mostly in the dependent areas, decreased lung aeration with alveolar collapse, and inflammatory lung edema resulting in elevated lung weight. As a result, lung imaging is a crucial tool for evaluating the mechanical and morphological traits of ARDS patients. Compared to traditional chest radiography, sensitivity and specificity of lung computed tomography (CT) and ultrasound are higher. The state of the art in the application of AI is summarized in this narrative review which focuses on CT and ultrasound techniques in patients with ARDS. A total of eighteen items were retrieved. The primary goals of using AI for lung imaging were to evaluate the risk of developing ARDS, the measurement of alveolar recruitment, potential alternative diagnoses, and outcome. While the physician must still be present to guarantee a high standard of examination, AI could help the clinical team provide the best care possible.

Keywords: artificial intelligence; lung imaging; CT; LUS; ARDS; COVID-19; deep learning; machine learning

1. Introduction

Broadly defined, artificial intelligence (AI) is a machine or computing platform that is capable of making intelligent decisions in a manner similar to the human mind [1]. In healthcare, AI could improve prognosis, diagnosis, treatment, and clinical workflow, particularly in the field of radiology, cardiovascular, and pathology [1,2]. Many of these medical tasks have been widely adopted in daily clinical practice [1]. During the last pandemic, significant progress was made in the development of AI resulting in more than 900 articles on COVID-19 and artificial intelligence [3]. Although the presence of a physician is still essential, AI could assist the clinical team in providing the best possible care.

During 2020, up to 30% of radiologic examinations were managed by AI with almost 20% planned for the following year [4,5], such as to detect intracranial hemorrhage, pulmonary embolism, and to monitor mammographic abnormalities. In addition, AI can improve scanning procedures, by reducing radiation exposure during scanning and acquisition, and then can optimize the sophisticated image reconstruction across magnetic resonance imaging, computed tomography (CT), and positron emission tomography modalities [4,5]. A recent survey found that radiologists would like to see AI improve anatomical measurements, lesion detection, and the quality of radiological imaging [4]. In particular, acute respiratory distress syndrome (ARDS) is a rather heterogeneous syndrome characterized by an inflammatory lung edema leading to an increased lung weight, decreased lung aeration with the presence of alveolar collapse, and interstitial opacities mainly in the dependent areas [6]. Lung imaging is an essential tool to assess not only the morphology but also the mechanical characteristics of ARDS patients. Lung CT and lung ultrasound (LUS) have a higher sensitivity and specificity than conventional chest radiography.

2. Machine Learning and Deep Learning

Machine learning (ML) is a subset of AI that focuses on developing algorithms and models that allow computers to learn from data and make predictions or decisions based on that data. These algorithms rely on manually engineered features. Developers write explicit instructions for the computer to follow. In ML, however, the computer learns patterns and relationships from data to make informed decisions or predictions. The primary goal of ML is to enable computers to improve their performance on a task over time by learning from examples rather than being explicitly programmed. ML algorithms are primarily designed to classify objects, detect patterns, predict outcomes, and make informed decisions [7].

In contrast, deep learning (DL) is a subfield of ML that focuses on training artificial neural networks with multiple layers (deep architectures) to learn complex patterns from data. In DL, models are based on deep artificial neural networks that can learn directly from data without the need for manual extraction. These neural networks are inspired by the structure and function of the human brain, where information is processed through interconnected neurons. The term "deep" in DL refers to the depth of the neural network, which consists of multiple hidden layers between the input and output layers. DL tends to work best with large datasets, as a large amount of data is required to successfully train deep neural networks. Certain neural network architectures such as the so-called convolutional neural networks (CNNs) are used specifically for image recognition. The potential applications of DL using lung CT and ultrasound may range from the early diagnosis, detection, and segmentation of specific lung regions to the prediction of the short- and long-term clinical outcomes [8].

3. Search Strategy

In this narrative review, we focus on the role of AI in the field of lung imaging in ARDS. Figure 1 shows the search strategy flowchart.

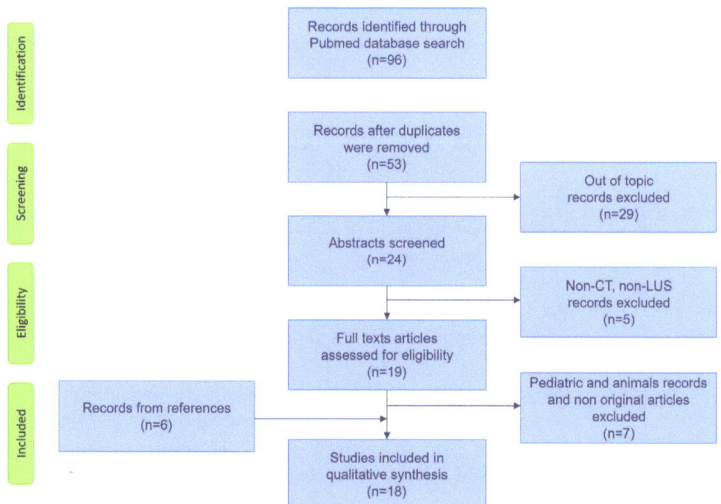

Figure 1. Flowchart of search strategy. CT: computed tomography; LUS: lung ultrasound.

We used PubMed and Embase databases performing two separate searches. For the first search, we used the following initial screening keywords: "lung CT scan AND artificial intelligence/machine learning AND ARDS/acute respiratory failure". For the second search, we used "lung ultrasound AND artificial intelligence/machine learning AND ARDS/acute respiratory failure". Then, the search was expanded using the following keywords: "lung imaging AND artificial intelligence/machine learning AND ARDS/acute respiratory failure", resulting in 96 articles. After excluding duplicates, we also excluded screened abstracts and articles that did not include artificial intelligence involving either CT imaging or lung ultrasound imaging. Nineteen articles were identified. We excluded articles on pediatric patients and animals, resulting in 12 papers. We included 6 articles from the references. We included a total number of 18 studies in the review, which are summarized in Table 1.

Table 1. Summary of the studies.

Author, Year	Study Design	Aim	Endpoints	AI Model	Results
Nishiyama, 2020 [9]	single center retrospective	prediction of prognosis	To evaluate the relationship between CT volume of well-aerated lung region and prognosis in ARDS patients.	An automated lung volumetry software of lung CT scan to identify lung region volumes by CT attenuation densities.	Well-aerated lung regions showed a positive correlation with 28-day survival. Survival outcome was better for percentage of well-aerated lung region/predicted total lung capacity ≥40% than <40%.
Gresser, 2021 [10]	single center retrospective	prediction of prognosis	To assess the potential of AI-based CT assessment and clinical score to predict the need for ECMO therapy in COVID-19 ARDS.	CT software provides segmentation of lung lobes providing a CT severity score.	AI-based assessment of lung involvement on CT scans at hospital admission and the SOFA scoring, especially if combined, can be used as risk stratification tools for subsequent ECMO requirement.
Hermann, 2021 [11]	multicenter retrospective	alveolar recruitment	To compare the accuracy in the computation of recruitability on CT scan between automatic lung segmentation performed by a properly trained neural network and manual segmentation in ARDS and COVID-19.	A DL algorithm to automatically segment ARDS injured lungs to calculate the lung recruitment.	The AI segmentation showed the same degree of inaccuracy of the manual segmentation. The recruitability measured with manual and AI segmentation had a bias of +0.3% and −0.5% expressed as change in well-aerated tissue fraction.
Kang, 2021 [12]	single center retrospective	differential diagnosis	To train a DL classifier model to differentiate between COVID-19 and bacterial pneumonia based on automatic segmentation of lung and lesion regions.	A DL model with deformable convolution neural network architecture trained to differentiate lesion patches of COVID-19 from those of bacterial pneumonia on CT scan.	DL lung CT scan analysis with constructed lesion clusters achieved an accuracy of 91.2% for classifying COVID-19 and bacterial pneumonia patients.

Table 1. *Cont.*

Author, Year	Study Design	Aim	Endpoints	AI Model	Results
Lanza, 2020 [13]	single center retrospective	prediction of prognosis	To test quantitative CT analysis using a semi-automated method as an outcome predictor in terms of need for oxygen support or intubation in COVID-19.	Quantitative CT analysis with a semi-automated segmentation algorithm that divides lungs into not aerated, poorly aerated, normally aerated and hyperinflated.	The amount of compromised lung volume can predict the need for oxygenation support (between 6–23% of compromised lung) and intubation (above 23%) and is a significant risk factor for in-hospital death.
Liu, 2020 [14]	single center retrospective	prediction of prognosis	To quantify pneumonia lesions by CT (% of ground-glass, semi-consolidation and consolidation volume) in the early days to predict progression to severe illness using AI algorithms in COVID-19.	CT quantitative analysis combines a fully convolutional network with adopting thresholding and morphological operations for segmentation of lung and pneumonia lesions.	CT features on day 0 and 4, and their changes from day 0 to day 4, showed predictive capability for severe illness within a 28-day follow up. CT quantification of pneumonia lesions can early and non-invasively predict the progression to severe illness.
Pennati, 2023 [2]	single center retrospective	alveolar recruitment	To develop and validate classifier models to identify patients with a high percentage of potentially recruitable lung from readily available clinical data and from a single CT scan quantitative analysis at ICU admission.	Four ML algorithms (Logistic regression, Support Vector Machine, Random Forest, XGboost) to predict lung recruitment starting from a single CT scan obtained at 5 cmH$_2$O at ICU admission.	The use of the four ML algorithms based on a CT scan at 5 cm H$_2$O were able to classify lung recruiter patients with similar AUC as the ML algorithm, based on the combination of lung mechanics, gas exchange and CT data.
Penarrubia, 2023 [15]	single center retrospective	alveolar recruitment	To assess both intra- and inter-observer smallest real difference exceeding measurement error of recruitment using both human and ML on low-dose CT scans acquired at 5 and 15 cm H$_2$O of PEEP in ARDS.	ML lung segmentation algorithm on CT scan to compute alveolar recruitment at 5 and 15 cm H$_2$O of PEEP.	Human–machine and human–human inter-observer measurement errors were similar, suggesting that ML segmentation algorithms are valid alternative to humans for quantifying alveolar recruitment on CT.

Table 1. *Cont.*

Author, Year	Study Design	Aim	Endpoints	AI Model	Results
Lopes, 2021 [16]	multicenter retrospective (study protocol)	prediction of prognosis	To develop a ML based on clinical, radiological and epidemiological data to predict the severity prognosis (ICU admission, intubation) in COVID-19.	A ML model receives a lung CT as input and outputs the stratification of lung parenchyma, discerning regions of the lungs with different densities.	Study in progress
Puhr-Westerheide, 2022 [17]	single center retrospective	diagnosis	To compare AI-based quantitative CT severity score to SOFA score in predicting in-hospital mortality at ICU admission in COVID-19 ARDS patients.	AI-based lung injury assessment on CT scan for the diagnostic performance to predict in-hospital mortality.	CT severity score was not associated to in-hospital mortality prediction, whereas the SOFA score showed a significant association.
Röhrich, 2021 [18]	single center prospective	prediction of prognosis	To develop a ML model for the early ARDS prediction from the first CT scan of trauma patients at hospital admission.	A ML model with convolutional neural network (radiomics) approach to automatically delineate the lung at lung CT to predict future ARDS.	The ML model with radiomics score resulted in a higher AUC (0.79) compared to injury severity score (0.66) and abbreviated injury score of the thorax (0.68) in prediction of ARDS. The radiomics score achieved a sensitivity and a specificity of 0.80 and 0.76.
Sarkar, 2023 [19]	single center retrospective	diagnosis and prediction of prognosis	To train and validate DL models to quantify pulmonary contusion as a percentage of total lung volume and assess the relationship between automated Lung Contusion Index and relevant clinical outcomes (ICU LoS and mechanical ventilation time).	DL model for automated CT scan segmentation to quantify the percent lung involvement indexed to total lung volumes.	Automated Lung Contusion Index was associated with ARDS, longer ICU LoS and longer mechanical ventilation time. Automated Lung Contusion Index and clinical variables predicted ARDS with an AUC of 0.70, while automated Lung Contusion Index alone predicted ARDS with an AUC of 0.68.

Table 1. *Cont.*

Author, Year	Study Design	Aim	Endpoints	AI Model	Results
Wang, 2020 [20]	retrospective study	diagnosis	To explore the relationship between the quantitative analysis results and the ARDS existence, using an automatic quantitative analysis model based on DL segmentation model in COVID-19.	DL model to provide an automatic quantitative analysis of infection regions on lung CT to assess their density and location.	The total volume and density of the lung infectious regions were not related to ARDS. The proportion of lesion density was associated with increased risk of ARDS in COVID-19.
Zhang, 2020 [21]	single center retrospective	diagnosis	To compare the performance of the three DL models and determine which model is more diagnostic.	Three DL models (VGG, Resnet and EfficientNet) are used to classify LUS images of pneumonia according to different clinical stages based on a self-made image dataset.	EfficientNet showed to be the best model providing the best accuracy for 3 and 4 clinical stages of pneumonia, with an accuracy of 94.62% and 91.18%, respectively. The best classification accuracy of 8 clinical features of pneumonia at LUS images was 82.75%.
Baloescu, 2020 [22]	single center retrospective	diagnosis	To test the DL algorithm to quantify the assessment of B lines in LUS images from a database of patients presenting at ED with dyspnea or chest pain and to compare the algorithm to expert human interpretation.	A DL model is trained and developed based on a dataset of LUS clips to assess presence/absence of B lines and severity classification.	The accuracy in detecting B lines was 94% with a kappa of 0.88; the accuracy of the severity assessment was 56% with a kappa of 0.65.

Table 1. Cont.

Author, Year	Study Design	Aim	Endpoints	AI Model	Results
Born, 2021 [23]	multicenter retrospective	differential diagnosis	To compare different AI models for the differential diagnosis of COVID-19 pneumonia and bacterial pneumonia.	Five AI models (VGG, VGG-CAM, NASNetMobile, VGG-segment, Segment-Enc) are tested on a dataset of LUS images and videos of healthy controls and patients affected by COVID-19 and bacterial pneumonia and compared in terms of recall, precision, specificity and F1 scores.	Two models (VGG and VGG-CAMI) had an accuracy of 88 ± 5% in distinguishing COVID-19 pneumonia and bacterial pneumonia.
Arntfield, 2021 [24]	multicenter retrospective	differential diagnosis	To compare the DL model and the surveyed LUS-competent physicians in the ability of discriminating pathological LUS imaging	A DL convolutional neural network model is trained on LUS images with B lines to discriminate between COVID-19 ARDS, non-COVID ARDS and hydrostatic pulmonary edema and compared with surveyed LUS-competent physicians.	The DL model showed an ability to discriminate between COVID-19 ARDS (AUC 1.0), non-COVID ARDS (AUC 0.934) and pulmonary edema (AUC 1.0) better than physician ability (AUCs 0.697, 0.704, 0.967).
Ebadi, 2021 [25]	multicenter retrospective	differential diagnosis	To compare the DL classifier model against ground truth classification provided by expert radiologists and clinicians.	A DL method based on the Kinetics-I3D network classifies an entire LUS scan, without the use of pre-processing or a frame-by-frame analysis, for automatic detection of ARDS features present in pneumonia and COVID-19 patients (A lines, B lines, consolidation and pleural effusion).	The DL model showed an accuracy of 90% and a precision score of 95% with the use of 5-fold cross validation.

AI: artificial intelligence; ARDS: acute respiratory distress syndrome; AUC: area under the curve; CT: computed tomography; DL: deep learning; ECMO: extracorporeal membrane oxygenation; ED: emergency department; ICU: intensive care unit; LoS: length of stay; LUS: lung ultrasound; ML: machine learning; PEEP: positive end-expiratory pressure; SOFA: Sequential Organ Failure Assessment.

4. Computed Tomography Scan

Lung CT scan has been used extensively for more than 20 years to improve our understanding of the pathophysiology of ARDS. In particular, the quantitative analysis of the ARDS lung CT scan has allowed the quantification of the amount of not aerated tissue, poorly aerated tissue, well-aerated tissue, and over inflated tissue, advancing the concept of the baby lung and of the lung as a "sponge model" [26]. This quantitative approach has shown the redistribution of the densities in prone position and the change in the not aerated tissue fraction at two airway pressures considered the gold standard for assessing recruitment in ARDS. In this context, CT scan has represented a useful tool to decide the better mechanical ventilation strategy [27]. Similarly, in the setting of chest trauma, the quantification of parenchyma damage, at hospital admission by CT scan, can help predict the evolution from the initial traumatic injuries to focal or diffuse alveolar hemorrhage followed by pulmonary edema and interstitial alterations typical of ARDS [28].

Then, recently during the COVID-19 pandemic, CT scan has played a relevant role as a screening tool due to its greater sensitivity for detecting early pneumonic changes. In fact, although COVID-19 is typically confirmed by viral nucleic acid detection, lung CT scan has been widely used to differentiate COVID-19 from other viral pneumoniae and to predict the severity of pneumonia even in the early stage [29].

The application of AI on CT scan lung images has been recently implemented in patients with COVID-19 disease to predict the evolution in ARDS, to stage and quantify the disease, and predict the outcome.

Similarly, in non-COVID-19 ARDS, AI has the potential to give a profound contribution, considering its ability to automatically and efficiently analyze and segment acutely injured lungs, to provide automated quantitative analysis, and to predict the development of ARDS, the alveolar recruitment, and the relationship between the quantitative analysis of lung tissue and specific outcomes.

4.1. Prediction of ARDS

The diagnosis and prediction of ARDS have been supported by various systems, tools, and techniques, both before and after the AI revolution. Imaging techniques such as chest radiography, CT, and LUS have played a critical role in the diagnosis and management of ARDS [30,31]. These lung imaging modalities have been essential in assessing lung aeration, predicting oxygenation response, and facilitating early diagnosis to prevent the progression of lung injury [32]. In addition, biomarkers have been explored for their potential in diagnosing ARDS and predicting its prognosis [33,34]. Recent advances in AI have significantly changed the landscape of traditional imaging techniques, allowing for more accurate and rapid analysis of medical imaging data for ARDS diagnosis and severity prediction [35].

AI-based diagnostic models combining clinical data and CT scans have been developed, providing accurate and explainable ARDS diagnostic models for real-life scenarios [36,37].

Recently, AI has facilitated the development of models to predict subsequent ARDS development using features identified at initial presentation with COVID-19, addressing the need for clinical decision support tools during the early stages of the COVID-19 pandemic [38,39].

In addition to COVID-19 pneumonia, blunt chest trauma is also currently associated with parenchymal lung injury to various extents, which may increase the risk of developing ARDS. Typically, the presence of an injury severity score (ISS) greater than 25 significantly increases the risk of developing ARDS [18]. Moreover, it has previously been shown that trauma patients with pulmonary contusions involving at least 20% of the total lung volume have a significantly higher risk of developing ARDS [40]. Thus, the ability to assess early information on lung CT that may be associated with the risk of developing ARDS could allow for timely supportive therapy. Röhrich et al. developed a ML method for the early prediction of ARDS based on CT in trauma patients at hospital admission. One hundred and twenty-three patients were enrolled. The model consisted of a fully automated ML and radiomics-based approach that showed a higher accuracy compared to an established score (ISS and abbreviated injury score of the thorax) to identify ARDS in trauma patients [18]. In this line, a rapid automated lung CT volumetry assessment of pulmonary contusions in trauma patients showed a good accuracy in assessing the risk of ARDS, length of intensive care stay, and time on mechanical ventilation [19].

4.2. Alveolar Recruitment

ARDS is characterized by widespread inflammation in the lung, leading to increased permeability of the alveolar–capillary barrier, impairment of pulmonary mechanical properties, and impaired gas exchange. There is often a phenomenon known as alveolar collapse or atelectasis, where some of the alveoli collapse and are not involved in gas exchange [41,42].

Mechanical ventilation itself can increase or cause lung damage known as ventilator-induced lung injury (VILI). Therefore, the therapeutic goal of mechanical ventilation in ARDS patients is not only to maintain "normal gas exchange" but also to protect the lung from VILI [43–45].

Lung protective strategies include low tidal volumes and adequate levels of positive end-expiratory pressure (PEEP) levels to keep the alveoli open and prevent them from collapsing. However, too high or too low levels of PEEP can lead to damage due to overdistension or cyclic collapse. Estimation of the percentage of lung that can be recruited or re-opened by applying transient increases in airway pressure has been demonstrated to be associated with the response to PEEP and prone position [27,46]. Thus, the quantification of alveolar recruitment can help the clinician optimize the protective ventilation strategy to avoid VILI.

The introduction of the lung CT quantitative analysis has allowed the assessment and quantification of the aerated and not aerated lung regions and the possible changes due to the mechanical ventilation and body position [6]. In particular, the application of the lung CT quantitative analysis performed at two different levels of airway pressure is considered the gold standard for the assessment of alveolar recruitment, because it can calculate the difference of not aerated tissue [47–49].

However, since the mid-1980's, the application of quantitative analysis was rarely used in clinical practice because it requires the manual segmentation of the lung by the physicians [48]. The assessment of lung recruitment can take up to 6–8 h with a certain degree of error [15]. To improve the ability to assess lung recruitment, a visual anatomical evaluation of recruitment has been proposed [48].

Moving from the successful application of DL to the segmentation process of CT lung images in ARDS [50,51], using two CNNs architectures, the Seg-Net and the U-Net, Herrmann et al. decided to implement the U-net to develop a DL algorithm to automatically segment injured lungs affected by ARDS and to calculate lung recruitment by performing two CT scans at 5 and 45 cmH$_2$O of airway pressure [11].

Training was performed on 15 healthy subjects (1302 slices), 100 ARDS patients (12,279 slices), and 20 COVID-19 patients (1817 slices): 80% of the patients were used for training and 20% for testing. The authors found that automatic lung segmentation performed by a properly trained neural network was reliable and closely matched the results obtained by manual segmentation. In fact, the total lung volume measured by AI and manual segmentation had a R^2 of 0.99 and a bias of -9.8 mL (CI $+56.0/-75.7$ mL). Although the model was not perfect, especially in the most damaged lung areas, which are difficult to identify even for a trained radiologist, but which did not exceed 10% of the lung parenchyma, the AI segmentation showed the same degree of inaccuracy as the manual segmentation. In fact, for recruitability measured using manual and AI segmentation, change in not aerated tissue fraction had a bias of $+0.3$% (CI $+6.2/-5.5$%) while -0.5% (CI $+2.3/-3.3$%) was expressed for change in well-aerated tissue fraction.

Subsequently, Penarrubia et al. in a single center study assessed both intra- and interobserver smallest real difference exceeding measurement error of recruitment using both human and ML lung segmentation on CT scan [15]. Low-dose CT scans were acquired at 5 and 15 cm H_2O of PEEP in 11 sedated and paralyzed ARDS patients and recruitment was computed as the change in weight of the not aerated lung regions. The intra-observer small real difference of recruitment was 3.5% of lung weight, while the human–human interobserver smallest real difference of recruitment was slightly higher amounting to 5.7% of lung weight, as also was the human–machine smallest real difference. Human–machine and human–human interobserver measurement errors were similar, suggesting that ML segmentation algorithms are a valid alternative to humans for quantifying alveolar recruitment on CT [15].

Furthermore, to overcome the difficulty in performing two CT scans at two different airway pressures, Pennati et al. developed a ML algorithm to predict lung recruitment in ARDS patients, starting from a single CT scan obtained at 5 cmH_2O upon admission to the intensive care unit (ICU) [2].

The authors demonstrated that in 221 retrospectively analyzed ARDS patients, the use of four ML algorithms (logistic regression, support vector machine, random forest, XGboost) based on a lung CT scan at 5 cmH_2O were able to classify lung recruiter patients with similar area under the curve (AUC) compared to a ML model based on the combination of lung mechanics, gas exchange, and CT data [2].

The application of this ML algorithm with an automatic lung segmentation and quantitative analysis could reduce the workload and ionizing radiation exposure of the traditional method of assessing lung recruitability.

4.3. Outcome

Concerning the outcome, hospital mortality has decreased over the decades, but has remained unchanged in recent years, despite advances in supportive care [52].

A small retrospective study of 42 patients with ARDS evaluated the relationship between the volume of well-aerated lung regions, calculated automatically by software, and outcome [9]. Total lung volumes and well-aerated lung regions were significantly higher in survivors. Estimates of the total volumetry and the regions of interest were obtained within three minutes with a very good reproducibility [9].

Several data have shown that lung volume and the amount of not aerated lung areas in COVID-19 are associated with respiratory severity and outcome [53]. Typical lung CT findings in COVID-19 patients include bilateral pulmonary ground-glass opacities and opacities with rounded edges usually localized in the peripheral lung regions [6].

Using a DL method to calculate the description of the CT, two clusters typically associated with COVID-19 and two clusters associated with bacterial pneumonia were found [12]. The clusters containing diffuse ground-glass opacities in the central and peripheral lung showed up to 91% accuracy in correctly classifying COVID 19 and pneumonia.

Liu et al. investigated the ability of quantitative lung CT analysis compared to traditional clinical biomarkers to predict progression to severe disease in the early stage of COVID-19 patients [14]. A group of 134 patients with COVID-19 who underwent lung CT scan and laboratory tests on day 0 and 4 were enrolled. All patients were followed up for 28 days until the first occurrence of severe disease or otherwise. Three AI-derived CT features were calculated according to Hounsfield units ($-700/-500$; $-500/-200$; and $-200/-60$ HU). The CT features at day 0 and day 4 and their changes from day 0 to day 4 showed the best discriminative ability to predict patient progression to severe disease. In this line, a retrospective study of COVID-19 patients used DL segmentation to assess lung volume and density composition [20]. The number of lung regions with a density between -549 and -450 of Hounsfield units was associated with an increased risk of ARDS. Although the results were not published, Lopes et al. proposed a multicenter retrospective longitudinal study to correlate the possible findings on lung CT in patients with COVID-19 infection and the course of the disease [16].

In COVID-19 patients, the use of the quantitative lung CT analysis at hospital admission, which calculates the volume of the affected lung as the sum of the poorly aerated and not aerated lung regions, predicted the need for oxygen support and intubation with good accuracy [13].

Regarding hospital mortality in COVID-19 ARDS based on AI quantification of lung involvement at hospital admission, the AI did not predict the outcome [17]. In contrast, the Sequential Organ Failure Assessment (SOFA) score resulted in an AUC for hospital mortality of 0.74 (95% CI 0.63–0.85), suggesting that other clinical parameters reflect the overall disease severity [54,55].

In severe COVID-19 ARDS patients with hypoxemia refractory to the conventional ventilation, veno-venous extracorporeal membrane oxygenation (ECMO) may be used to improve the outcome. However, the potential improvement in outcome is higher when ECMO support is applied in the early phase. Therefore, a possible early stratification should be considered. The use of an AI-based quantification of lung involvement was able to predict the need for ECMO with an acceptable AUC [0.83 (95% CI 0.73–0.94)] [10]. In addition, combining the SOFA score with CT lung involvement at ICU admission improved the AUC to 0.91 (95% CI 0.84–0.97) [10].

In summary, while the extent of lung involvement on imaging is an important consideration in assessing the severity of ARDS, there is not a specific "critical amount" that universally predicts outcome or guides the need for repeat imaging or ECMO use [10]. The decision to use ECMO is multifactorial and is based on clinical judgment, including considerations of the patient's overall health, the underlying cause of ARDS, and the potential for recovery. Similarly, the timing and need for repeat imaging are individualized based on the clinical course of the patient and the judgment of the healthcare provider. In fact, the early clinical course of the disease may be more predictive of the outcome than the assessment at time of admission to the ICU [56].

5. Lung Ultrasound

LUS has been shown to be a useful tool in the assessment of numerous lung diseases and, in recent years, has proven to be also effective in the emergency care setting to screen patients with suspected COVID-19 pneumonia [57–59]. In fact, compared to traditional imaging, LUS has many advantages: it is radiation-free, inexpensive, rapid, bedside feasible, non-invasive, and lacks the laborious workflow of a CT scan. Considering all these features and its good accuracy as compared with lung CT scan, LUS is commonly used in the ICU to screen patients for ARDS [60–64]. Indeed, LUS has the potential to predict mortality in ARDS patients with a high level of accuracy (AUC 0.85). These findings also exhibit a strong correlation with the prognostic value derived from the invasively measured extravascular lung water index. Furthermore, in this condition, LUS is able to assess the likelihood of post-extubation distress after a successful spontaneous breathing trial, with an AUC of 0.86, and is also able to assess regional and global lung aeration [64–67]. LUS images in ARDS are characterized by the presence of a non-homogeneously distributed alveolar sonographic interstitial syndrome characterized by the presence of vertical artifacts (including the so-called "B lines" and the "white lung"), along with pleural thickening and consolidation in dependent regions [68,69]. However, these features, especially the vertical artifacts, are not specific for ARDS as they can be detected in many other pathological conditions (i.e., pulmonary edema, pneumonia, and pulmonary fibrosis). In addition, LUS interpretation can be limited by operator confidence in image acquisition and interpretation, which can lead to intra-reader variability and a limited inter-reader agreement [70,71].

To overcome these limitations and to curb operator-related variability, AI has recently been employed in different medical areas to aid LUS image analysis and interpretation [14,72], such as emergency and intensive care settings [3,73].

DL has the ability to directly process and gather intermediate and advanced features obtained from raw data, such as ultrasound images, and then make intelligent decisions based on the learned features. The absence of cognitive bias or the need for spatial pixel connections allows DL to treat images as numerical sequences, enabling the evaluation of quantitative patterns that could unveil insights beyond human interpretation thereby enhancing human diagnostic capability. According to the type of the skill requested (i.e., classification, detection, and segmentation), there are mainly three types of DL architecture: supervised deep networks or deep discriminative models, unsupervised deep networks or deep generative models, and hybrid deep networks. Supervised deep networks are the most widely used in ultrasound imaging, the major methodology of interest being the CNN [14,74,75].

Few studies are currently available regarding the use of DL in LUS for the evaluation of ARDS in non-COVID-19 patients. During the recent COVID-19 pandemic, LUS disease-specific patterns showed a higher sensitivity compared to chest X-ray in the identification of COVID-19 pneumonia [76,77], making this disease model the predominant focus of DL application. Indeed, the automated assessment enabled by DL ensures a prompt diagnosis in situations where resources and trained personnel are scarce, ideally addressing such challenges.

5.1. Prediction of ARDS Diagnosis

Two studies investigated the possibility of introducing DL modalities to discriminate different stages of parenchymal changes secondary to pneumonia [21] by grading vertical artifacts [22] of LUS.

Baloescu et al. designed a new custom DL that operated on dynamic ultrasound data for automated assessment of sonographic lung B lines. The DL consisted of a CNN developed using 2415 sub-clips of 12 frames each from 400 emergency department patients. Each sub-clip was evaluated by two emergency physicians with expertise in LUS, using a predeterminate ordinal scale from 0 (none) to 4 (severe). In addition, a binary classification was performed pooling together as "normal" the images with score 0 or 1 and as "abnormal" the images with score 2–4. The experts' rating was used as ground truth and compared with the interpretations given by the new DL model using 100 sub-clips not used during the DL training. Considering the assessment of presence/absence of B lines, the new DL model showed an overall accuracy of 94% with kappa of 0.88; however, for the severity assessment, the overall accuracy was only 56% with kappa of 0.65, showing that the new algorithm is better at distinguishing B lines but not their severity [22].

Zhang et al. investigated the feasibility of computer-assisted ultrasound diagnosis using three CNN-based DL models—VGG, ResNet, and EfficientNet—for the detection and classification of pneumonia based on a self-made LUS image dataset built on a total of 10,350 LUS images. Each image of the dataset was manually classified into eight clinical features of pneumonia (0 = normal; 1 = B lines < 3; 2 = B lines > 3; 3 = area of merging B line is less than half; 4 = area of merging B line is more than half; 5 = depth of pieces is less than 1 cm; 6 = air bronchogram and depth of parenchymal hepatization is less than 3 cm; 7 = pleural effusion and depth of parenchymal hepatization is more than 3 cm). Since for some of the features evaluated by Baloescu there were not enough images for training and testing sets, several clinical features were manually grouped together into different "classes" resulting in three different datasets: one including three classes (class 1: feature 0; class 2: features 1–4; class 3: features 5–7), one including four classes (class 1: feature 0; class 2: features 1–4; class 3: features 5–6; class 4: feature 7), and the last one encompassing eight classes, i.e., a class for each of the eight features. All of the three datasets were compared across classification models and the EfficientNet showed to be the best model providing for the three and four classes datasets an accuracy of 94.62% and 91.18%, respectively, whilst the best classification accuracy of the eight classes dataset was only 82.75% [21].

5.2. Differential Diagnosis

AI has been applied to LUS imaging for its potential role in differentiating healthy subjects from COVID-19 pneumonia and ARDS, hydrostatic pulmonary edema, and bacterial pneumonia and ARDS.

Born et al. proposed another DL LUS model able to distinguish COVID-19 from healthy subjects and bacterial pneumonia with a sensitivity of 0.90 ± 0.08 and a specificity of 0.96 ± 0.04. The model was developed using a dataset made by 261 recordings from a total of 216 patients affected with COVID-19, bacterial pneumonia, non-COVID-19 viral pneumonia, and healthy controls. Due to data availability, the three non-COVID-19 viral pneumonia videos were excluded. Five DL models were then compared in terms of recall, precision, specificity, and F1 scores. Overall, both VGG and VGG-CAM showed encouraging results, achieving an accuracy of 88 ± 5% in the detection of COVID-19 pneumonia, across a 5-fold cross-validation with 3234 frames [23]. Arntfield et al. developed another CNN able to discriminate between similar appearing LUS images with pathological B lines of three different origins (COVID-19 ARDS, non-COVID ARDS, and hydrostatic pulmonary edema) using a total of 612 LUS videos from 243 patients (84 COVID-19 ARDS, 78 non-COVID-19 ARDS, and 81 hydrostatic pulmonary edema). To assess the CNN performance, a subset of 10% of the total data was used, not previously used during the training process. The evaluation made by CNN was then compared to the LUS interpretation given by experienced physicians completing an online interpretation exercise. The trained CNN performance on the independent dataset showed an ability to discriminate between COVID-19 (AUC 1.0), non-COVID-19 ARDS (AUC 0.934), and pulmonary edema (AUC 1.0) pathologies. This was significantly better than the physicians' ability (AUCs 0.697, 0.704, and 0.967 for the COVID-19 ARDS, non-COVID-19 ARDS, and pulmonary edema classes, respectively; $p < 0.01$), showing that a trained neural network is able to detect subvisible features within LUS images [24].

Ebadi et al. proposed a fast and reliable DL model, specifically the Kinetics-I3D network, using LUS scans to explore the possibility of detecting and differentiating ARDS from pneumonia. Compared to other DL models, this trained model was able to classify an entire LUS scan obtained at the point-of-care, eliminating the need for preprocessing or analyzing frames individually, since the neural network could be retrained with new data to adapt the model to the needs of specific LUS applications. The results obtained with the new DL methods were benchmarked against ground truth assessed by expert radiologists showing an accuracy of 90% and a precision score of 95%. Moreover, the proposed model was very rapid as it was able to process the entire scan with a single forward pass into the network, avoiding time-consuming frame-by-frame analysis [25].

5.3. Limitations of AI in LUS

To date, the application of DL in thoracic echography has been very limited as compared to other imaging techniques. One of the reasons is the limited availability of organized LUS databases. In fact, to reach an optimal learning performance, a wide number of labeled LUS images is needed. This requirement can be challenging as LUS is an evolving technique, and currently, there are only a limited number of experts capable of providing a suitable interpretation.

Indeed, to date, LUS training for ARDS has often been the prerogative of emergency department and ICU staff, lacking the structured, shared, and formal reporting typical of other radiologic tests such as lung CT, which may limit standardization and uniform informative input for DL. On the other hand, the majority of the radiology training programs do not include education in LUS interpretation.

The prevalent issue arising from a deep model with limited training samples is overfitting that can be addressed by two different approaches: model optimization and transfer learning. Model optimization focuses on making the DL model itself to work better with available data using different types of strategies (e.g., well-designed initialization/momentum strategies, efficient activation functions, dropout, and batch normalization, stack/denoising), whereas transfer learning utilizes knowledge from one domain to enhance the performance in another domain with limited data.

Another limitation is that many of the shared LUS databases lack a complete interpretation of the thorax (since the evaluations are mostly performed with a focused approach) and important information such as patient details and technical or setting data. Collecting these data should help differentiate similar LUS patterns that are only apparently non-disease specific, such as those observed in patients with ARDS.

6. Conclusions

The application of ML technique to lung CT scan image processing can represent a valid tool to provide a broader adoption of CT scan quantitative analysis in the clinical practice of ARDS management, in particular the prediction of the alveolar recruitment and patient outcomes. Similarly, the application of AI to LUS imaging may implement clinician performance in distinguishing and interpreting similar LUS patterns deriving from different pathological etiologies with the potential to provide an accurate diagnosis (Figure 2). Indeed, there are several areas that could benefit from the application of AI in this field, including diagnosis, assessment of severity, progression, and response to treatment. However, AI is not ready for widespread use and models may not be as accurate because progression to advanced respiratory failure is not as common and predictable. In fact, part of the ML-based algorithms described in this review were based on image datasets collected during the COVID-19 pandemic. Nonetheless, updated algorithms have already been defined thanks to the ability to re-train those same algorithms with new image datasets. In this sense, AI is an evolving technology and an ongoing process of refinement and several biases should be overcome in the development of further models to guarantee sufficient robustness and reproducibility to be competitive compared with current standard methods and thus to support clinical judgment, starting from high quality imaging datasets.

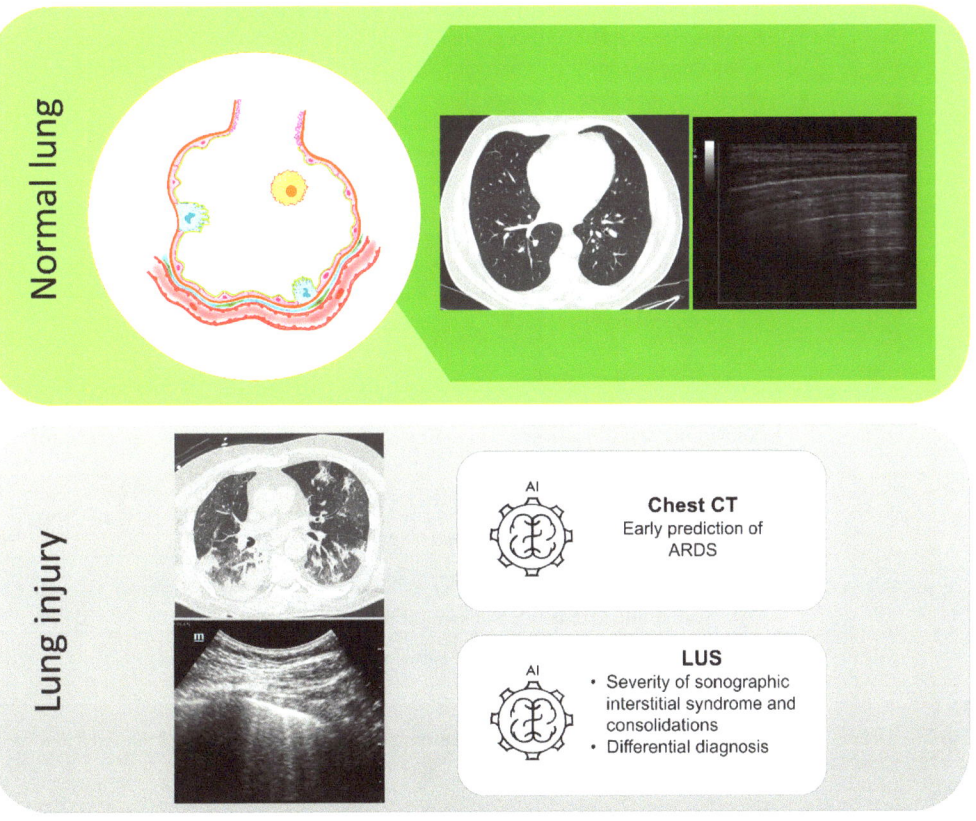

Figure 2. *Cont.*

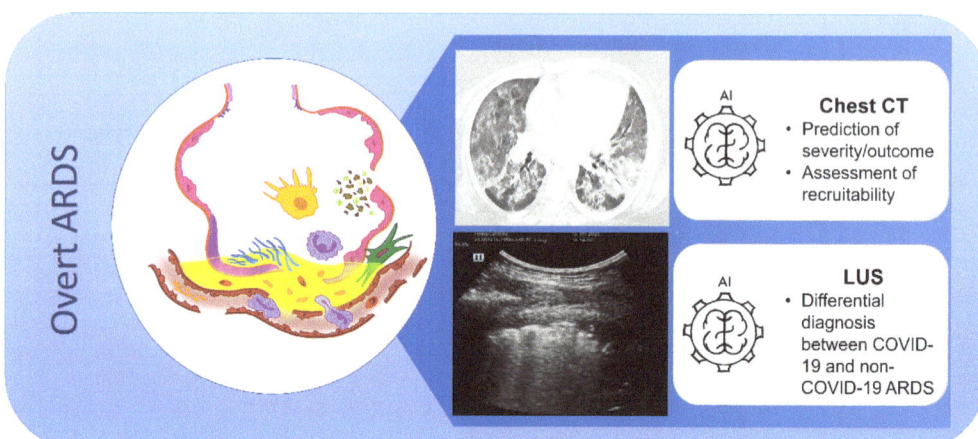

Figure 2. Current potential areas of application for artificial intelligence applied to lung computed tomography and lung ultrasound imaging in different stages of lung disease. Green upper box: normal lung histology (drawing **on the left**), axial projection of a lung CT scan (image **in the middle**), and a LUS scan showing normal pleural findings with repetitive physiological horizontal artifacts (A lines), a typical sign indicating a normal aerated lung. Grey box in the middle: a lung CT scan (**upper image**) and LUS scan (**lower image**) in a patient with acute lung injury. Note the presence of vertical artifacts arising from the pleural line (B lines), indicating the presence of a sonographic interstitial syndrome. Blue box at the bottom: overt ARDS (drawing on the left) with alveolar–capillary damage, alveolar edema, cellular debris, neutrophilic migration (in violet), activated macrophages (in yellow), fibroblast activation, and fibrin deposition (in green). The lung CT scan (**upper figure in the middle**) and the LUS scan (**lower figure in the middle**) represent the typical radiological findings in a representative patient with ARDS. Note the inhomogeneity of aerated and not aerated parenchyma at the axial projection of the lung CT and the irregular pleural profile, with areas of high lung density (white lung) interspersed by parenchymal subpleural infiltrates. The two different imaging approaches carry different qualitative and quantitative information of the same pathological pattern. AI: artificial intelligence; ARDS: acute respiratory distress syndrome; CT: computed tomography; LUS: lung ultrasound.

Author Contributions: Conceptualization, D.C., S.C. and D.R.; methodology, S.C., G.C., F.D. and D.R.; software, G.C. and F.D.; writing-original draft preparation, S.C. and D.R.; writing-review and editing, S.C. and D.R.; supervision, D.C. and P.S. All authors have read and agreed to the published version of the manuscript.

Funding: This research received no external funding.

Institutional Review Board Statement: Not applicable.

Informed Consent Statement: Not applicable.

Data Availability Statement: Not applicable.

Conflicts of Interest: The authors declare no conflicts of interest.

References

1. Haug, C.J.; Drazen, J.M. Artificial Intelligence and Machine Learning in Clinical Medicine, 2023. *N. Engl. J. Med.* **2023**, *388*, 1201–1208. [CrossRef] [PubMed]
2. Pennati, F.; Aliverti, A.; Pozzi, T.; Gattarello, S.; Lombardo, F.; Coppola, S.; Chiumello, D. Machine Learning Predicts Lung Recruitment in Acute Respiratory Distress Syndrome Using Single Lung CT Scan. *Ann. Intensive Care* **2023**, *13*, 60. [CrossRef]

3. Suri, J.S.; Agarwal, S.; Gupta, S.K.; Puvvula, A.; Biswas, M.; Saba, L.; Bit, A.; Tandel, G.S.; Agarwal, M.; Patrick, A.; et al. A Narrative Review on Characterization of Acute Respiratory Distress Syndrome in COVID-19-Infected Lungs Using Artificial Intelligence. *Comput. Biol. Med.* **2021**, *130*, 104210. [CrossRef] [PubMed]
4. Allen, B.; Agarwal, S.; Coombs, L.; Wald, C.; Dreyer, K. 2020 ACR Data Science Institute Artificial Intelligence Survey. *J. Am. Coll. Radiol.* **2021**, *18*, 1153–1159. [CrossRef] [PubMed]
5. Najjar, R. Redefining Radiology: A Review of Artificial Intelligence Integration in Medical Imaging. *Diagnostics* **2023**, *13*, 2760. [CrossRef] [PubMed]
6. Chiumello, D.; Papa, G.F.S.; Artigas, A.; Bouhemad, B.; Grgic, A.; Heunks, L.; Markstaller, K.; Pellegrino, G.M.; Pisani, L.; Rigau, D.; et al. ERS Statement on Chest Imaging in Acute Respiratory Failure. *Eur. Respir. J.* **2019**, *54*, 1900435. [CrossRef] [PubMed]
7. Seo, H.; Badiei Khuzani, M.; Vasudevan, V.; Huang, C.; Ren, H.; Xiao, R.; Jia, X.; Xing, L. Machine Learning Techniques for Biomedical Image Segmentation: An Overview of Technical Aspects and Introduction to State-of-Art Applications. *Med. Phys.* **2020**, *47*, e148–e167. [CrossRef]
8. Hinton, G.E.; Osindero, S.; Teh, Y.W. A Fast Learning Algorithm for Deep Belief Nets. *Neural Comput.* **2006**, *18*, 1527–1554. [CrossRef]
9. Nishiyama, A.; Kawata, N.; Yokota, H.; Sugiura, T.; Matsumura, Y.; Higashide, T.; Horikoshi, T.; Oda, S.; Tatsumi, K.; Uno, T. A Predictive Factor for Patients with Acute Respiratory Distress Syndrome: CT Lung Volumetry of the Well-Aerated Region as an Automated Method. *Eur. J. Radiol.* **2020**, *122*, 108748. [CrossRef]
10. Gresser, E.; Reich, J.; Sabel, B.O.; Kunz, W.G.; Fabritius, M.P.; Rübenthaler, J.; Ingrisch, M.; Wassilowsky, D.; Irlbeck, M.; Ricke, J.; et al. Risk Stratification for Ecmo Requirement in Covid-19 Icu Patients Using Quantitative Imaging Features in Ct Scans on Admission. *Diagnostics* **2021**, *11*, 1029. [CrossRef]
11. Herrmann, P.; Busana, M.; Cressoni, M.; Lotz, J.; Moerer, O.; Saager, L.; Meissner, K.; Quintel, M.; Gattinoni, L. Using Artificial Intelligence for Automatic Segmentation of CT Lung Images in Acute Respiratory Distress Syndrome. *Front. Physiol.* **2021**, *12*, 676118. [CrossRef] [PubMed]
12. Kang, M.; Hong, K.S.; Chikontwe, P.; Luna, M.; Jang, J.G.; Park, J.; Shin, K.C.; Park, S.H.; Ahn, J.H. Quantitative Assessment of Chest CT Patterns in COVID-19 and Bacterial Pneumonia Patients: A Deep Learning Perspective. *J. Korean Med. Sci.* **2021**, *36*, e46. [CrossRef] [PubMed]
13. Lanza, E.; Muglia, R.; Bolengo, I.; Santonocito, O.G.; Lisi, C.; Angelotti, G.; Morandini, P.; Savevski, V.; Politi, L.S.; Balzarini, L. Quantitative Chest CT Analysis in COVID-19 to Predict the Need for Oxygenation Support and Intubation. *Eur. Radiol.* **2020**, *30*, 6770–6778. [CrossRef] [PubMed]
14. Liu, S.; Wang, Y.; Yang, X.; Lei, B.; Liu, L.; Li, S.X.; Ni, D.; Wang, T. Deep Learning in Medical Ultrasound Analysis: A Review. *Engineering* **2019**, *5*, 261–275. [CrossRef]
15. Penarrubia, L.; Verstraete, A.; Orkisz, M.; Davila, E.; Boussel, L.; Yonis, H.; Mezidi, M.; Dhelft, F.; Danjou, W.; Bazzani, A.; et al. Precision of CT-Derived Alveolar Recruitment Assessed by Human Observers and a Machine Learning Algorithm in Moderate and Severe ARDS. *Intensive Care Med. Exp.* **2023**, *11*, 8. [CrossRef] [PubMed]
16. Lopes, F.P.P.L.; Kitamura, F.C.; Prado, G.F.; de Aguiar Kuriki, P.E.; Garcia, M.R.T. Machine Learning Model for Predicting Severity Prognosis in Patients Infected with COVID-19: Study Protocol from COVID-AI Brasil. *PLoS ONE* **2021**, *16*, e0245384. [CrossRef]
17. Puhr-Westerheide, D.; Reich, J.; Sabel, B.O.; Kunz, W.G.; Fabritius, M.P.; Reidler, P.; Rübenthaler, J.; Ingrisch, M.; Wassilowsky, D.; Irlbeck, M.; et al. Article Sequential Organ Failure Assessment Outperforms Quantitative Chest Ct Imaging Parameters for Mortality Prediction in Covid-19 Ards. *Diagnostics* **2022**, *12*, 10. [CrossRef]
18. Röhrich, S.; Hofmanninger, J.; Negrin, L.; Langs, G.; Prosch, H. Radiomics Score Predicts Acute Respiratory Distress Syndrome Based on the Initial CT Scan after Trauma. *Eur. Radiol.* **2021**, *31*, 5443–5453. [CrossRef]
19. Sarkar, N.; Zhang, L.; Campbell, P.; Liang, Y.; Li, G.; Khedr, M.; Khetan, U.; Dreizin, D. Pulmonary Contusion: Automated Deep Learning-Based Quantitative Visualization. *Emerg. Radiol.* **2023**, *30*, 435–441. [CrossRef]
20. Wang, Y.; Chen, Y.; Wei, Y.; Li, M.; Zhang, Y.; Zhang, N.; Zhao, S.; Zeng, H.; Deng, W.; Huang, Z.; et al. Quantitative Analysis of Chest CT Imaging Findings with the Risk of ARDS in COVID-19 Patients: A Preliminary Study. *Ann. Transl. Med.* **2020**, *8*, 594. [CrossRef]
21. Zhang, J.; Chng, C.B.; Chen, X.; Wu, C.; Zhang, M.; Xue, Y.; Jiang, J.; Chui, C.K. Detection and Classification of Pneumonia from Lung Ultrasound Images. In Proceedings of the 2020 5th International Conference on Communication, Image and Signal Processing, CCISP 2020, Chengdu, China, 13–15 November 2020.
22. Baloescu, C.; Toporek, G.; Kim, S.; McNamara, K.; Liu, R.; Shaw, M.M.; McNamara, R.L.; Raju, B.I.; Moore, C.L. Automated Lung Ultrasound B-Line Assessment Using a Deep Learning Algorithm. *IEEE Trans. Ultrason. Ferroelectr. Freq. Control* **2020**, *67*, 2312–2320. [CrossRef] [PubMed]
23. Born, J.; Wiedemann, N.; Cossio, M.; Buhre, C.; Brändle, G.; Leidermann, K.; Goulet, J.; Aujayeb, A.; Moor, M.; Rieck, B.; et al. Accelerating Detection of Lung Pathologies with Explainable Ultrasound Image Analysis. *Appl. Sci.* **2021**, *11*, 672. [CrossRef]
24. Arntfield, R.; VanBerlo, B.; Alaifan, T.; Phelps, N.; White, M.; Chaudhary, R.; Ho, J.; Wu, D. Development of a Convolutional Neural Network to Differentiate among the Etiology of Similar Appearing Pathological b Lines on Lung Ultrasound: A Deep Learning Study. *BMJ Open* **2021**, *11*, e045120. [CrossRef] [PubMed]

25. Erfanian Ebadi, S.; Krishnaswamy, D.; Bolouri, S.E.S.; Zonoobi, D.; Greiner, R.; Meuser-Herr, N.; Jaremko, J.L.; Kapur, J.; Noga, M.; Punithakumar, K. Automated Detection of Pneumonia in Lung Ultrasound Using Deep Video Classification for COVID-19. *Inform. Med. Unlocked* **2021**, *25*, 100687. [CrossRef] [PubMed]
26. Gattinoni, L.; Pesenti, A. The Concept of "Baby Lung". *Intensive Care Med.* **2005**, *31*, 776–784. [CrossRef] [PubMed]
27. Gattinoni, L.; Caironi, P.; Pelosi, P.; Goodman, L.R. What Has Computed Tomography Taught Us about the Acute Respiratory Distress Syndrome? *Am. J. Respir. Crit. Care Med.* **2001**, *164*, 1701–1711. [CrossRef]
28. Raghavendran, K.; Davidson, B.A.; Woytash, J.A.; Helinski, J.D.; Marschke, C.J.; Manderscheid, P.A.; Notter, R.H.; Knight, P.R. The Evolution Of Isolated Bilateral Lung Contusion from Blunt Chest Trauma In Rats: Cellular and Cytokine Responses. *Shock* **2005**, *24*, 132. [CrossRef]
29. Ko, J.P.; Liu, G.; Klein, J.S.; Mossa-Basha, M.; Azadi, J.R. Pulmonary COVID-19: Multimodality Imaging Examples. *RadioGraphics* **2020**, *40*, 1893–1894. [CrossRef]
30. Sheard, S.; Rao, P.; Devaraj, A. Imaging of Acute Respiratory Distress Syndrome. *Respir. Care* **2012**, *57*, 607. [CrossRef]
31. Ball, L.; Vercesi, V.; Costantino, F.; Chandrapatham, K.; Pelosi, P. Lung Imaging: How to Get Better Look inside the Lung. *Ann. Transl. Med.* **2017**, *5*, 294. [CrossRef]
32. Pierrakos, C.; Smit, M.R.; Hagens, L.A.; Heijnen, N.F.L.; Hollmann, M.W.; Schultz, M.J.; Paulus, F.; Bos, L.D.J. Assessment of the Effect of Recruitment Maneuver on Lung Aeration Through Imaging Analysis in Invasively Ventilated Patients: A Systematic Review. *Front. Physiol.* **2021**, *12*, 666941. [CrossRef]
33. Butt, Y.; Kurdowska, A.; Allen, T.C. Acute Lung Injury: A Clinical and Molecular Review. *Arch. Pathol. Lab. Med.* **2016**, *140*, 345–350. [CrossRef]
34. Isabel García-Laorden, M.; Lorente, J.A.; Flores, C.; Slutsky, A.S.; Villar, J. Biomarkers for the Acute Respiratory Distress Syndrome: How to Make the Diagnosis More Precise. *Ann. Transl. Med.* **2017**, *5*, 283. [CrossRef] [PubMed]
35. Shi, F.; Wang, J.; Shi, J.; Wu, Z.; Wang, Q.; Tang, Z.; He, K.; Shi, Y.; Shen, D. Review of Artificial Intelligence Techniques in Imaging Data Acquisition, Segmentation, and Diagnosis for COVID-19. *IEEE Rev. Biomed. Eng.* **2021**, *14*, 4–15. [CrossRef] [PubMed]
36. Farzaneh, N.; Ansari, S.; Lee, E.; Ward, K.R.; Sjoding, M.W. Collaborative Strategies for Deploying Artificial Intelligence to Complement Physician Diagnoses of Acute Respiratory Distress Syndrome. *NPJ Digit. Med.* **2023**, *6*, 62. [CrossRef] [PubMed]
37. Pai, K.-C.; Chao, W.-C.; Huang, Y.-L.; Sheu, R.-K.; Chen, L.-C.; Wang, M.-S.; Lin, S.-H.; Yu, Y.-Y.; Wu, C.-L.; Chan, M.-C. Artificial Intelligence–Aided Diagnosis Model for Acute Respiratory Distress Syndrome Combining Clinical Data and Chest Radiographs. *Digit. Health* **2022**, *8*, 20552076221120316. [CrossRef] [PubMed]
38. Jiang, Z.; He, C.; Wang, D.; Shen, H.; Sun, J.; Gan, W.; Lu, J.; Liu, X. The Role of Imaging Techniques in Management of COVID-19 in China: From Diagnosis to Monitoring and Follow-Up. *Med. Sci. Monit.* **2020**, *26*, e924582. [CrossRef] [PubMed]
39. Lam, C.; Tso, C.F.; Green-Saxena, A.; Pellegrini, E.; Iqbal, Z.; Evans, D.; Hoffman, J.; Calvert, J.; Mao, Q.; Das, R. Semisupervised Deep Learning Techniques for Predicting Acute Respiratory Distress Syndrome From Time-Series Clinical Data: Model Development and Validation Study. *JMIR Form. Res.* **2021**, *5*, e28028. [CrossRef]
40. Miller, P.R.; Croce, M.A.; Bee, T.K.; Qaisi, W.G.; Smith, C.P.; Collins, G.L.; Fabian, T.C. Ards after Pulmonary Contusion: Accurate Measurement of Contusion Volume Identifies High-Risk Patients. *J. Trauma* **2001**, *51*, 223–228, discussion 229–230. [CrossRef]
41. Ashbaugh, D.G.; Boyd Bigelow, D.; Petty, T.L.; Levine, B.E. Acute Respiratory Distress In Adults. *Lancet* **1967**, *290*, 319–323. [CrossRef]
42. Ware, L.B.; Matthay, M.A. The Acute Respiratory Distress Syndrome. *N. Engl. J. Med.* **2000**, *342*, 1334–1349. [CrossRef]
43. Gattinoni, L.; Pesenti, A.; Rossi, G.P.; Vesconi, S.; Fox, U.; Kolobow, T.; Agostoni, A.; Pelizzola, A.; Langer, M.; Uziel, L.; et al. Treatment of Acute Respiratory Failure with Low-Frequency Positive-Pressure Ventilation and Extracorporeal Removal of CO_2. *Lancet* **1980**, *316*, 292–294. [CrossRef] [PubMed]
44. Kolobow, T.; Moretti, M.P.; Fumagalli, R.; Mascheroni, D.; Prato, P.; Chen, V.; Joris, M. Severe Impairment in Lung Function Induced by High Peak Airway Pressure during Mechanical Ventilation. *Am. Rev. Respir. Dis.* **1987**, *135*, 312–315.
45. Hickling, K.G.; Henderson, S.J.; Jackson, R. Low Mortality Associated with Low Volume Pressure Limited Ventilation with Permissive Hypercapnia in Severe Adult Respiratory Distress Syndrome. *Intensive Care Med.* **1990**, *16*, 372–377. [CrossRef] [PubMed]
46. Gattinoni, L.; D'Andrea, L.; Pelosi, P.; Vitale, G.; Pesenti, A.; Fumagalli, R. Regional Effects and Mechanism of Positive End-Expiratory Pressure in Early Adult Respiratory Distress Syndrome. *JAMA* **1993**, *269*, 2122–2127. [CrossRef] [PubMed]
47. Gattinoni, L.; Caironi, P.; Cressoni, M.; Chiumello, D.; Ranieri, V.M.; Quintel, M.; Russo, S.; Patroniti, N.; Cornejo, R.; Bugedo, G. Lung Recruitment in Patients with the Acute Respiratory Distress Syndrome. *N. Engl. J. Med.* **2006**, *354*, 1775–1786. [CrossRef]
48. Chiumello, D.; Marino, A.; Brioni, M.; Menga, F.; Cigada, I.; Lazzerini, M.; Andrisani, M.C.; Biondetti, P.; Cesana, B.; Gattinoni, L. Visual Anatomical Lung CT Scan Assessment of Lung Recruitability. *Intensive Care Med.* **2013**, *39*, 66–73. [CrossRef]
49. Chiumello, D.; Formenti, P.; Coppola, S. Lung Recruitment: What Has Computed Tomography Taught Us in the Last Decade? *Ann. Intensive Care* **2019**, *9*, 12. [CrossRef]
50. Badrinarayanan, V.; Kendall, A.; Cipolla, R. SegNet: A Deep Convolutional Encoder-Decoder Architecture for Image Segmentation. *IEEE Trans. Pattern Anal. Mach. Intell.* **2017**, *39*, 2481–2495. [CrossRef]

51. Ronneberger, O.; Fischer, P.; Brox, T. U-Net: Convolutional Networks for Biomedical Image Segmentation. In Proceedings of the International Conference on Medical Image Computing and Computer-Assisted Intervention, Munich, Germany, 5–9 October 2015; Lecture Notes in Computer Science (including subseries Lecture Notes in Artificial Intelligence and Lecture Notes in Bioinformatics). Volume 9351.
52. Bellani, G.; Laffey, J.G.; Pham, T.; Fan, E.; Brochard, L.; Esteban, A.; Gattinoni, L.; Van Haren, F.M.P.; Larsson, A.; McAuley, D.F.; et al. Epidemiology, Patterns of Care, and Mortality for Patients with Acute Respiratory Distress Syndrome in Intensive Care Units in 50 Countries. *JAMA—J. Am. Med. Assoc.* **2016**, *315*, 788–800. [CrossRef]
53. Chiumello, D.; Busana, M.; Coppola, S.; Romitti, F.; Formenti, P.; Bonifazi, M.; Pozzi, T.; Palumbo, M.M.; Cressoni, M.; Herrmann, P.; et al. Physiological and Quantitative CT-Scan Characterization of COVID-19 and Typical ARDS: A Matched Cohort Study. *Intensive Care Med.* **2020**, *46*, 2187–2196. [CrossRef] [PubMed]
54. Chiumello, D.; Modafferi, L.; Fratti, I. Risk Factors and Mortality in Elderly ARDS COVID-19 Compared to Patients without COVID-19. *J. Clin. Med.* **2022**, *11*, 5180. [CrossRef] [PubMed]
55. Coppola, S.; Chiumello, D.; Busana, M.; Giola, E.; Palermo, P.; Pozzi, T.; Steinberg, I.; Roli, S.; Romitti, F.; Lazzari, S.; et al. Role of Total Lung Stress on the Progression of Early COVID-19 Pneumonia. *Intensive Care Med.* **2021**, *47*, 1130–1139. [CrossRef]
56. Pozzi, T.; Fratti, I.; Tomarchio, E.; Bruno, G.; Catozzi, G.; Monte, A.; Chiumello, D.; Coppola, S. Early Time-Course of Respiratory Mechanics, Mechanical Power and Gas Exchange in ARDS Patients. *J. Crit. Care* **2024**, *79*, 154444. [CrossRef] [PubMed]
57. Soldati, G.; Smargiassi, A.; Inchingolo, R.; Buonsenso, D.; Perrone, T.; Briganti, D.F.; Perlini, S.; Torri, E.; Mariani, A.; Mossolani, E.E.; et al. Proposal for International Standardization of the Use of Lung Ultrasound for Patients with COVID-19. *J. Ultrasound Med.* **2020**, *39*, 1413–1419. [CrossRef] [PubMed]
58. Smith, M.J.; Hayward, S.A.; Innes, S.M.; Miller, A.S.C. Point-of-Care Lung Ultrasound in Patients with COVID-19—A Narrative Review. *Anaesthesia* **2020**, *75*, 1096–1104. [CrossRef]
59. Kulkarni, S.; Down, B.; Jha, S. Point-of-Care Lung Ultrasound in Intensive Care during the COVID-19 Pandemic. *Clin. Radiol.* **2020**, *75*, 710.e1–710.e4. [CrossRef]
60. Li, L.; Yang, Q.; Li, L.; Guan, J.; Liu, Z.; Han, J.; Chao, Y.; Wang, Z.; Yu, X. The Value of Lung Ultrasound Score on Evaluating Clinical Severity and Prognosis in Patients with Acute Respiratory Distress Syndrome. *Chin. Crit. Care Med.* **2015**, *27*, 579–584. [CrossRef]
61. Haddam, M.; Zieleskiewicz, L.; Perbet, S.; Baldovini, A.; Guervilly, C.; Arbelot, C.; Noel, A.; Vigne, C.; Hammad, E.; Antonini, F.; et al. Lung Ultrasonography for Assessment of Oxygenation Response to Prone Position Ventilation in ARDS. *Intensive Care Med.* **2016**, *42*, 1546–1556. [CrossRef]
62. Caltabeloti, F.P.; Monsel, A.; Arbelot, C.; Brisson, H.; Lu, Q.; Gu, W.J.; Zhou, G.J.; Auler, J.O.C.; Rouby, J.J. Early Fluid Loading in Acute Respiratory Distress Syndrome with Septic Shock Deteriorates Lung Aeration without Impairing Arterial Oxygenation: A Lung Ultrasound Observational Study. *Crit. Care* **2014**, *18*, R91. [CrossRef]
63. Bouhemad, B.; Brisson, H.; Le-Guen, M.; Arbelot, C.; Lu, Q.; Rouby, J.J. Bedside Ultrasound Assessment of Positive End-Expiratory Pressure-Induced Lung Recruitment. *Am. J. Respir. Crit. Care Med.* **2011**, *183*, 341–347. [CrossRef] [PubMed]
64. Breitkopf, R.; Treml, B.; Rajsic, S. Lung Sonography in Critical Care Medicine. *Diagnostics* **2022**, *12*, 1405. [CrossRef] [PubMed]
65. Zhao, Z.; Jiang, L.; Xi, X.; Jiang, Q.; Zhu, B.; Wang, M.; Xing, J.; Zhang, D. Prognostic Value of Extravascular Lung Water Assessed with Lung Ultrasound Score by Chest Sonography in Patients with Acute Respiratory Distress Syndrome. *BMC Pulm. Med.* **2015**, *15*, 98. [CrossRef] [PubMed]
66. Soummer, A.; Perbet, S.; Brisson, H.; Arbelot, C.; Constantin, J.M.; Lu, Q.; Rouby, J.J. Ultrasound Assessment of Lung Aeration Loss during a Successful Weaning Trial Predicts Postextubation Distress. *Crit. Care Med.* **2012**, *40*, 2064–2072. [CrossRef] [PubMed]
67. Chiumello, D.; Umbrello, M.; Papa, G.F.S.; Angileri, A.; Gurgitano, M.; Formenti, P.; Coppola, S.; Froio, S.; Cammaroto, A.; Carrafiello, G. Global and Regional Diagnostic Accuracy of Lung Ultrasound Compared to CT in Patients with Acute Respiratory Distress Syndrome. *Crit. Care Med.* **2019**, *47*, 1599–1606. [CrossRef]
68. Corradi, F.; Brusasco, C.; Pelosi, P. Chest Ultrasound in Acute Respiratory Distress Syndrome. *Curr. Opin. Crit. Care* **2014**, *20*, 98–103. [CrossRef]
69. Volpicelli, G.; Mussa, A.; Garofalo, G.; Cardinale, L.; Casoli, G.; Perotto, F.; Fava, C.; Frascisco, M. Bedside Lung Ultrasound in the Assessment of Alveolar-Interstitial Syndrome. *Am. J. Emerg. Med.* **2006**, *24*, 689–696. [CrossRef]
70. Corradi, F.; Via, G.; Forfori, F.; Brusasco, C.; Tavazzi, G. Lung Ultrasound and B-Lines Quantification Inaccuracy: B Sure to Have the Right Solution. *Intensive Care Med.* **2020**, *46*, 1081–1083. [CrossRef]
71. Millington, S.J.; Arntfield, R.T.; Guo, R.J.; Koenig, S.; Kory, P.; Noble, V.; Mallemat, H.; Schoenherr, J.R. Expert Agreement in the Interpretation of Lung Ultrasound Studies Performed on Mechanically Ventilated Patients. *J. Ultrasound Med.* **2018**, *37*, 2659–2665. [CrossRef]
72. Muse, E.D.; Topol, E.J. Guiding Ultrasound Image Capture with Artificial Intelligence. *Lancet* **2020**, *396*, 749. [CrossRef]
73. Suri, J.; Agarwal, S.; Gupta, S.; Puvvula, A.; Viskovic, K.; Suri, N.; Alizad, A.; El-Baz, A.; Saba, L.; Fatemi, M.; et al. Systematic Review of Artificial Intelligence in Acute Respiratory Distress Syndrome for COVID-19 Lung Patients: A Biomedical Imaging Perspective. *IEEE J. Biomed. Health Inform.* **2021**, *25*, 4128–4139. [CrossRef] [PubMed]
74. LeCun, Y.; Bengio, Y.; Hinton, G. Deep Learning. *Nature* **2015**, *521*, 436–444. [CrossRef] [PubMed]
75. Deng, L.; Yu, D. Deep Learning: Methods and Applications. *Found. Trends Signal Process.* **2013**, *7*, 197–387. [CrossRef]

76. Gibbons, R.C.; Magee, M.; Goett, H.; Murrett, J.; Genninger, J.; Mendez, K.; Tripod, M.; Tyner, N.; Costantino, T.G. Lung Ultrasound vs. Chest X-Ray Study for the Radiographic Diagnosis of COVID-19 Pneumonia in a High-Prevalence Population. *J. Emerg. Med.* **2021**, *60*, 615–625. [CrossRef]
77. Pare, J.R.; Camelo, I.; Mayo, K.C.; Leo, M.M.; Dugas, J.N.; Nelson, K.P.; Baker, W.E.; Shareef, F.; Mitchell, P.M.; Schechter-Perkins, E.M. Point-of-Care Lung Ultrasound Is More Sensitive than Chest Radiograph for Evaluation of COVID-19. *West. J. Emerg. Med.* **2020**, *21*, 771–778. [CrossRef]

Disclaimer/Publisher's Note: The statements, opinions and data contained in all publications are solely those of the individual author(s) and contributor(s) and not of MDPI and/or the editor(s). MDPI and/or the editor(s) disclaim responsibility for any injury to people or property resulting from any ideas, methods, instructions or products referred to in the content.

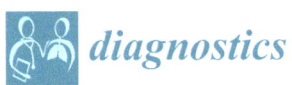

Article

Categorizing Acute Respiratory Distress Syndrome with Different Severities by Oxygen Saturation Index

Shin-Hwar Wu [1,*], Chew-Teng Kor [2,3], Shu-Hua Chi [4] and Chun-Yu Li [4]

[1] Division of Critical Care Internal Medicine, Department of Emergency Medicine and Critical Care, Changhua Christian Hospital, Changhua 50006, Taiwan

[2] Big Data Center, Changhua Christian Hospital, Changhua 50006, Taiwan; 179297@cch.org.tw

[3] Graduate Institute of Statistics and Information Science, National Changhua University of Education, Changhua 50006, Taiwan

[4] Section of Respiratory Therapy, Department of Emergency Medicine and Critical Care, Changhua Christian Hospital, Changhua 31940, Taiwan; S.-H.C.); 181285@cch.org.tw (C.-Y.L.)

* Correspondence: 126366@cch.org.tw; Tel.: +886-4-7238595 (ext. 3971)

Abstract: The oxygen saturation index (OSI), defined by F_IO_2/S_pO_2 multiplied by the mean airway pressure, has been reported to exceed the Berlin definition in predicting the mortality of acute respiratory distress syndrome (ARDS). The OSI has served as an alternative to the Berlin definition in categorizing pediatric ARDS. However, the use of the OSI for the stratification of adult ARDS has not been reported. A total of 379 invasively ventilated adult ARDS patients were retrospectively studied. The ARDS patients were classified into three groups by their incidence rate of mortality: mild (OSI < 14.69), moderate (14.69 < OSI < 23.08) and severe (OSI > 23.08). OSI-based categorization was highly correlated with the Berlin definition by a Kendall's tau of 0.578 ($p < 0.001$). The Kaplan–Meier curves of the three OSI-based groups were significantly different ($p < 0.001$). By the Berlin definition, the hazard ratio for 28-day mortality was 0.58 (0.33–1.05) and 0.95 (0.55–1.67) for the moderate and severe groups, respectively (compared to the mild group). In contrast, the corresponding hazard ratio was 1.01 (0.69–1.47) and 2.39 (1.71–3.35) for the moderate and severe groups defined by the OSI. By multivariate analysis, OSI-based severe ARDS was independently associated with 28-D or 90-D mortality. In conclusion, we report the first OSI-based stratification for adult ARDS and find that it serves well as an alternative to the Berlin definition.

Keywords: acute respiratory distress syndrome; classification; mortality; oxygen saturation index

1. Introduction

The Berlin definition is currently the most widely accepted standard for the diagnosis and classification of acute respiratory distress syndrome (ARDS). However, there are some shortcomings to this definition.

First, its prognostic prediction ability is far from satisfactory. The area under the receiver operating characteristic (AUROC) of mortality prediction was only around 0.57 [1,2], which was just slightly larger than that under chance. The severity classification of the Berlin definition is based solely on the initial P_aO_2/F_IO_2, which has been found to be poorly associated with mortality in patients with ARDS in many studies [3–5]. Several important factors with potential prognostic implications are neglected in the Berlin definition. For one thing, high inflation airway pressure can increase mechanical stress on the lung and the chances of ventilator-induced lung injury [6–8]. Lower airway pressure has been shown to be associated with survival benefits of ventilated patients with ARDS [9,10]. By incorporating mean airway pressure (MAP) into P_aO_2/F_IO_2, the oxygenation index (OI) is calculated using the equation

$$OI = \frac{F_IO_2 \times MAP \times 100}{P_aO_2}$$

The OI has been found to be better than P_aO_2/F_IO_2 in predicting the mortality of ARDS patients [11,12].

Another drawback of the Berlin definition is that its application is confined to settings when P_aO_2 is available. P_aO_2 can only be obtained sporadically by arterial puncture, which is painful and potentially harmful to patients. The absence of arterial blood gas data during crucial hypoxemic episodes may lead to a misclassification of the severity of ARDS in a patient. In areas where arterial blood analysis is unavailable, the prevalence of ARDS is inevitably under-reported. On the contrary, S_aO_2 can be continuously monitored by noninvasive pulse oximeters, which are ubiquitous in most ICUs. The S_aO_2/F_IO_2 and P_aO_2/F_IO_2 ratios are highly correlated [13] and provide similar prognostic information [14]. They also have similar cut-off points to identify mild and moderate ARDS [15,16]. The S_aO_2/F_IO_2 ratio has served as an alternative to the P_aO_2/F_IO_2 ratio in defining pediatric ARDS [17] and adult ARDS in resource-limited settings [18,19].

The oxygen saturation index (OSI) is generated by adding MAP to the S_aO_2/F_IO_2 ratio and is calculated using the equation

$$OSI = \frac{F_IO_2 \times MAP \times 100}{S_pO_2}$$

The OSI can be non-invasively obtained and performs better than S_aO_2/F_IO_2, P_aO_2/F_IO_2 or the OI in predicting the mortality rate of ARDS [20,21]. The OSI can also be helpful in stratifying mortality risk for ARDS patients. The AUROCs to diagnose the P_aO_2/F_IO_2 ratio of less than 100, 200 and 300 with the OSI were 0.922, 0.869 and 0.787, respectively [22]. Using the OSI instead of P_aO_2/F_IO_2 to define and categorize ARDS can bypass the aforementioned drawbacks of the Berlin definition. The OSI has already been used to define and categorize pediatric ARDS with different severities [17]. For adults, the role of the OSI in the stratification of risk in patients with ARDS has not been studied enough. In this study, we tried to evaluate using the OSI to categorize adult ARDS patients with different severities.

2. Materials and Methods

2.1. Patient Enrollment

We retrospectively collected the data of invasively ventilated patients with ARDS admitted to Changhua Christian Hospital, a medical center with a total of 130 ICU beds distributed in 5 separate wards, between January 2012 and November 2018. These patients were identified by screening discharge diagnoses of ARDS and acute respiratory failure in electronic archives. Each diagnosis of ARDS was defined by the Berlin definition [1] and was reconfirmed by a pulmonologist. Exclusion criteria included age less than 20 or over 90 years old, body weight less than 40 or over 100 Kg, a total duration of invasive ventilation less than 48 h, absence of retrievable data of arterial blood gas or MAP in the first 3 days of ARDS diagnosis, using airway pressure release ventilation or high-frequency oscillation ventilation or extracorporeal membrane oxygenation during the ARDS period, co-morbidities of metastatic malignancy, congestive heart failure (left ventricular ejection fraction less than 35%) or ventilator dependence (invasive ventilation for 21 days or more before the onset of ARDS), having been transferred to other hospital or discharged against medical advice (without traceable clinical outcome), having been withdrawn from the life-support due to hospice, having been enrolled in other ARDS-related clinical studies and absence of need for lung-protective ventilation, which was defined by $F_IO_2 \geq 50\%$ and PEEP > 5 cmH$_2$O [23]. The patients' data were traced until death or the 90th day after the diagnosis of ARDS. This study was approved by the institutional review board of Changhua Christian Hospital (approval number 191228).

2.2. Data Collection

Baseline variables when ARDS was diagnosed for the first time were collected. They include age, sex, body mass index (BMI), acute physiology and chronic health evaluation II (APACHE II) score, sequential organ failure assessment (SOFA) score, comorbidity, risk factors for ARDS and type of ICU admitted. Whether patients received sedation, muscle relaxant, systemic steroid, vasopressor, hemodialysis, prone position or total parenteral nutrition during the ARDS period was recorded. If the patients were under pressure-targeted ventilation and plateau pressures were not measured directly, the peak airway pressure or the sum of PEEP and the set increment of inspiratory pressure were used to represent plateau pressure [23].

2.3. Derivation of OI, OSI and Other Indices

The highest MAP and lowest P_aO_2/F_IO_2 and S_aO_2/F_IO_2 in the initial 3 days after ARDS diagnosis were used to calculate OI and OSI. The equation for calculating OI and OSI was mentioned in the previous section. We also adopt the lowest P_aO_2/F_IO_2 and S_aO_2/F_IO_2 of the initial 3 days as the commonly used predictor of ARDS mortality. Categorization according to Berlin definition was based on the lowest P_aO_2/F_IO_2 of the initial 3 days.

2.4. Statistical Analysis

Scatter plots and Spearman's rho correlation analysis were used to present the linear correlation of OI and OSI. Categorical and continuous variables were expressed as numbers (proportions), mean ± standard deviation (SD) and median and interquartile range (IQR), respectively. The discriminating abilities of OI, OSI, S_pO_2/F_IO_2, P_aO_2/F_IO_2, APACHE II score and Berlin definition regarding mortality were assessed using receiver operating characteristic (ROC) curves and the corresponding AUROCs. Furthermore, ROC was also used to evaluate the OI and OSI categories with respect to P_aO_2/F_IO_2 of less than 200 or 100, respectively. The incidence rate per 100 person–days was used to visualize the trend of the hazard ratio for death over continuous values of OSI and OI. OI and OSI values were classified into low, moderate and high groups based on similar magnitudes of hazard according to the incidence rate per 100 person-days. Kendall's tau correlation was calculated to evaluate the correlation between the categorizations by P_aO_2/F_IO_2 ratio-based Berlin definition, OI category and OSI category. Kaplan–Meier curves of estimated 28-day and 90-day survival were plotted and differences between the three groups were compared using the log-rank test. Survival analyses were performed to assess the association of OI, OSI levels and groups with mortality, using the low group category as the reference. According to the OI and OSI groups, crude and multivariate Cox proportional hazard models were constructed to estimate the mortality risk during the follow-up period. Statistical analyses were performed using SAS, and a visualization plot was performed using the R software (version 4.1.0 accessed on 18 May 2021; The Comprehensive R Archive Network: http://cran.r-project.org). All two-sided *p*-values less than 0.05 were considered statistically significant.

3. Results

3.1. Clinical Characteristics of Patients with ARDS

A total of 786 patients were found with invasive ventilation for ARDS and acute respiratory failure. Four hundred and seven patients were excluded due to extreme body weight for 20 of them, absence of traceable clinical outcomes for 19 of them, having been invasively ventilated for less than 48 h for 175 of them, other terminal comorbidities for 102 of them, absence of arterial blood gas data in the initial 3 days for 3 of them, having been ventilated by special modes for 2 of them, having received extracorporeal membrane oxygenation during the ARDS period for 70 of them, absence of ventilator settings eligible for lung-protective ventilation for 12 of them and having been withdrawn from a life-sustaining machine for hospice for 4 of them. Therefore, 379 patients were analyzed. The clinical characteristics of these patients are summarized in Table 1.

Table 1. Clinical characteristics of the patients with ARDS (n = 379).

	Value
Age (year), mean ± SD	64 ± 16
Male, No. (%)	262 (69)
BMI, median (IQR), (Kg/m^2)	23 (20–26)
APACHE II Score, median (IQR)	24 (18–30)
SOFA score, median (IQR)	7 (5–10)
Lung injury score, median (IQR)	11 (10–12)
Severity by Berlin definition	
Mild, No. (%)	23 (6)
Moderate, No. (%)	145 (38)
Severe, No. (%)	189 (50)
Missing, No. (%)	22 (6)
Comorbidity	
Chronic obstructive pulmonary disease, No. (%)	126 (33)
Diabetes mellitus, No. (%)	137 (36)
Hypertension, No. (%)	178 (47)
Chronic kidney disease, No. (%)	50 (13)
Heart failure, No. (%)	117 (31)
Cerebral vascular accident, No. (%)	90 (24)
Liver cirrhosis, No. (%)	44 (12)
Malignancy, No. (%)	88 (23)
Surgical ICU Admission, No. (%)	57 (15)
Treatment received during ARDS period	
Sedation, No. (%)	350 (92)
Muscle relaxant, No. (%)	356 (94)
Vasopressor, No. (%)	294 (78)
Total parenteral nutrition, No. (%)	75 (20)
Systemic steroid, No. (%)	320 (84)
Prone position, No. (%)	42 (11)
Hemodialysis, No. (%)	50 (13)
Continuous hemofiltration, No. (%)	126 (33)
Oxygenation index, median (IQR)	21 (15–31)
Oxygen saturation index, median (IQR)	19 (14–24)
V_T/PBW [1] (mL/Kg), median (IQR)	9 (8–10)
P_aO_2/F_IO_2 ratio, median (IQR)	96 (71–133)
C_{RS} [2] (mL/cmH$_2$O), median (IQR)	26 (22–31)
Plateau Pressure [3] (cmH$_2$O), median (IQR)	32 (30–35)
PEEP (cmH$_2$O), median (IQR)	10 (10–12)
Driving Pressure [3] (cmH$_2$O), median (IQR)	21 (19–24)
28-day Mortality, No. (%)	186 (49)
90-day Mortality, No. (%)	233 (61)
Ventilator-free days, day 1–28 [4], median (IQR)	16 (6–22)

[1] V_T/PBW: tidal volume/predicted body weight. [2] C_{RS}: respiratory system compliance. [3] Putative numbers, subject to over-estimation. See Section 2 or details. [4] In patients surviving by day 28.

3.2. Correlation between OI and OSI

The OI and OSI were correlated by OI = −4.449 + 1.406 OSI and Spearman's rho of 0.844 ($p < 0.001$) (Figure S1).

3.3. Comparison of ROC Curves of Commonly Used Indices in the Prediction of Mortality

The ROC curves of six commonly used indices, i.e., OI, OSI, S_pO_2/F_IO_2, P_aO_2/F_IO_2, APACHE II score and the Berlin definition, for predicting the mortality of ARDS patients, are depicted in Figure 1. The AUROC of the OSI was 0.630 (95% CI: 0.57–0.69) in predicting mortality at 28 days. This value was higher than that of any other index. In terms of predicting 90-day mortality, the AUROC of the OSI was 0.621 (95% CI: 0.56–0.68). Again, this AUROC was the largest among the six commonly used indices.

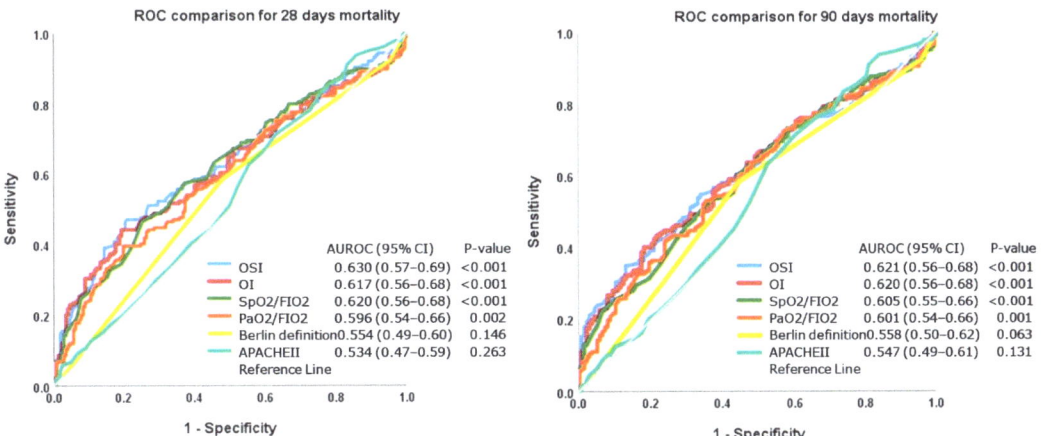

Figure 1. Comparison of ROC curves of six commonly used predictors of ARDS mortality. AUROCs of OSI were the highest for mortality at 28 days or 90 days.

3.4. Using the OI or OSI Category to Diagnose P_aO_2/F_IO_2 Less Than 200 or 100

The AUROC of the OI category for diagnosing P_aO_2/F_IO_2 of less than 200 and 100 was 0.79 (0.72–0.87) and 0.94 (0.92–0.97), respectively. The AUROCs of the OSI category in diagnosing P_aO_2/F_IO_2 of less than 200 and 100 were 0.76 (0.68–0.84) and 0.84 (0.79–0.88), respectively (Figure S2).

3.5. Using the OI and OSI Values to Categorize ARDS with Different Severities

The incidence rates of mortality for every 100-person-day were plotted against continuous OI and OSI values divided by each 10 percentiles, as seen in Figure 2. Based on incidence rates of mortality, the types of ARDS were categorized into three mutually exclusive groups: mild (OI < 15.91, or OSI < 14.69), moderate (15.91 < OI < 28.78 or 14.69 < OSI < 23.08) and severe (OI > 28.78, or OSI > 23.08).

3.6. Correlations between OI/OSI-Based and P_aO_2/F_IO_2-Based (Berlin Definition) Categorization

OI or OSI-based categorization was highly correlated with P_aO_2/F_IO_2 ratio categorization by a Kendall's tau of 0.754 ($p < 0.001$) (for the OI) or 0.578 ($p < 0.001$) (for the OSI) (Figure 3).

3.7. Mortality of Various OI/OSI-Based Severity Categories

The Kaplan–Meier curves of ARDS patients with various OI or OSI-based severity categories were significantly different for 28-day or 90-day mortality. All of these log-rank p-values were less than 0.001 (Figure 4). The mortality rate for each OI- or OSI-based severity category is presented in Table S1.

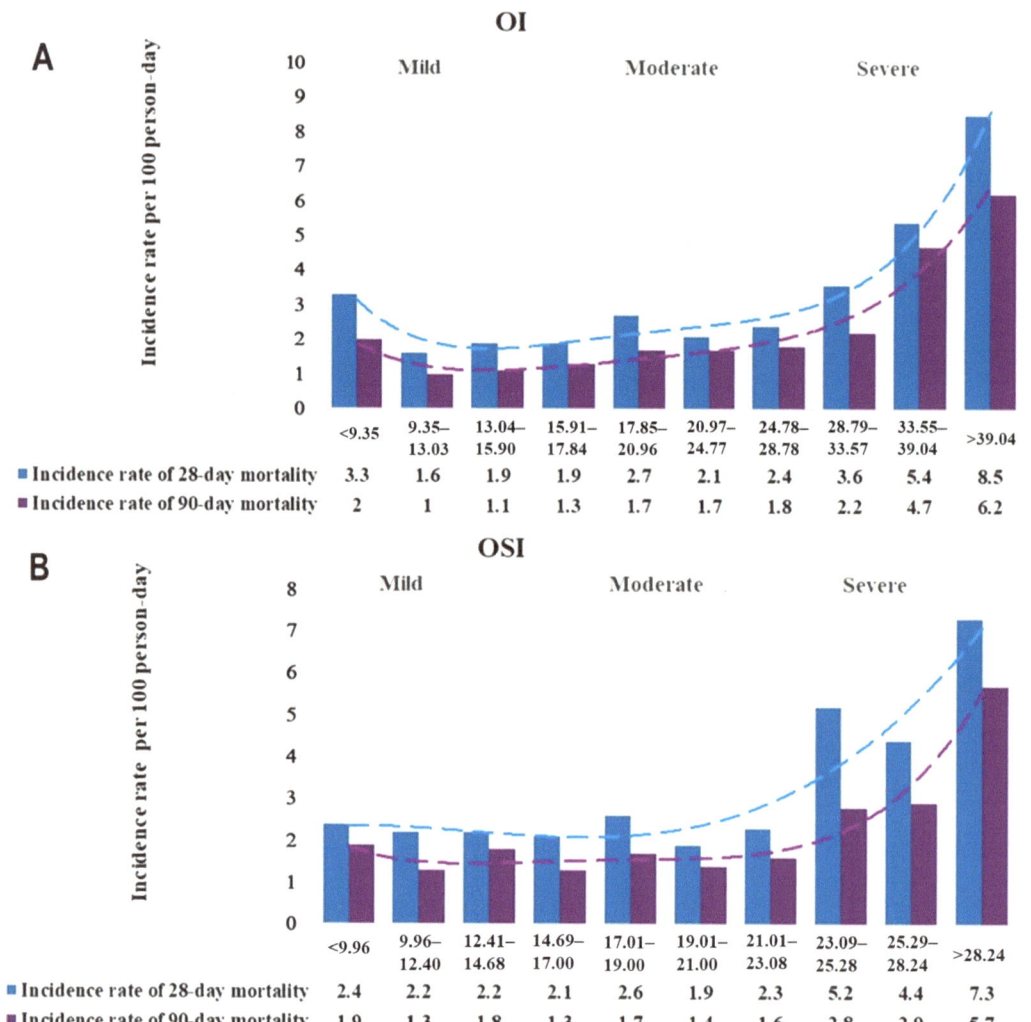

Figure 2. Incidence rate of mortality per 100-person-day stratified by the 10th percentiles of OI (**A**) and OSI (**B**). ARDS were classified into 3 groups: mild (OI < 15.91, or OSI < 14.69), moderate (15.91 < OI < 28.78 or 14.69 < OSI < 23.08) and severe (OI > 28.78, or OSI > 23.08).

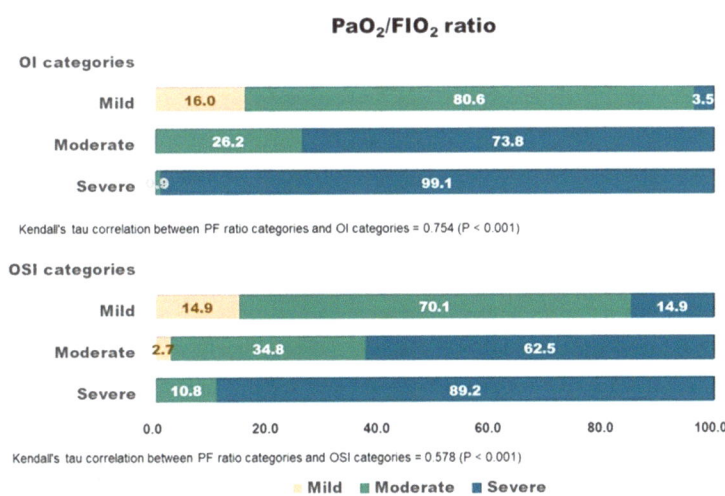

Figure 3. Correlation between OI/OSI-based and P_aO_2/F_IO_2-based categorizations by Kendall's tau. Both were highly correlated by a Kendall's tau of 0.754 ($p < 0.001$) (for OI) or 0.578 ($p < 0.001$) (for OSI).

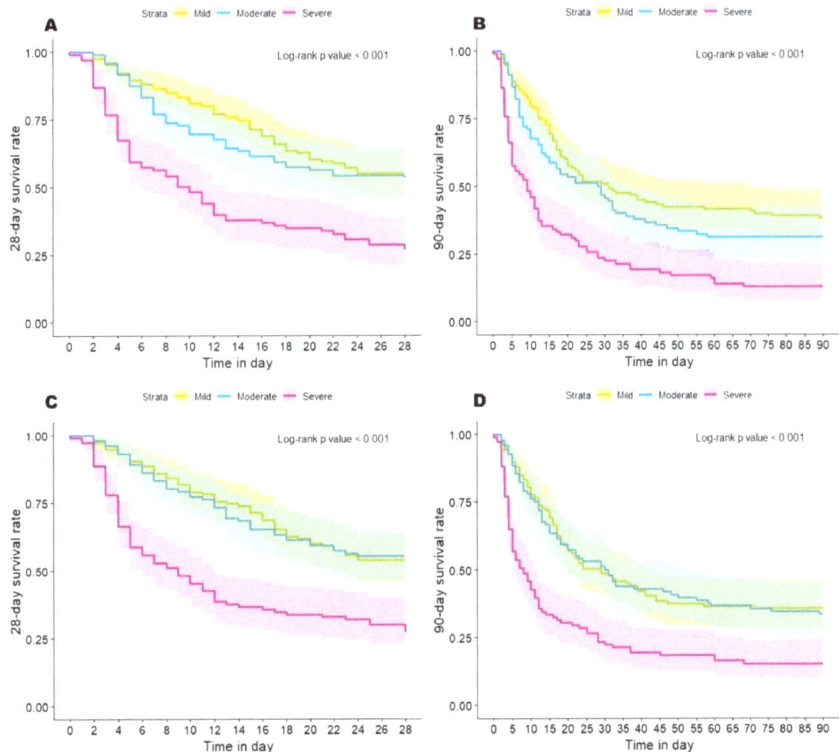

Figure 4. Kaplan–Meier curves of ARDS patients with various OI/OSI-based categories. ARDS patients categorized by OI for 28-day (**A**) or 90-day (**B**) survival. Kaplan–Meier curves of ARDS patients categorized by OSI for 28-day (**C**) or 90-day (**D**) survival.

3.8. Univariate Analyses of Variables Associated with Mortality

By univariate analysis, the selected variables potentially associated with mortality at 28 days are presented in Table 2.

Table 2. Univariate analysis of selected variables potentially associated with 28-day mortality.

	Survival	Death	HR (95% CI)	p-Value
Age (year), mean ± SD	62.4 ± 16.6	65.3 ± 15	1.00 (0.99–1.01)	0.40
Male, No. (%)	126 (65)	136 (73)	1.37 (0.99–1.90)	0.06
BMI, median (IQR), (Kg/m^2)	23 (21–27)	23 (20–26)	0.97 (0.94–1.00)	0.07
APACHE II Score, median (IQR)	24 (18–30)	24 (19–29)	1.00 (0.99–1.02)	0.57
SOFA score, median (IQR)	7 (5–10)	7 (5–10)	1.02 (0.98–1.06)	0.29
Lung injury score, median (IQR)	11 (10–12)	11 (10–12)	1.01 (0.94–1.09)	0.82
Severity by Berlin definition				
Mild, No. (%)	9 (5)	14 (8)	1	1
Moderate, No. (%)	87 (48)	58 (33)	0.58 (0.33–1.05)	0.07
Severe, No. (%)	87 (48)	102 (59)	0.95 (0.55–1.67)	0.87
OI, median (IQR)	18 (13–27)	24 (16–35)	1.03 (1.02–1.05)	<0.01 *
Mild, No. (%)	87 (47)	57 (33)	1	
Moderate, No. (%)	62 (34)	45 (26)	1.11 (0.75–1.64)	0.60
Severe, No. (%)	35 (19)	72 (41)	2.45 (1.73–3.47)	<0.01 *
OSI, median (IQR)	18 (13–22)	21 (14–26)	1.05 (1.03–1.07)	<0.01 *
Mild, No. (%)	90 (47)	63 (34)	1	
Moderate, No. (%)	67 (35)	47 (25)	1.01 (0.69–1.47)	0.96
Severe, No. (%)	36 (19)	76 (41)	2.39 (1.71–3.35)	<0.01 *
Comorbidity				
Hypertension, No. (%)	98 (51)	80 (43)	0.74 (0.55–0.98)	0.04 *
Liver cirrhosis, No. (%)	15 (8)	29 (16)	1.61 (1.08–2.39)	0.02 *
Malignancy, No. (%)	32 (17)	56 (30)	1.54 (1.13–2.11)	0.01 *
Treatment received				
Vasopressor, No. (%)	128 (66)	166 (89)	3.12 (1.96–4.97)	<0.01 *
Hemodialysis, No. (%)	30 (16)	20 (11)	0.61 (0.38–0.97)	0.04 *
Continuous hemofiltration, No. (%)	42 (22)	84 (45)	1.99 (1.49–2.66)	<0.01 *
V_T/PBW [1] (ml/Kg)	9 (8–10)	9 (8–10)	0.86 (0.8–0.94)	<0.01 *
C_{RS} [2] (ml/cmH$_2$O)	28 (25–33)	24 (20–28)	0.94 (0.92–0.96)	<0.01 *
PEEP (cmH$_2$O)	10 (9–12)	11 (10–13)	1.13 (1.06–1.22)	<0.01 *
Driving pressure [3] (cmH$_2$O)	20 (18–23)	22 (20–25)	1.07 (1.03–1.10)	<0.01 *

[1] V_T/PBW: Tidal volume/predicted body weight. [2] C_{RS}: Compliance of respiratory system. [3] Putative numbers, subject to over-estimation. See Section 2 for details. * $p < 0.05$.

The OI and OSI were both associated with increased mortality. However, the traditional ICU severity index (APACHE II score, SOFA score) or lung injury score was not associated with mortality at 28 days. Severe ARDS classified by OI > 28.78 had a 28-D mortality hazard ratio (HR) of 2.37 (1.73–3.26) over the mild counterpart (OI < 15.91) ($p < 0.01$). Severe ARDS classified by OSI > 23.08 had a 28-D mortality HR of 2.14 (1.58–2.91) over the mild counterpart (OSI < 14.69) ($p < 0.01$). In contrast, the 28-D mortality HR of severe ARDS classified by the Berlin definition was 0.89 (0.53–1.47) over the mild counterpart, which was not significantly different ($p = 0.64$). The contributors to 90-day mortality are presented in Table S2. The data are similar to those of mortality at 28 days.

3.9. Multivariate Cox Proportional Hazard Analyses of Variables Associated with Mortality

Multivariate Cox proportional hazard analyses found that the OI (or OSI) as a continuous value and respiratory system compliance (C_{RS}) were independently associated with mortality at 28 days. When patients were divided into three groups of severity based on the OI (or OSI), the severe group (versus mild) and C_{RS} were independent factors associated with mortality at 28 days. The OI (or OSI) was also independently associated with mortality at 90 days (Table 3).

Table 3. Multivariate Cox proportional hazard analysis of factors associated with mortality.

	28-Day Mortality [1]				90-Day Mortality [2]			
	aHR [3] (95% CI)	p	aHR (95% CI)	p	aHR (95% CI)	p	aHR (95% CI)	p
	OI or OSI as continuous values							
OI	1.03 (1.01–1.04)	<0.01	-	-	1.04 (1.02–1.06)	<0.001	-	-
OSI	-	-	1.03 (1.01–1.05)	<0.01	-	-	1.04 (1.02–1.06)	<0.01
C_{RS}	0.93 (0.91–0.96)	<0.01	0.94 (0.92–0.97)	<0.01	0.93 (0.90–0.95)	<0.001	0.93 (0.91–0.95)	<0.01
V_T/PBW	1.06 (0.95–1.17)	0.31	1.06 (0.96–1.17)	0.26	1.15 (1.04–1.27)	0.007	1.12 (1.01–1.23)	0.03
	OI or OSI as 3 groups							
OI group								
Mild	1	-	-	-	1	-	-	-
Moderate	1.05 (0.71–1.57)	0.80	-	-	1.47 (0.95–2.30)	0.09	-	-
Severe	2.24 (1.54–3.26)	<0.01	-	-	3.03 (1.85–4.95)	<0.01	-	-
OSI group								
Mild	-	-	1	-	-	-	1	-
Moderate	-	-	0.98 (0.67–1.44)	0.94	-	-	0.96 (0.66–1.41)	0.84
Severe	-	-	2.26 (1.58–3.24)	<0.01	-	-	2.15 (1.43–3.24)	<0.01
C_{RS}	0.93 (0.91–0.96)	<0.01	0.93 (0.91–0.96)	<0.01	0.93 (0.90–0.95)	<0.01	0.93 (0.90–0.95)	<0.01
V_T/PBW	1.07 (0.96–1.19)	0.22	1.06 (0.96–1.17)	0.25	1.16 (1.06–1.28)	0.01	1.15 (1.05–1.26)	<0.01

[1] Model was adjusted for gender, BMI, hypertension, liver cirrhosis, malignancy, vasopressor, hemodialysis and continuous hemofiltration. [2] Model was adjusted for age, gender, BMI, P_aO_2/F_IO_2 ratio, hypertension, liver cirrhosis, malignancy, vasopressor, systemic steroid, prone position and continuous hemofiltration. [3] Adjusted hazard ratio.

4. Discussion

In this study, we report the first OSI-based mortality risk stratification in adult ARDS patients. This novel categorization showed a good correlation the with P_aO_2/F_IO_2-based Berlin definition (Figure 3), but it did not require an invasive technique and could be conveniently obtained. Furthermore, this OSI-based categorization was found to be superior to the P_aO_2/F_IO_2-based Berlin definition in discriminating the risk of mortality at 28 or 90 days (Tables 2, S1 and S2). Therefore, we think that the OSI could be an alternative to the P_aO_2/F_IO_2-based Berlin definition in categorizing adult ARDS with different severities.

Our study also demonstrates that the OSI has the largest AUROC in discriminating either 28-day or 90-day mortality, better than the other five commonly used predictors, i.e., OI, S_pO_2/F_IO_2, P_aO_2/F_IO_2, APACHE II score and the Berlin definition in this study (Figure 1). This result was in congruence with several previous reports [20,21]. For the detection of hypoxemia, S_aO_2 (or S_pO_2) is less sensitive than P_aO_2 when S_aO_2 is above 97%, but S_pO_2 is a reliable predictor of P_aO_2 in most other clinical circumstances [24]. Unlike sporadically sampled P_aO_2, S_pO_2 is continuously monitored and less likely to miss any hypoxemic episode. Missing P_aO_2/F_IO_2 data during significant hypoxemia may lead to the underestimation of severity and inaccurate prognostic prediction. We think that this may be the main reason why S_pO_2-based OSI outperforms other P_aO_2-based indices in prognostic prediction. Our speculation gains support from a large retrospective study including more than 35,000 patients. This study found that substituting missing P_aO_2/F_IO_2 data in the Sequential Organ Failure Assessment score with S_pO_2/F_IO_2 has greater discrimination ability for mortality than the miss-as-normal technique. The difference was most prominent in a subgroup of patients without baseline P_aO_2/F_IO_2 data [25].

Incorporating airway pressure into the equation may be another explanation for the OSI's superior prognostic prediction ability compared to S_pO_2/F_IO_2, P_aO_2/F_IO_2 or the Berlin definition. Airway pressure is associated with lung compliance and ventilator settings, which surely contribute to outcomes of ARDS, as we have demonstrated in our multivariate analysis (Table 3). Barotrauma is the first well-studied mechanism of ventilator-induced lung injury [26]. Animal and clinical studies have shown that high airway pressure can induce pulmonary alveolar damage [6–8]. On the contrary, lower airway pressure has been shown to have a survival benefit in several large clinical trials [9,10].

DesPres et al. found that, when the OSI of their ARDS patients was greater than 19, the hospital mortality risk was greater than 30% [20]. Another study reported an adjusted odds ratio of 5.22 for mortality when the OSI was greater than 12 [21]. However, the above information is too indistinct to be applied in stratifying clinical ARDS cases. Here, we suggest unequivocal cut-off points (14.69 and 23.08) for defining three categories of ARDS, which are in line with usual clinical practice and the Berlin definition. The cutoff points that we suggested reflect the specific population group we collected in this study. This needs further verification by more studies with larger case numbers.

The outcomes of our mild and moderate groups are not significantly different no matter whether they are defined by the OI, OSI or Berlin definition. The hazard ratios of 28-D mortality for the moderate group (vs. mild) are 1.11, 1.01 and 0.58 by the OI, OSI and Berlin definition, respectively (Table 2). Since the discriminative ability of the Berlin definition has been proved [1], the failure to differentiate the two may be due to sampling-related type II error rather than the test itself. The inadequate number of mild ARDS cases (by the Berlin definition) may contribute to this error (Table 1). The correlation between the mild OI/OSI and P_aO_2/F_IO_2 ratio is not as significant as in the severe cases (Figure 3) can also be explained by this underrepresentation of the mild group. That is the first limitation of this study.

The second limitation of this study is that the patients were all collected from one medical center. To make the result of this study more relevant to patients with ARDS from other areas, we need more research with broader demographics.

Another limitation of this study is that only intubated patients with ARDS were enrolled. Non-invasive ventilators or high flow nasal oxygen are now more frequently applied to ARDS patients with a condition not severe enough to be intubated. The definition of pediatric ARDS has been broadened to include non-intubated patients [17]. The newly released global definition of ARDS also includes non-intubated adult patients [19]. We hope that future OSI or OI studies can incorporate this cohort of patients. However, accurately measuring airway pressure for OSI/OI calculation in non-intubated ARDS patients is an obstacle to overcome.

ARDS patients with COVID-19 were not included in our study. We are not confident that the results obtained from this study are applicable to this specific group of patients.

5. Conclusions

We present the first OSI-based severity stratification for adult patients with ARDS and find that it serves well as an alternative to the Berlin definition. The cut-off values we proposed need verification in future studies.

Supplementary Materials: The following supporting information can be downloaded at: https://www.mdpi.com/article/10.3390/diagnostics14010037/s1, Figure S1:The correlation between OI and OSI by scatter plots and Spearman's rho correlation analysis; Figure S2: Using the OI or OSI category to diagnose P_aO_2/F_IO_2 less than 200 or 100 by ROC; Table S1: Mortality of various category of ARDS patient defined by Berlin definition, OI and OSI; Table S2: Univariate analysis of selected variables potentially associated with 90-day mortality.

Author Contributions: S.-H.W. drafted the manuscript. C.-T.K. analyzed the data and performed statistical calculations. S.-H.C. and C.-Y.L. collected clinical data from study patients. All authors have read and agreed to the published version of the manuscript.

Funding: This study was supported by Grant Number 109-CCH-IRP-111 (Changhua Christian Hospital).

Institutional Review Board Statement: This study was approved by the Institutional Review Board of Changhua Christian Hospital (Approval No. 191228).

Informed Consent Statement: The Board has waived the requirement for informed consent from participants.

Data Availability Statement: The data presented in this study are available upon reasonable request from the corresponding author.

Conflicts of Interest: The authors declared that they had no competing interests.

References

1. Ranieri, V.M.; Rubenfeld, G.D.; Thompson, B.T.; Ferguson, N.D.; Caldwell, E.; Fan, E.; Camporota, L.; Slutsky, A.S. Acute respiratory distress syndrome: The Berlin Definition. *Jama* **2012**, *307*, 2526–2533. [CrossRef] [PubMed]
2. Caser, E.B.; Zandonade, E.; Pereira, E.; Gama, A.M.; Barbas, C.S. Impact of distinct definitions of acute lung injury on its incidence and outcomes in Brazilian ICUs: Prospective evaluation of 7133 patients. *Crit. Care Med.* **2014**, *42*, 574–582. [CrossRef] [PubMed]
3. Ware, L.B. Prognostic determinants of acute respiratory distress syndrome in adults: Impact on clinical trial design. *Crit. Care Med.* **2005**, *33*, S217–S222. [CrossRef] [PubMed]
4. Venet, C.; Guyomarc'h, S.; Pingat, J.; Michard, C.; Laporte, S.; Bertrand, M.; Gery, P.; Page, D.; Vermesch, R.; Bertrand, J.C.; et al. Prognostic factors in acute respiratory distress syndrome: A retrospective multivariate analysis including prone positioning in management strategy. *Intensive Care Med.* **2003**, *29*, 1435–1441. [CrossRef] [PubMed]
5. Luhr, O.R.; Karlsson, M.; Thorsteinsson, A.; Rylander, C.; Frostell, C.G. The impact of respiratory variables on mortality in non-ARDS and ARDS patients requiring mechanical ventilation. *Intensive Care Med.* **2000**, *26*, 508–517. [CrossRef] [PubMed]
6. Tsuno, K.; Miura, K.; Takeya, M.; Kolobow, T.; Morioka, T. Histopathologic pulmonary changes from mechanical ventilation at high peak airway pressures. *Am. Rev. Respir. Dis.* **1991**, *143 Pt 1*, 1115–1120. [CrossRef]
7. Kolobow, T.; Moretti, M.P.; Fumagalli, R.; Mascheroni, D.; Prato, P.; Chen, V.; Joris, M. Severe impairment in lung function induced by high peak airway pressure during mechanical ventilation. An experimental study. *Am. Rev. Respir. Dis.* **1987**, *135*, 312–315. [CrossRef]
8. Parker, J.C.; Hernandez, L.A.; Peevy, K.J. Mechanisms of ventilator-induced lung injury. *Crit. Care Med.* **1993**, *21*, 131–143. [CrossRef]
9. Amato, M.B.; Meade, M.O.; Slutsky, A.S.; Brochard, L.; Costa, E.L.; Schoenfeld, D.A.; Stewart, T.E.; Briel, M.; Talmor, D.; Mercat, A.; et al. Driving pressure and survival in the acute respiratory distress syndrome. *N. Engl. J. Med.* **2015**, *372*, 747–755. [CrossRef]
10. Brower, R.G.; Matthay, M.A.; Morris, A.; Schoenfeld, D.; Thompson, B.T.; Wheeler, A. Ventilation with lower tidal volumes as compared with traditional tidal volumes for acute lung injury and the acute respiratory distress syndrome. *N. Engl. J. Med.* **2000**, *342*, 1301–1308. [CrossRef]
11. Seeley, E.; McAuley, D.F.; Eisner, M.; Miletin, M.; Matthay, M.A.; Kallet, R.H. Predictors of mortality in acute lung injury during the era of lung protective ventilation. *Thorax* **2008**, *63*, 994–998. [CrossRef] [PubMed]
12. Monchi, M.; Bellenfant, F.; Cariou, A.; Joly, L.M.; Thebert, D.; Laurent, I.; Dhainaut, J.F.; Brunet, F. Early predictive factors of survival in the acute respiratory distress syndrome. A multivariate analysis. *Am. J. Respir. Crit. Care Med.* **1998**, *158*, 1076–1081. [CrossRef] [PubMed]
13. Pisani, L.; Roozeman, J.P.; Simonis, F.D.; Giangregorio, A.; van der Hoeven, S.M.; Schouten, L.R.; Horn, J.; Neto, A.S.; Festic, E.; Dondorp, A.M.; et al. Risk stratification using SpO(2)/FiO(2) and PEEP at initial ARDS diagnosis and after 24 h in patients with moderate or severe ARDS. *Ann. Intensive Care* **2017**, *7*, 108. [CrossRef] [PubMed]
14. Chen, W.; Janz, D.R.; Shaver, C.M.; Bernard, G.R.; Bastarache, J.A.; Ware, L.B. Clinical Characteristics and Outcomes Are Similar in ARDS Diagnosed by Oxygen Saturation/Fio$_2$ Ratio Compared with Pao$_2$/Fio$_2$ Ratio. *Chest* **2015**, *148*, 1477–1483. [CrossRef] [PubMed]
15. Bashar, F.R.; Vahedian-Azimi, A.; Farzanegan, B.; Goharani, R.; Shojaei, S.; Hatamian, S.; Mosavinasab, S.M.M.; Khoshfetrat, M.; Khatir, M.A.K.; Tomdio, A.; et al. Comparison of non-invasive to invasive oxygenation ratios for diagnosing acute respiratory distress syndrome following coronary artery bypass graft surgery: A prospective derivation-validation cohort study. *J. Cardiothorac. Surg.* **2018**, *13*, 123. [CrossRef] [PubMed]
16. Babu, S.; Abhilash, K.P.; Kandasamy, S.; Gowri, M. Association between SpO(2)/FiO(2) Ratio and PaO(2)/FiO(2) Ratio in Different Modes of Oxygen Supplementation. *Indian J. Crit. Care Med.* **2021**, *25*, 1001–1005. [CrossRef] [PubMed]
17. Khemani, R.G.; Smith, L.S.; Zimmerman, J.J.; Erickson, S. Pediatric acute respiratory distress syndrome: Definition, incidence, and epidemiology: Proceedings from the Pediatric Acute Lung Injury Consensus Conference. *Pediatr. Crit. Care Med.* **2015**, *16* (Suppl. S1), S23–S40. [CrossRef] [PubMed]

18. Riviello, E.D.; Kiviri, W.; Twagirumugabe, T.; Mueller, A.; Banner-Goodspeed, V.M.; Officer, L.; Novack, V.; Mutumwinka, M.; Talmor, D.S.; Fowler, R.A. Hospital Incidence and Outcomes of the Acute Respiratory Distress Syndrome Using the Kigali Modification of the Berlin Definition. *Am. J. Respir. Crit. Care Med.* **2016**, *193*, 52–59. [CrossRef]
19. Matthay, M.A.; Arabi, Y.; Arroliga, A.C.; Bernard, G.; Bersten, A.D.; Brochard, L.J.; Calfee, C.S.; Combes, A.; Daniel, B.M.; Ferguson, N.D.; et al. A New Global Definition of Acute Respiratory Distress Syndrome. *Am. J. Respir. Crit. Care Med.* **2023**. *published online ahead of print*. [CrossRef]
20. DesPrez, K.; McNeil, J.B.; Wang, C.; Bastarache, J.A.; Shaver, C.M.; Ware, L.B. Oxygenation Saturation Index Predicts Clinical Outcomes in ARDS. *Chest* **2017**, *152*, 1151–1158. [CrossRef]
21. Chen, W.L.; Lin, W.T.; Kung, S.C.; Lai, C.C.; Chao, C.M. The Value of Oxygenation Saturation Index in Predicting the Outcomes of Patients with Acute Respiratory Distress Syndrome. *J. Clin. Med.* **2018**, *7*, 205. [CrossRef] [PubMed]
22. Otekeiwebia, A.; Ajao, O.; Ingrid, P.; Foreman, M. 668: Performance of Oxygen Saturation Index among Adults with Type I Respiratory Failure. *Crit. Care Med.* **2014**, *42*, A1521. [CrossRef]
23. Needham, D.M.; Colantuoni, E.; Mendez-Tellez, P.A.; Dinglas, V.D.; Sevransky, J.E.; Dennison Himmelfarb, C.R.; Desai, S.V.; Shanholtz, C.; Brower, R.G.; Pronovost, P.J. Lung protective mechanical ventilation and two year survival in patients with acute lung injury: Prospective cohort study. *Bmj* **2012**, *344*, e2124. [CrossRef] [PubMed]
24. Wick, K.D.; Matthay, M.A.; Ware, L.B. Pulse oximetry for the diagnosis and management of acute respiratory distress syndrome. *Lancet Respir. Med.* **2022**, *10*, 1086–1098. [CrossRef]
25. Schenck, E.J.; Hoffman, K.L.; Oromendia, C.; Sanchez, E.; Finkelsztein, E.J.; Hong, K.S.; Kabariti, J.; Torres, L.K.; Harrington, J.S.; Siempos, I.I.; et al. A Comparative Analysis of the Respiratory Subscore of the Sequential Organ Failure Assessment Scoring System. *Ann. Am. Thorac. Soc.* **2021**, *18*, 1849–1860. [CrossRef]
26. Tonetti, T.; Vasques, F.; Rapetti, F.; Maiolo, G.; Collino, F.; Romitti, F.; Camporota, L.; Cressoni, M.; Cadringher, P.; Quintel, M.; et al. Driving pressure and mechanical power: New targets for VILI prevention. *Ann. Transl. Med.* **2017**, *5*, 286. [CrossRef]

Disclaimer/Publisher's Note: The statements, opinions and data contained in all publications are solely those of the individual author(s) and contributor(s) and not of MDPI and/or the editor(s). MDPI and/or the editor(s) disclaim responsibility for any injury to people or property resulting from any ideas, methods, instructions or products referred to in the content.

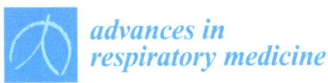

Article

COVID-19 Acute Respiratory Distress Syndrome: Treatment with Helmet CPAP in Respiratory Intermediate Care Unit by Pulmonologists in the Three Italian Pandemic Waves

Martina Piluso [1], Clarissa Ferrari [2], Silvia Pagani [1,*], Pierfranco Usai [1], Stefania Raschi [1], Luca Parachini [1], Elisa Oggionni [1], Chiara Melacini [1], Francesca D'Arcangelo [1], Roberta Cattaneo [1], Cristiano Bonacina [1], Monica Bernareggi [1], Serena Bencini [1], Marta Nadalin [3,4], Mara Borelli [3,4], Roberto Bellini [1], Maria Chiara Salandini [1] and Paolo Scarpazza [1]

1. Lung Unit, Cardiothoracic Vascular Department, Vimercate Hospital, 20871 Vimercate, Italy; martina.piluso@asst-brianza.it (M.P.); pierfranco.usai@asst-brianza.it (P.U.); stefania.raschi@asst-brianza.it (S.R.); luca.parachini@asst-brianza.it (L.P.); elisa.oggionni@asst-brianza.it (E.O.); chiara.melacini@asst-brianza.it (C.M.); francesca.darcangelo@asst-brianza.it (F.D.); roberta.cattaneo@asst-brianza.it (R.C.); cristiano.bonacina@asst-brianza.it (C.B.); monica.bernareggi@asst-brianza.it (M.B.); serena.bencini@asst-brianza.it (S.B.); roberto.bellini@asst-brianza.it (R.B.); mariachiara.salandini@asst-brianza.it (M.C.S.); paolo.scarpazza@asst-brianza.it (P.S.)
2. Research and Clinical Trials Office, Poliambulanza Foundation Hospital, 25124 Brescia, Italy; claclafer@gmail.com
3. School of Medicine and Surgery, University of Milano-Bicocca, 20126 Milan, Italy; maartanadalin@gmail.com (M.N.); maraborelli123@gmail.com (M.B.)
4. Cardiothoracic Vascular Department, Respiratory Unit, Fondazione IRCCS San Gerardo dei Tintori, 20900 Monza, Italy
* Correspondence: silvia.pagani91@gmail.com; Tel.: +39-0396657090

Highlights:

What are the main findings?

- Good clinical outcomes with H-CPAP in RICU, especially in mild and moderate CARDS.
- Significant improvement of prognosis in the three different waves: patients' diseases were found to be progressively slightly less severe. (No patient had yet received at least one dose of vaccination against COVID-19.)

What is the implication of the main finding?

- H-CPAP success strongly correlates with worst PaO_2/FiO_2 ratio and D-dimer level at admission.
- Relevance of proper management during hospitalization by pulmonologists in RICU.

Abstract: COVID-19 Acute Respiratory Distress Syndrome (CARDS) is the most serious complication of COVID-19. The SARS-CoV-2 outbreaks rapidly saturated intensive care unit (ICU), forcing the application of non-invasive respiratory support (NIRS) in respiratory intermediate care unit (RICU). The primary aim of this study is to compare the patients' clinical characteristics and outcomes (Helmet-Continuous Positive Airway Pressure (H-CPAP) success/failure and survival/death). The secondary aim is to evaluate and detect the main predictors of H-CPAP success and survival/death. A total of 515 patients were enrolled in our observational prospective study based on CARDS developed in RICU during the three Italian pandemic waves. All selected patients were treated with H-CPAP. The worst ratio of arterial partial pressure of oxygen (PaO_2) and fraction of inspired oxygen (FiO_2) PaO_2/FiO_2 during H-CPAP stratified the subjects into mild, moderate and severe CARDS. H-CPAP success has increased during the three waves (62%, 69% and 77%, respectively) and the mortality rate has decreased (28%, 21% and 13%). H-CPAP success/failure and survival/death were related to the PaO_2/FiO_2 (worst score) ratio in H-CPAP and to steroids' administration. D-dimer at admission, FiO_2 and positive end expiratory pressure (PEEP) were also associated with H-CPAP success. Our study suggests good outcomes with H-CPAP in CARDS in RICU. A widespread use of steroids could play a role.

Citation: Piluso, M.; Ferrari, C.; Pagani, S.; Usai, P.; Raschi, S.; Parachini, L.; Oggionni, E.; Melacini, C.; D'Arcangelo, F.; Cattaneo, R.; et al. COVID-19 Acute Respiratory Distress Syndrome: Treatment with Helmet CPAP in Respiratory Intermediate Care Unit by Pulmonologists in the Three Italian Pandemic Waves. *Adv. Respir. Med.* 2023, *91*, 383–396. https://doi.org/10.3390/arm91050030

Academic Editor: Monika Franczuk

Received: 8 August 2023
Revised: 14 September 2023
Accepted: 15 September 2023
Published: 20 September 2023

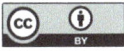

Copyright: © 2023 by the authors. Licensee MDPI, Basel, Switzerland. This article is an open access article distributed under the terms and conditions of the Creative Commons Attribution (CC BY) license (https:// creativecommons.org/licenses/by/ 4.0/).

Keywords: COVID-19 ARDS; Helmet CPAP; RICU; corticosteroids; pulmonologist

1. Introduction

Acute hypoxemic respiratory failure (AHRF) is the most common cause of intensive care unit (ICU) admission in adult patients, often leading to endotracheal intubation and invasive mechanical ventilation (IMV). Although COVID-19 causes very mild symptoms in most cases, approximately 20% of the patients develop acute hypoxemic respiratory failure (AHRF) with bilateral interstitial pneumonia [1]. Acute respiratory distress syndrome (ARDS) is the most serious complication of COVID-19 that occurs in 20–41% of patients with AHRF [2]. Despite the progress achieved in supportive care, the mortality rate of ARDS in ICU is still high (35–40%) and it increases with the severity of hypoxemia (27% in mild, 32% in moderate, 45% in severe ARDS, as defined by the Berlin Definition) [3].

In COVID-19 acute respiratory distress syndrome (CARDS) treated with IMV in ICU, prognosis seems to be even worse than that associated with non-COVID-19-related ARDS, and it varies widely [4–7]. In Lombardy, northern Italy, the COVID-19 pandemic has led to a substantial increase in the number of patients admitted to hospital with CARDS. In particular, in the first wave, this produced a heavy burden on the healthcare system, especially on ICUs, which easily ran out of resources since almost 10% of the hospitalized COVID-19 patients needed IMV. Until the outbreak of COVID-19 pandemic, evidence suggested the limiting of non-invasive respiratory support (NIRS) to carefully selected patients with mild-to-moderate ARDS and to apply it in experienced centers with close monitoring of blood gases and respiratory mechanics in order to avoid delayed intubation in case of failure [8,9].

The frequent lack of ICU beds has pushed authorities to create respiratory intermediate care units (RICU) in order to face the increasing number of patients with CARDS who need respiratory support and monitoring [10]. This can be carried out by pulmonologists with good previous experience in treating severe community-acquired pneumonia with helmet continuous positive airway pressure (H-CPAP) [11] where H-CPAP had previously demonstrated good efficacy [11,12]. Concerning NIRS, CPAP was significantly associated with a lower risk of mortality [13–15], and the H-CPAP has been proposed as an alternative to facemask [16]. In addition, for healthcare workers' protection from SARS-CoV-2 infection, the helmet has negligible air dispersion [17]. Applying a single level of pressure during the entire respiratory cycle, CPAP enables a reduction in the risk of excessive transpulmonary pressure and contributes to lung protection (reducing the risk of patient self-induced lung injury (P-SILI)). In addition, H-CPAP was available for all treated patients and it was easier to manage than pressure support ventilation (PSV) with Helmet. Other forms of NIRS, such as high flow nasal cannula (HFNC), were numerically unavailable.

The primary aim of this study is to compare the patients' clinical characteristics and outcomes (H-CPAP success defined as direct discharge from RICU without intubation and survival/death) during the three different waves. The secondary aim is to evaluate and detect the main predictors of H-CPAP success and survival/death in patients selected according to CARDS criteria.

2. Materials and Methods

2.1. Sample Selection

During the three waves of COVID-19 pandemic, 2159 patients with COVID-19 pneumonia, defined as the presence of interstitial pulmonary infiltrates and a positive SARS-CoV-2 nasal-pharyngeal swab, were admitted at Vimercate Hospital, Lombardy, Italy between March 2020 and May 2021. Of these, 871 patients were hospitalized in the Pulmonology Division. Among these, 515 were enrolled in our observational prospective study based on the development of CARDS defined by the Berlin Definition (ratio of arterial partial pressure of oxygen (PaO_2) and fraction of inspired oxygen (FiO_2) $PaO_2/FiO_2 \leq 300$ with positive end-expiratory pressure (PEEP) $\geq$ 5 cm H_2O and bilateral interstitial pneumonia) during hospital stay [3]. The exclusion criteria were as follows: age higher than 81 (patients older than 81 were rarely admitted to ICU, and there were none in our case study) and patients who did not develop CARDS during hospitalization. All selected patients (ages 18–80) were treated with H-CPAP in RICU. No patient had yet received one dose of vaccination against COVID-19.

2.2. Clinical Procedures and Monitoring

In our hospital, the ad hoc RICU dedicated to COVID-19 patients with AHRF (implemented from 6 to 50 beds) was characterized by continuous multi-parametric monitors, access to high-flow oxygen and air sources with systems to obtain adequate values of delivered FiO_2, onsite life support and intubation kit, a nurse patient ratio between 1:6 and 1:10, and full day shifts run by pulmonologists.

All patients included in the study were hemodynamically stable, with a normal Glasgow Coma Scale (GCS) score, (GCS = 15) and did not show multi-organ system failure, acidosis or hypercapnia [18]. They poorly responded to treatment with high-flow oxygen therapy with a Venturi mask or a non-rebreathing oxygen mask (oxygen saturation (SpO_2) $\leq$ 92%, respiratory rate > 24, Breaths Per Minute, thoraco-abdominal dyssynchrony).

H-CPAP was delivered with a pressure between 5 and 15 cm H_2O. and FiO_2 between 50 and 100%, with a target oxygen saturation of 92–98%; if reducing the FiO_2 up to 50%, the saturation remained above 98%, and the PEEP also progressively decreased. During H-CPAP therapy, the patients were moved, when feasible, into prone position, which was maintained for at least two hours. After two hours, the blood gas control PaO_2/FiO_2 ratio was re-calculated. The most critical patients were selected by pulmonologists and evaluated by intensivists to decide on ICU transfer.

The indication for IMV included the following criteria: (1) a reduced level of consciousness, (2) persistent hypoxemia with altered mechanical breathing, (3) H-CPAP intolerance, (4) hemodynamic instability, and (5) multi-organ failure.

The Do-Not-Intubate (DNI) order was the decision to withhold intubation and to use H-CPAP as the "ceiling" treatment considering the patient's characteristics and the reduced availability of ICU beds. DNI criteria was considered by intensivists only in cases in which intubation was necessary, not at the admission stage.

Unless contraindicated, prophylactic low-molecular-weight heparin was administered to all patients, except those already on home anticoagulation therapy. In the first wave, Computed Tomography (CT) Angiography (Revolution 128S, General Electric Company, Boston, MA, USA) was performed as soon as the clinical condition worsened in association with a significant increase in D-dimer (immunoturbidimetric method - Instrument: ACLTOP550, Instrumentation Laboratory, Bedford, MA, USA; Reagent: Instrumentation Laboratory, Bedford, MA, USA). With D-dimer >1000 and CT Angiography negative for pulmonary embolism, 100 units/kg of low-molecular-weight heparin was administered daily [19]. In the second and third waves, the D-dimer dosage was performed daily for the first week of hospital stay and, in case of a significant increase even without clinical worsening, CT Angiography was performed. Therapeutic low-molecular-weight heparin (100 unit/kg twice a day) was administered in case of confirmed pulmonary embolism.

In the first wave, most patients were treated with systemic corticosteroids (methylprednisolone at a dose of 1 mg/kg per day) for 10 days gradually reduced in case of positive outcome. In the second and third waves, all patients received corticosteroids.

2.3. Statistical Analysis

Descriptive statistics for the socio-demographic, clinical and outcome variables are given in terms of mean, median and standard deviation for numerical variables and percentage distribution for categorical variables. Normality assumption was assessed using the Shapiro–Wilk test and the graphical inspection via QQ-plots. ANOVA or corresponding nonparametric Kruskal–Wallis tests were applied for comparing numerical variables across three categories of pandemic waves. Chi-squared tests were applied for analyzing the association between categorical variables and waves.

Associations among socio-demographic and clinical variables with the three outcomes (one at a time) were evaluated using univariate logistic regression models. Subsequently, multiple logistic models, including, as covariates and factors, all the significant variables detected through univariate models, were performed. The choice of the best model, in terms of significant predictors which better explain the outcome, was carried out by following the stepwise procedure [20].

Finally, the survival analysis through the Kaplan–Meier (KM) curve was used to analyze the survival time in hospital. Differences in KM-curves between different groups were evaluated using the Log-rank test.

The analyses were carried out using SPSS Statistics for Windows, (Version 26.0) and the software R (R Core Team (2020), https://www.R-project.org/ (accessed on 28 February 2022)). The stepwise procedure was performed using the stepAIC function of the R library MASS. Statistical significance was set at level 0.05.

3. Results

3.1. Socio-Demographic, Clinical and Outcomes Assessments across the Three Waves

Sample characteristics and features' descriptions of this prospective observational study are reported in Tables 1–3. The sample did not show differences among waves for the socio-demographic features except for the categorical variable 'smoke'. With regard to the comorbidities, differences among waves were found for patients with diabetes, tumor and chronic renal failure: a higher percentage of patients with such comorbidities were detected in the second and the third waves.

Table 1. Socio-demographic features, comorbidity and prognostic score of the whole sample by waves.

Variables			Wave1 Mean [Median] (SD) N = 150	Wave2 Mean [Median] (SD) N = 180	Wave3 Mean [Median] (SD) N = 185	Tot	p-Value	Post Hoc
			Socio-demographic features					
Age			61.9 [63.3] (10.8)	63.5 [65] (10.9)	62.2 [64] (11.2)	515	0.316	
Sex		Females	N = 27; 24.3%	N = 38; 34.2%	N = 46; 41.4%	111	0.310	
		Males	N = 123; 30.4%	N = 142; 35.1%	N = 139; 34.7%	404		
Body Mass Index (BMI)			29.4 [29.4] (4.7)	30.2 [29] (6.6)	29.7 [29] (4.7)	361	0.847	
Smoke		No	N = 104; 39.2%	N = 69; 26%	N = 92; 34.7%	265	<0.001	1 vs. 2,3
		Yes	N = 1; 4.2%	N = 8; 33.5%	N = 15; 62.5%	24		
		Ex-smokers	N = 45; 26%	N= 65; 37.6%	N = 63; 36.4%	173		
			Comorbidity and prognostic score					
Hypertension		No	N = 78; 32.9%	N = 74; 31.2%	N = 85; 35.9%	237	0.142	
		Yes	N = 72; 25.9%	N = 106; 38.1%	N = 100; 36%	278		
Ischemic cardiac disease		No	N = 132; 29.7%	N = 150; 33.8%	N = 163; 36.5%	445	0.349	
		Yes	N = 15; 25%	N = 26; 43.3%	N = 19; 31.7%	60		
Cardiovascular disease		No	N = 129; 30.3%	N = 144; 33.8%	N = 153; 35.9%	426	0.357	
		Yes	N = 21; 23.6%	N = 36; 40.4%	N = 32; 36%	89		
Hypercholesterolemia		No	N = 122; 28.3%	N = 152; 35.3%	N = 157; 36.4%	431	0.646	
		Yes	N = 28; 33.3%	N = 28; 33.3%	N = 28; 33.3%	84		
Diabetes		No	N = 139; 32.7%	N = 136; 32%	N = 150; 35.3%	425	<0.001	1 vs. 2,3
		Yes	N = 11; 12.2%	N = 44; 48.9%	N = 35; 38.9%	90		

Table 1. Cont.

Variables			Wave1 Mean [Median] (SD) N = 150	Wave2 Mean [Median] (SD) N = 180	Wave3 Mean [Median] (SD) N = 185	Tot	p-Value	Post Hoc
Neoplasia								
		No	N = 144; 31%	N = 149; 32.1%	N = 171; 36.9%	464	<0.001	2 vs. 1,3
		Yes	N = 6; 11.8%	N = 31; 60.8%	N = 14; 27.5%	51		
Chronic obstructive pulmonary disease (COPD)/asthma								
		No	N = 136; 29.4%	N = 158; 34.2%	N = 168; 36.4%	462	0.571	
		Yes	N = 14; 26.4%	N = 22; 41.5%	N = 17; 32.1%	53		
Chronic renal failure								
		No	N = 149; 30.5%	N = 164; 33.6%	N = 175; 35.9%	488	0.004	1 vs. 2,3
		Yes	N = 1; 3.7%	N = 16; 59.3%	N = 10; 37%	27		
Apache II score			10.6 [10] (3.6)	10.3 [11] (5.0)	9.7 [10] (4.3)	513	0.110	

Percentages are reported by row, i.e., the percentages are expressed in terms of total across waves; percentage by column can be obtained considering the patient numbers by wave reported in the table head. N: number of patients.

Table 2. Pharmacological treatment, blood tests, CARDS classes at admission and ICU transfer of the whole sample by waves.

Variables			Wave1 Mean [Median] (SD) N = 150	Wave2 Mean [Median] (SD) N = 180	Wave3 Mean [Median] (SD) N = 185	Tot	p-Value	Post Hoc
			Pharmacological treatment during hospitalization					
Antivirals								
		No	N = 46; 11.3%	N = 176; 43.3%	N = 184; 45.3%	406	<0.001	1 vs. 2,3
		Yes	N = 104; 95.4%	N = 4; 3.7%	N = 1; 0.9%	109		
Remdesivir								
		No	N = 146; 29%	N = 177; 35.1%	N = 181; 35.9%	504	0.822	
		Yes	N = 4; 36.4%	N = 3; 27.3%	N = 4; 36.4%	11		
Azithromycin								
		No	N = 113; 43.6%	N = 70; 27.0%	N = 76; 29.3%	259	<0.001	1 vs. 2,3
		Yes	N = 37; 14.5%	N = 110; 43%	N = 109; 42.6%	256		
Tocilizumab								
		No	N = 139; 27.6%	N= 180; 35.7%	N = 185; 36.7%	504	<0.001	1 vs. 2,3
		Yes	N = 11; 100%	N = 0; 0%	N = 0; 0%	11		
Plaquenil								
		No	N = 5; 1.4%	N= 180; 48.6%	N = 185; 50%	370	<0.001	1 vs. 2,3
		Yes	N = 145; 100%	N = 0; 0%	N = 0; 0%	145		
Steroids								
		No	N = 32; 86.5%	N = 4; 10.8%	N = 1; 2.7%	37	<0.001	1 vs. 2,3
		Yes	N = 118; 24.7%	N = 176; 36.8%	N = 184; 38.5%	478		
			COVID-19 Acute Respiratory Distress Syndrome (CARDS) classes at admission and Intensive Care Unit (ICU) transfer					
CARDS classes (admission)								
	Pre-CARDS		N = 25; 33.3%	N = 29; 38.7%	N = 21; 28%	75		
	Mild		N = 50; 28.1%	N = 61; 34.3%	N = 67; 37.6%	178	0.486	
	Moderate		N = 60; 27.1%	N = 74; 33.5%	N= 87; 39.4%	221		
	Severe		N = 15; 36.6%	N = 16; 39%	N = 10; 24.4%	41		
Intensive Care Unit								
		No	N = 118; 28.6%	N = 143; 34.7%	N = 151; 36.7%	412	0.777	
		Yes	N = 32; 31.1%	N = 37; 35.9%	N = 34; 33%	103		
			Blood tests					
D-dimer test (admission) (ng/mL)			3629.8 [630] (9423)	586.6 [296] (1521)	443.2 [288] (919)	502	<0.001	1 vs. 2,3
D-dimer test (worst) (ng/mL)			6939.2 [2067] (12382)	3571.9 [1049] (9468)	2447 [719] (5054)	503	<0.001	1 vs. 2,3

Table 2. Cont.

Variables	Wave1 Mean [Median] (SD) N = 150	Wave2 Mean [Median] (SD) N = 180	Wave3 Mean [Median] (SD) N = 185	Tot	p-Value	Post Hoc
Ferritin (admission) (ng/mL)	1993.3 [1283] (1943)	1894.4 [1027] (2542)	3551.1 [1712] (4384)	186	0.183	
Ferritin (worst)(ng/mL)	2750.4 [1631] (3115)	2368.9 [1274] (2864)	2008.9 [1540] (1498	205	0.290	
Interleukin-6 (admission) (pg/mL)	64.8 [32] (83.4)	60.8 [33] (78.0)	58.8 [34] (73.4)	377	0.925	
Interleukin-6 (worst)(pg/mL)	338.2 [89] (950.5)	171.8 [103.5] (235.7)	113.1 [65.5] (164.5)	398	0.029	2 vs. 3

Percentages are reported by row, i.e., the percentages are expressed in terms of total across waves; percentages by column can be obtained considering the patient numbers by wave reported in the table head. N: number of patients.

Table 3. CPAP treatments and outcomes of the whole sample by waves.

Variables		Wave1 Mean [Median] (SD) N = 150	Wave2 Mean [Median] (SD) N = 180	Wave3 Mean [Median] (SD) N = 185	Tot	p-Value	Post Hoc
		Helmet Continuous Positive Air Pressure (H-CPAP) treatments					
Positive End Expiratory Pressure (PEEP)		12.8 [12] (2.0)	9.7 [9] (7.0)	8.1 [8] (1.2)	512	<0.001	1 vs. 2 vs. 3
FiO_2		81.3 [80] (12.4)	70.2 [70] (11.6)	71.8 [70] (9.4)	514	<0.001	1 vs. 2,3
PaO_2/FiO_2 (in oxygen)		132.3 [115.5] (64.4)	159.6 [137] (53.8)	147.5 [130] (64.0)	514	0.001	1 vs. 2,3
First PaO_2/FiO_2 (in H-CPAP)		217.8 [203.5] (105.8)	212.1 [199.5] (91.8)	202.8 [195] (77.4)	515	0.747	
Worst PaO_2/FiO_2 (in H-CPAP)		100.5 [80] (56.5)	116.7 [100.5] (53.8)	147.0 [135] (64.5)	477	<0.001	1 vs. 2 vs. 3
PaO_2/FiO_2 post-pronation (in H-CPAP)		242.4 [227.5] (119.6)	273.3 [227.5] (108.6)	249.7 [240] (97.1)	396	0.051	
Proned	No	N = 54; 50.9%	N = 24; 22.6%	N = 28; 26.4%	106	<0.001	1 vs. 2,3
	Yes	N = 96; 23.5%	N = 156; 38.1%	N= 157; 38.4%	409		
Do Not Intubate (DNI)	No	N = 128; 27.2%	N = 164; 34.9%	N = 178; 37.9%	470	0.002	3 vs. 1,2
	Yes	N = 22; 48.9%	N = 16; 35.6%	N = 7; 15.6%	45		
			Outcomes				
Death	No	N = 108; 26.2%	N = 143; 34.7%	N = 161; 39.1%	412	0.003	1 vs. 3
	Yes	N = 42; 40.8%	N = 37; 35.9%	N = 24; 23.3%	103		
H-CPAP success	No	N = 57; 36.8%	N = 55; 35.5%	N = 43; 27.7%	155	0.014	1 vs. 3
	Yes	N = 93; 25.8%	N = 125; 34.7%	N = 142; 39.4%	360		

Percentages are reported by row, i.e., the percentages are expressed in terms of total across waves; percentages by column can be obtained considering the patient numbers by wave reported in the table head. PEEP: Positive end expiratory pressure; PaO_2/FiO_2: ratio of arterial partial pressure of oxygen (PaO_2) and fraction of inspired oxygen (FiO_2). N: number of patients.

Regarding the pharmacological treatments, there was a reduction in the administration of antivirals, tocilizumab and hydroxychloroquine over the course of the waves, while there was an increase in the administration of azithromycin and steroids. Remdesivir was rarely used in all waves (only in 11 patients, 2%).

Additionally, the choice to prone patients increased significantly over the course of the waves.

D-dimer test was higher in wave 1 with respect to wave 2 and 3, while interleukin-6 (IL-6 worst) was lower in wave 3 with respect to the previous waves. Interleukin-6 was dosed using the sandwich electrochemiluminescence immunoassay method (ECLIA) (by ACLTOP550, Instrumentation Laboratory, Bedford, MA, USA; Reagent: Instrumentation Laboratory, Bedford, MA, USA). Concerning H-CPAP treatment, PEEP and FiO_2 were statistically higher in wave 1 with respect to the subsequent waves, whereas PaO_2/FiO_2 in oxygen and PaO_2/FiO_2 (worst) were significantly lower in the first wave with respect to waves 2 and 3.

General improvements over the course of the waves have also been noticed for the main outcomes: mortality, H-CPAP success and DNI. In particular, the mortality rate was, respectively, 28% in the first wave, 20.5% in the second and 12.9% in the third wave. H-CPAP success increased from 62% (93/150) to 69.4% (125/180) and to 78.4% (142/185), and DNI decreased from 22 (14.6%) to 16 (8.8%) and to 7 (3.8%) (Tables 1–3).

Most patients at admission presented a CARDS pattern. CARDS was mild in 178 (34.6%), moderate in 221 (42.9%) and severe in 41 (7.9%). There are a number of patients (n = 75, 14.6%) who did not fulfill CARDS criteria at admission (pre-CARDS) but all of them developed CARDS during hospital stay (Figure 1). The worst PaO_2/FiO_2 ratio during H-CPAP stratified the subjects into mild (82–15.9%), moderate (202–39.2%) and severe (231–44.9%) CARDS (Figure 1).

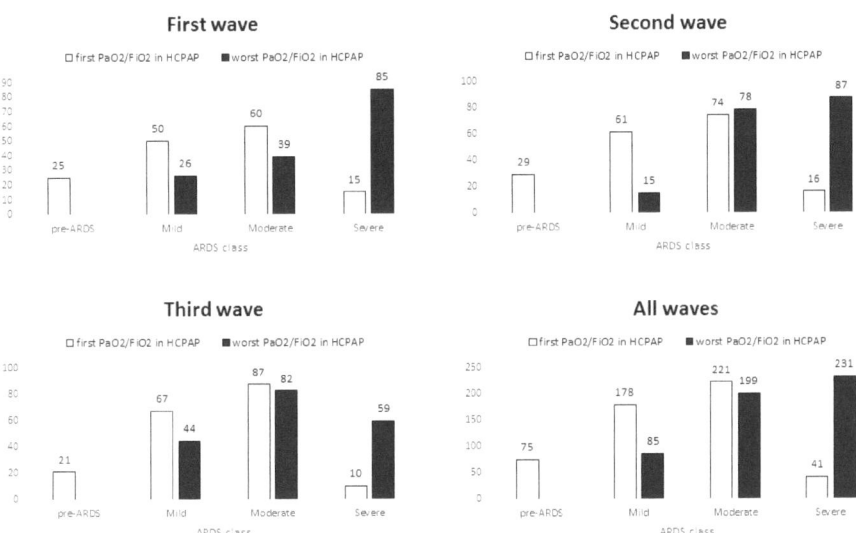

Figure 1. CARDS classes at different waves: number of patients by CARDS class for the parameter PaO_2/FiO_2 taken at two time points (first and worst in H-CPAP).

3.2. Complications

Among the 515 patients, 360 (70%) were successfully discharged without IMV; 104 were transferred to ICU to receive IMV and, of these, 52 finally survived. A total of 45 received the DNI order. Of the 53 patients who died in the RICU ward, 43 had DNI orders, 1 acute myocardial infarction, 2 massive pulmonary embolism, 3 cardio-circulatory arrests, 1 stroke in paroxysmal atrial fibrillation, 1 respiratory arrest and 2 sepsis after ICU discharge.

The main complications (Table S1) that developed during hospital stays included the following: 54 pulmonary embolism, 8 thrombosis, 10 bleedings, 15 pneumomediastinum, 5 pneumothoraxes, 15 supraventricular tackyarrhythmias, and 12 severe bacterial superinfections. The rate of patients with pulmonary embolism (on the total number of patients) was statistically different across the waves (p-values < 0.001), as well as the rate of deaths with pulmonary embolisms on the total of deaths (p-values = 0.033).

3.3. Predictors of the H-CPAP Success and Survival/Death Outcomes

For each of the two outcomes, the most prominent predictors are reported in Tables S2 and S3 in the Supplementary Materials.

Considering all the statistically significant variables, multiple logistic models (with stepwise procedure for the variable selections) were applied in order to obtain the best predictors of each outcome. The results are reported in Table 4. The most important factors for the H-CPAP success were as follows: the worst PaO_2/FiO_2 ratio during H-CPAP and FiO_2 (both with p-values < 0.001), as high levels of PaO_2/FiO_2 and FiO_2 were associated with better (Odds Ratio (OR) = 1.038) and worse (OR = 0.944) H-CPAP success, respectively. Additionally, the administration of steroids had a relevant impact (p-values = 0.001) on H-CPAP success: the administration of steroids increases the probability of H-CPAP success by almost 14 times with respect to non-administration (OR = 13.92). In addition, D-dimer at admission and the level of PEEP were also found to be significantly associated with H-CPAP success: an increase of 1000 unit in D-dimer level reduced H-CPAP success by 9.5% (OR = 0.905), while an increase of 1 unit in PEEP decreased the probability of H-CPAP success by about 12% (OR = 0.88). Regarding survival/death, the worst PaO_2/FiO_2 ratio during H-CPAP and the administration of steroids were also the best predictors for this second outcome: a high level of PaO_2/FiO_2 was associated with a lower probability of death (OR = 0.96), while patients treated with steroids showed a lower probability (of about 77%: OR = 0.23) of death with respect to patients who did not undergo steroid therapy.

Table 4. Multiple logistic regression models outputs for each of the two outcomes.

Outcome (Dependent) Variable	Independent Variables	Coeff (b)	exp(b) = Odds Ratio (OR) #	Lower Lim OR 95% CI	Upper Lim OR 95% CI	p-Value	Nagelkerke R2
H-CPAP success (yes vs. no)	Worst PaO_2/FiO_2 (in H-CPAP)	0.037	1.038	1.028	1.048	<0.001	0.54
	FiO_2 in H-CPAP	−0.057	0.944	0.915	0.974	<0.001	
	Steroids (yes vs. no)	2.63	13.915	2.611	74.207	0.001	
	D-dimer at admission (×1000)	−0.1	0.905	0.980	1	0.031	
	average PEEP	−0.13	0.878	−0.260	−0.001	0.048	
Death (yes vs. no)	Worst PaO_2/FiO_2 (in H-CPAP)	−0.038	0.963	0.951	0.974	<0.001	0.41
	Steroids (yes vs. no)	−1.45	0.233	0.075	0.730	0.012	
	Lactate dehydrogenase (LDH) at admission	0.001	1.001	0.999	1.003	0.088	

OR larger than 1 indicate large probability to belong to H-CPAP success or dead for a unit increase (or to pass from first specified category to second specified reference category) in the independent variable. E.g., an increase of 1 in FiO_2 in H-CPAP produced a reduced probability (of 1 − 0.944 = 5.6%) of H-CPAP success; similarly, the administration of steroids increases the probability of H-CPAP success by almost 14 times with respect to non-administration. PEEP: Positive end expiratory pressure; PaO_2/FiO_2: ratio of arterial partial pressure of oxygen (PaO_2) and fraction of inspired oxygen (FiO_2).

3.4. Survival Analysis

An exhaustive survival analysis was carried out by considering the waves and the predictors of the two outcomes highlighted in the previous analyses as predictors (groups) of the KM curves. In Figure 2, KM curves for the three waves are depicted. Interestingly, the curves for waves 1 and 2 are not statistically different (Log rank test p-values = 0.196), while the curve for wave 3 is different from the previous ones (p-values = 0.004). KM curves were also estimated for different levels of worst PaO_2/FiO_2 ratio during H-CPAP (less than first quartile = 77; ≥77), and for steroid therapy (yes vs. no). All these factors were statistically associated with survival and all the KM curves were statistically different among the predictor groups (p-values < 0.025 for worst PaO_2/FiO_2; p-values < 0.001 for steroid therapy).

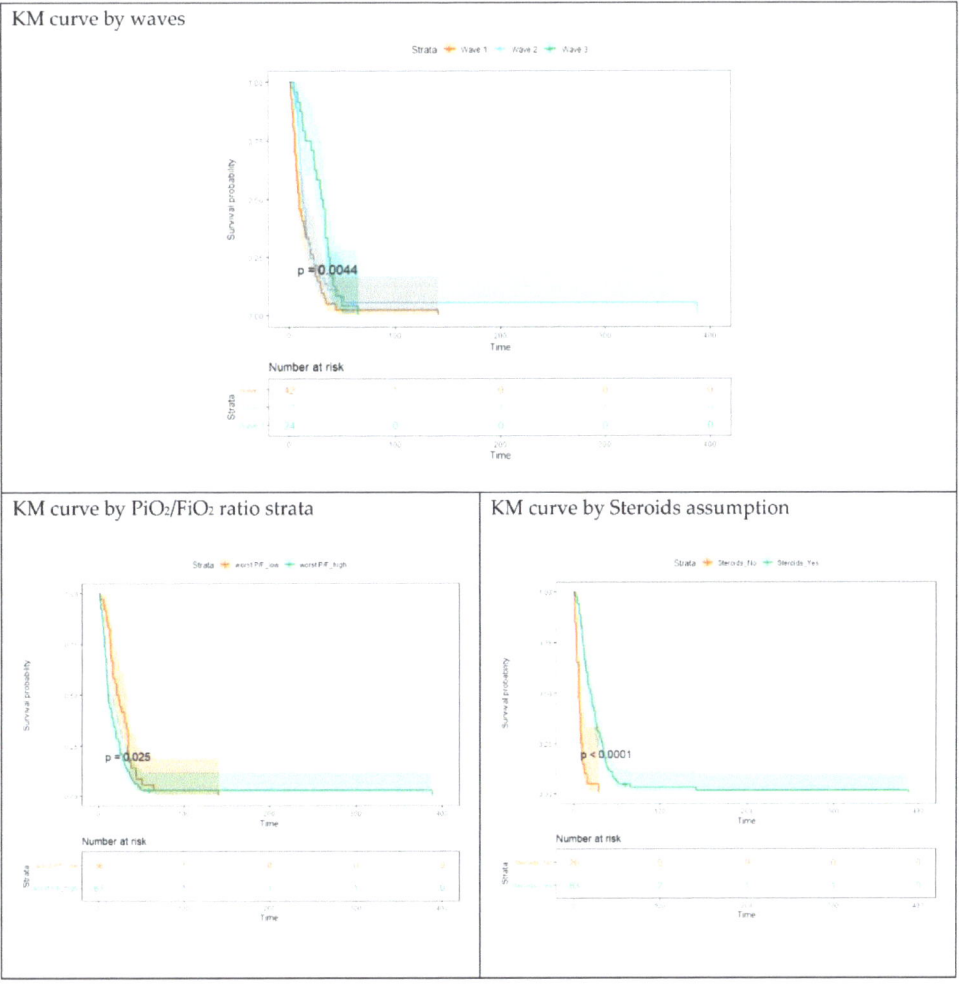

Figure 2. Survival analysis output: Kaplan–Meier survival curves.

4. Discussion

This prospective observational study aims to better understand the effectiveness of H-CPAP in patients who developed CARDS during hospitalization in RICU.

The patient samples did not show differences among waves for socio-demographic features (Table 1). In the first wave, less compromised patients (fewer patients with diabetes and chronic renal failure and fewer smokers) presented a worse trend. During the second and third pandemic waves, the hospital mortality for patients admitted with CARDS was significantly reduced compared to that registered in the first pandemic period. H-CPAP success increased and DNI numbers decreased.

In the first wave, most patients were treated with systemic corticosteroids. In contrast, in the second and third waves, practically all patients received corticosteroids following new clinical trials [21] and our previous experience with steroid use in severe community-acquired pneumonia [11,22]. In the first wave, PaO_2/FiO_2 in oxygen was significantly lower and D-dimer significantly higher. These were demonstrated to be independent risk factors for adverse outcomes [23,24] and the result is also confirmed in our study. In addition, D-dimer at admission, worst D-dimer and worst IL-6 were significantly higher in the first wave, suggesting more severe inflammation. Worst PaO_2/FiO_2 in H-CPAP was significantly lower in the first wave. No differences were found between the first PaO_2/FiO_2 in H-CPAP among the three waves and the patients with preARDS and mild, moderate, and severe ARDS at admission were equally distributed during the different waves; however, this parameter was obtained with PEEP progressively decreasing.

Helmet success and survival/death outcomes progressively improved over the course of the three waves reflecting a slight progressive reduction in patient severity associated with improved clinical management (practically 100% steroid in the second and third waves; daily D-dimer monitoring for pulmonary embolism diagnosis; progressive increase in prone position).

DNI order was considered only in cases that needed intubation and decreased during the three waves due to the higher availability of ICU beds (equal percentage of patients transferred to ICU in the different waves despite higher patient severity in the first period).

CARDS has a biphasic trend confirmed in all three waves (Figure 1). The two stages of the disease correspond to the initially worsening trend of most of our patients, from admission to subsequent days of hospitalization, and they are likely to switch from L (low elastance, low lung weight, low recruitability—ground glass opacities at CT, preserved lung compliance) to H (high elastance, high lung weight, high recruitability—extensive densification at CT) CARDS [25–27]. Probably, in the first stage of the disease, improvement in oxygenation through the application of PEEP or pronation is mainly not due to the recruitment, but to the redistribution of perfusion in the lungs [25,28]. In the second stage of the disease, the application of PEEP recruits non-aerated alveoli in dependent pulmonary regions stabilizes the airways and reduces the inhomogeneity of lung volume distribution [18]. PEEP can be applied in spontaneously breathing patients in the form of CPAP [29].

The most important complications are shown in Table S1. The increased frequency of pulmonary embolism diagnosis in the second and third waves is explained by daily D-dimer monitoring and a higher use of CT Angiography.

Low PaO_2/FiO_2 ratio during H-CPAP, high FiO_2 and average helmet PEEP were important factors of H-CPAP failure as a result of more severe AHRF; as already known, the mortality rate of ARDS increases with the severity of hypoxemia [3].

An increase of 1000 unit in D-dimer level (more severe "cytokine storm") reduces the H-CPAP success by 9.5% [24].

A widespread use of steroids in our center could play a role in good clinical outcomes. Our study shows that the administration of steroids increases the chance to H-CPAP success of almost 14 times, confirming what has been demonstrated in the RECOVERY TRIAL [21], a large multicenter randomized controlled trial where patients receiving dexamethasone had a reduced death rate especially on mechanical ventilation.

Additionally, for the second outcome, survival/death, the worst PaO_2/FiO_2 ratio during H-CPAP and the administration of steroids were the best predictors. In our study there is a lower probability of death (77%) with respect to patients who did not undergo steroid therapy (Table 4).

Prone position in non-intubated spontaneously breathing patients is widely applied alongside NIRS. Its effectiveness in reducing intubation rates and mortality and its tolerability, timing and optimal duration are still not completely clear [30]. Prone position has gradually been increased over the course of the three waves based on early suggestions in the literature [30,31]. In our patients, prone position determined a meaningful increase in PaO_2/FiO_2 value, although this improvement does not represent a good prognostic factor in itself. This response could give patients a chance to overcome the critical phase of CARDS and avoid intubation. We want to emphasize the fact that, despite the extremely low values of worst PaO_2/FiO_2 ratio recorded, 82 (15.9%) mild, 202 (39.2%) moderate, 231 (44.9%) severe CARDS, 70% of our patients were finally discharged without a need for IMV. In mild patients, H-CPAP had a success of 98.8%; in moderate patients, of 93%; and in severe patients, of 41%. In addition, 89 out of 231 patients in the "severe CARDS" group were transferred to ICU and, of these, 44 finally survived, with a final mortality rate of 39.8%, in agreement with the mortality rate described for patients with severe non-COVID-19 ARDS in the ICU (45%). We underline that, in our group of patients, mortality rates in mild and moderate ARDS are inferior to those reported in literature [3,8], considering the different features of patients admitted to ICUs (i.e., multiorgan failure).

Many management models for noninvasive treatment of CARDS in RICU have been proposed in the literature [31–33]. To our knowledge, to date, this is the only study entirely carried out in RICU on patients who all presented with CARDS and were all treated with H-CPAP in the three COVID-19 waves. We may therefore assume that the proper management in RICU, the use of H-CPAP as NIRS, prone position, and large steroid use affect the prognosis of patients with CARDS [34].

A constant clinical and parametric monitoring during hospitalization by the pulmonologist in RICU is critical in the prompt recognition and treatment of every possible worsening in clinical conditions, an event than can arise even later in the course of the disease. In fact, the majority of patients moved to a worse CARDS class during hospitalization (Figure 1). Furthermore, our data seem to exclude a possible delay in intubation timing due to H-CPAP treatment and this is remarked by a mortality rate of almost 50% in patients finally admitted to the ICU, substantially comparable with 55% of all Lombardy ICUs [7] and other countries' experiences [35]. In addition, we must remember that even if delayed intubation is associated with increased mortality in patients with AHRF [35,36], it is also true that premature intubation when NIRS is adequate exposes patients to potentially unnecessary risks associated with IMV [16,37].

Our study has several limitations that can limit the generalizability of our results, including being monocentric, the lack of a control group and the peculiar setting of the study, characterized by an emergency pandemic situation with continuous changes in scientific evidence. Nevertheless, further multicentric trials are needed in order to confirm these data. In addition, the Berlin Definition of ARDS required that patients must be in IMV in moderate and severe ARDS, with the exception of mild ARDS, in which patients can receive CPAP ≥ 5 cm H_2O. In our study, ARDS was classified as moderate or severe during H-CPAP; however, the new recently published ARDS definition [38] allows for classification as moderate and severe in H-CPAP too.

5. Conclusions

Our study suggests good clinical outcomes with H-CPAP in RICU, especially in mild and moderate CARDS.

We observed a significant improvement in prognosis in the three different waves, as the patients' conditions are found to be progressively slightly less severe.

CARDS has a biphasic trend confirmed in all three waves, with a trend of worsening the patients' conditions from admission to subsequent days of hospitalization.

The CARDS severity (worst PaO_2/FiO_2 in H-CPAP, FiO_2 in H-CPAP, average PEEP and D-dimer at admission) strongly correlates with the first outcome (H-CPAP success). Worst PaO_2/FiO_2 in H-CPAP also strongly correlates with the second outcome (survival/death).

There was a significant prognosis improvement in subjects who received corticosteroids.

Pulmonologists' proper management during hospitalization in RICU may affect these patients' trend.

Supplementary Materials: The following supporting information can be downloaded at: https://www.mdpi.com/article/10.3390/arm91050030/s1, Table S1: Complication across the three waves; Table S2: Univariate logistic regression models with H-CPAP success (yes vs. no) as dependent variable (only significant variables/predictors are reported); Table S3: Univariate Logistic regression models with Death (yes vs. no) as dependent variable (only significant variables/predictors are reported).

Author Contributions: Conceptualization, M.P., C.F., S.P. and P.S.; Data Curation, M.P., P.U., S.R., L.P., E.O., C.M., F.D., R.C., C.B., M.B. (Monica Bernareggi), S.B., M.N., M.B. (Mara Borelli), R.B., M.C.S. and P.S.; Methodology, M.P., C.F., S.P. and P.S.; Writing—Original Draft, M.P., C.F., S.P. and P.S.; Writing—Review and Editing, M.P., C.F., S.P. and P.S. All authors have read and agreed to the published version of the manuscript.

Funding: This research received funding for publication from our hospital: Vimercate Hospital, C.F. and VAT number 09314320962.

Institutional Review Board Statement: Human participants were involved in this research; the study was conducted in accordance with the Declaration of Helsinki. Our study was approved by the local institution, Vimercate Hospital, ASST-Brianza, according to the legal requirements concerning observational studies (Resolution 0000573). Patient consent was waived.

Informed Consent Statement: Due to the nature of the present observational study and data anonymization, the patients' consent to participate was not required, as declared by the ASST Brianza Ethic Committee.

Data Availability Statement: The datasets analyzed during the current study are available from the corresponding author on reasonable request.

Acknowledgments: All nurses and healthcare support workers in RICU for their assistance to the patients.

Conflicts of Interest: The authors declare that the research was conducted in the absence of any commercial or financial relationships that could be construed as potential conflict of interest.

References

1. Ren, L.-L.; Wang, Y.-M.; Wu, Z.-Q.; Xiang, Z.-C.; Guo, L.; Xu, T.; Jiang, Y.-Z.; Xiong, Y.; Li, Y.-J.; Li, X.-W.; et al. Identification of a novel coronavirus causing severe pneumonia in human: A descriptive study. *Chin. Med. J.* **2020**, *133*, 1015–1024. [CrossRef] [PubMed]
2. Wang, D.; Hu, B.; Hu, C.; Zhu, F.; Liu, X.; Zhang, J.; Wang, B.; Xiang, H.; Cheng, Z.; Xiong, Y.; et al. Clinical Characteristics of 138 Hospitalized Patients With 2019 NovelCoronavirus–Infected Pneumonia in Wuhan, China. *JAMA* **2020**, *323*, 1061. [CrossRef] [PubMed]
3. Ranieri, V.M.; Rubenfeld, G.D.; Thompson, B.T.; Ferguson, N.D.; Caldwell, E.; Fan, E.; Camporota, L.; Slutsky, A.S. Acute respiratory distress syndrome: The Berlin Definition. *JAMA* **2012**, *307*, 2526–2533. [PubMed]
4. Yang, X.; Yu, Y.; Xu, J.; Shu, H.; Xia, J.; Liu, H.; Wu, Y.; Zhang, L.; Yu, Z.; Fang, M.; et al. Clinical course and outcomes of critically ill patients with SARS-CoV-2 pneumonia in Wuhan, China: A single-centered, retrospective, observational study. *Lancet Respir. Med.* **2020**, *8*, 475–481. [CrossRef] [PubMed]
5. Bhatraju, P.K.; Ghassemieh, B.J.; Nichols, M.; Kim, R.; Jerome, K.R.; Nalla, A.K.; Greninger, A.L.; Pipavath, S.; Wurfel, M.M.; Evans, L.; et al. Covid-19 in Critically Ill Patients in the Seattle Region—Case Series. *N. Engl. J. Med.* **2020**, *382*, 2012–2022. [CrossRef]
6. Richardson, S.; Hirsch, J.S.; Narasimhan, M.; Crawford, J.M.; McGinn, T.; Davidson, K.W.; The Northwell COVID-19 Research Consortium. Presenting Characteristics, Comorbidities, and Outcomes among 5700 Patients Hospitalized with COVID-19 in the New York City Area. *JAMA* **2020**, *323*, 2052–2059. [CrossRef]
7. Grasselli, G.; Greco, M.; Zanella, A.; Albano, G.; Antonelli, M.; Bellani, G.; Bonanomi, E.; Cabrini, L.; Carlesso, E.; Castelli, G.; et al. Risk Factors Associated with Mortality Among Patients with COVID-19 in Intensive Care Units in Lombardy, Italy. *JAMA Intern. Med.* **2020**, *180*, 1345–1355. [CrossRef]
8. Grassi, A.; Foti, G.; Laffey, J.G.; Bellani, G. Noninvasive mechanical ventilation in early acute respiratory distress syndrome. *Pol. Arch. Intern. Med.* **2017**, *127*, 614–620. [CrossRef]
9. Demoule, A.; Hill, N.; Navalesi, P. Can we prevent intubation in patients with ARDS? *Intensive Care Med.* **2016**, *42*, 768–771. [CrossRef]
10. Grasselli, G.; Zangrillo, A.; Zanella, A.; Antonelli, M.; Cabrini, L.; Castelli, A.; Cereda, D.; Coluccello, A.; Foti, G.; Fumagalli, R.; et al. Baseline Characteristics and Outcomes of 1591 Patients Infected with SARS-CoV-2 Admitted to ICUs of the Lombardy Region, Italy. *JAMA* **2020**, *323*, 1574–1581. [CrossRef]
11. Brambilla, A.M.; Aliberti, S.; Prina, E.; Nicoli, F.; Del Forno, M.; Nava, S.; Ferrari, G.; Corradi, F.; Pesoli, P.; Bignamini, A.; et al. Helmet CPAP vs. oxygen therapy in severe hypoxemic respiratory failure due to pneumonia. *Intensiv. Care Med.* **2014**, *40*, 942–949. [CrossRef] [PubMed]
12. Cosentini, R.; Brambilla, A.M.; Aliberti, S.; Bignamini, A.; Nava, S.; Maffei, A.; Martinotti, R.; Tarsia, P.; Monzani, V.; Pelosi, P. Faculty Opinions recommendation of Helmet continuous positive airway pressure vs oxygen therapy to improve oxygenation in community-acquired pneumonia: A randomized, controlled trial. *Chest* **2010**, *138*, 114–120. [CrossRef] [PubMed]

13. Chiumello, D.; Brochard, L.; Marini, J.J.; Slutsky, A.S.; Mancebo, J.; Ranieri, V.M.; Thompson, B.T.; Papazian, L.; Schultz, M.J.; Amato, M.; et al. Respiratory support in patients with acute respiratory distress syndrome: An expert opinion. *Crit. Care* **2017**, *21*, 240. [CrossRef] [PubMed]
14. Sakuraya, M.; Okano, H.; Masuyama, T.; Kimata, S.; Hokari, S. Efficacy of non-invasive and invasive respiratory management strategies in adult patients with acute hypoxaemic respiratory failure: A systematic review and network meta-analysis. *Crit. Care* **2021**, *25*, 414. [CrossRef]
15. Ferreyro, B.L.; Angriman, F.; Munshi, L.; Del Sorbo, L.; Ferguson, N.D.; Rochwerg, B.; Ryu, M.J.; Saskin, R.; Wunsch, H.; da Costa, B.R.; et al. Association of Noninvasive Oxygenation Strategies with All-Cause Mortality in Adults with Acute Hypoxemic Respiratory Failure: A Systematic Review and Me-ta-analysis. *JAMA* **2020**, *324*, 57–67. [CrossRef]
16. Patel, B.K.; Wolfe, K.S.; Pohlman, A.S.; Hall, J.B.; Kress, J.P. Effect of Noninvasive Ventilation Delivered by Helmet vs Face Mask on the Rate of Endotracheal Intubation in Patients with Acute Respiratory Distress Syndrome: A Randomized Clinical Trial. *JAMA* **2016**, *315*, 2435–2441. [CrossRef]
17. Ferioli, M.; Cisternino, C.; Leo, V.; Pisani, L.; Palange, P.; Nava, S. Protecting healthcare workers from SARS-CoV-2 infection: Practical indications. *Eur. Respir. Rev.* **2020**, *29*, 200068. [CrossRef]
18. Ferrer, M.; Esquinas, A.; Leon, M.; Gonzalez, G.; Alarcon, A.; Torres, A. Noninvasive ventilation in severe hypoxemic respiratory failure: A randomized clinical trial. *Am. J. Respir. Crit. Care Med.* **2003**, *168*, 1438–1444. [CrossRef]
19. Tang, N.; Bai, H.; Chen, X.; Gong, J.; Li, D.; Sun, Z. Anticoagulant treatment is associated with decreased mortality in severe coronavirus disease 2019 patients with coagulopathy. *J. Thromb. Haemost.* **2020**, *18*, 1094–1099. [CrossRef]
20. Venables, W.N.; Ripley, B.D. *Modern Applied Statistics with S*; Springer: Berlin, Germany, 2002. [CrossRef]
21. The Recovery Collaborative Group; Horby, P.; Lim, W.S.; Emberson, J.R.; Mafham, M.; Bell, J.L.; Linsell, L.; Staplin, N.; Brightling, C.; Ustianowski, A.; et al. Dexamethasone in Hospitalized Patients with Covid. *N. Engl. J. Med.* **2021**, *384*, 693–704.
22. Confalonieri, M.; Urbino, R.; Potena, A.; Piattella, M.; Parigi, P.; Puccio, G.; Della Porta, R.; Giorgio, C.; Blasi, F.; Umberger, R.; et al. Hydrocortisone infusion for severe communi-ty-acquired pneumonia: A preliminary randomized study. *Am. J. Respir. Crit. Care Med.* **2005**, *171*, 242–248. [CrossRef] [PubMed]
23. Santus, P.; Radovanovic, D.; Saderi, L.; Marino, P.; Cogliati, C.; De Filippis, G.; Rizzi, M.; Franceschi, E.; Pini, S.; Giuliani, F.; et al. Severity of respiratory failure at admission and in-hospital mortality in patients with COVID-19: A prospective observational multicentre study. *BMJ Open* **2020**, *10*, e043651. [CrossRef] [PubMed]
24. Yao, Y.; Cao, J.; Wang, Q.; Shi, Q.; Liu, K.; Luo, Z.; Chen, X.; Chen, S.; Yu, K.; Huang, Z.; et al. D-dimer as a biomarker for disease severity and mortality in COVID-19 patients: A case control study. *J. Intensiv. Care* **2020**, *8*, 49. [CrossRef]
25. Gattinoni, L.; Coppola, S.; Cressoni, M.; Busana, M.; Rossi, S.; Chiumello, D. COVID-19 Does Not Lead to a "Typical" Acute Res-piratory Distress Syndrome. *Am. J. Respir. Crit. Care Med.* **2020**, *201*, 1299–1300. [CrossRef] [PubMed]
26. Dhont, S.; Derom, E.; Van Braeckel, E.; Depuydt, P.; Lambrecht, B.N. The pathophysiology of "happy" hypoxemia in COVID. *Respir. Res.* **2020**, *21*, 198. [CrossRef]
27. Han, R.; Huang, L.; Jiang, H.; Dong, J.; Peng, H.; Zhang, D. Early Clinical and CT Manifestations of Coronavirus Disease 2019 (COVID-19) Pneumonia. *Am. J. Roentgenol.* **2020**, *215*, 338–343. [CrossRef]
28. Gattinoni, L.; Chiumello, D.; Caironi, P.; Busana, M.; Romitti, F.; Brazzi, L.; Camporota, L. COVID-19 pneumonia: Different respiratory treatments for different phenotypes? *Intensive Care Med.* **2020**, *46*, 1099–1102. [CrossRef]
29. Chiumello, D.; Esquinas, A.M.; Moerer, O.; Terzi, N. A systematic technical review of the systems for the continuous positive airway pressure. *Minerva Anestesiol.* **2012**, *78*, 1385–1393.
30. Fazzini, B.; Page, A.; Pearse, R.; Puthucheary, Z. Prone positioning for non-intubated spontaneously breathing patients with acute hypoxaemic respiratory failure: A systematic review and meta-analysis. *Br. J. Anaesth.* **2021**, *128*, 352–362. [CrossRef]
31. Longhini, F.; Bruni, A.; Garofalo, E.; Navalesi, P.; Grasselli, G.; Cosentini, R.; Foti, G.; Mattei, A.; Ippolito, M.; Accurso, G.; et al. Helmet continuous positive airway pressure and prone positioning: A proposal for an early management of COVID-19 patients. *Pulmonology* **2020**, *26*, 186–191. [CrossRef]
32. Radovanovic, D.; Rizzi, M.; Pini, S.; Saad, M.; Chiumello, D.A.; Santus, P. Helmet CPAP to Treat Acute Hypoxemic Respiratory Failure in Patients with COVID-19: A Management Strategy Proposal. *J. Clin. Med.* **2020**, *9*, 1191. [CrossRef] [PubMed]
33. Ing, R.J.; Bills, C.; Merritt, G.; Ragusa, R.; Bremner, R.M.; Bellia, F. Role of Helmet-Delivered Noninvasive Pressure Support Ventilation in COVID-19 Patients. *J. Cardiothorac. Vasc. Anesthesia* **2020**, *34*, 2575–2579. [CrossRef]
34. Piluso, M.; Scarpazza, P.; Oggionni, E.; Celeste, A.; Bencini, S.; Bernareggi, M.; Bonacina, C.; Cattaneo, R.; Melacini, C.; Raschi, S.; et al. Helmet Continuous Positive Airway Pressure in COVID-19 Related Acute Respiratory Distress Syndrome in Respiratory Intermediate Care Unit. *Austin J. Infect. Dis.* **2021**, *8*, 1061. [CrossRef]
35. Karagiannidis, C.; Hentschker, C.; Westhoff, M.; Weber-Carstens, S.; Janssens, U.; Kluge, S.; Pfeifer, M.; Spies, C.; Welte, T.; Rossaint, R.; et al. Observational study of changes in utilization and outcomes in mechanical ventilation in COVID-19. *PLoS ONE* **2022**, *17*, e0262315. [CrossRef] [PubMed]
36. Brochard, L.; Slutsky, A.; Pesenti, A. Mechanical Ventilation to Minimize Progression of Lung Injury in Acute Respiratory Failure. *Am. J. Respir. Crit. Care Med.* **2017**, *195*, 438–442. [CrossRef] [PubMed]

37. Tobin, M.J. Basing Respiratory Management of COVID-19 on Physiological Principles. *Am. J. Respir. Crit. Care Med.* **2020**, *201*, 1319–1320. [CrossRef]
38. Matthay, M.A.; Arabi, Y.; Arroliga, A.C.; Bernard, G.; Bersten, A.D.; Brochard, L.J.; Calfee, C.S.; Combes, A.; Daniel, B.M.; Ferguson, N.D.; et al. A New Global Definition of Acute Respiratory Distress Syndrome. *Am. J. Respir. Crit. Care Med.* **2023**; *ahead of print*. [CrossRef]

Disclaimer/Publisher's Note: The statements, opinions and data contained in all publications are solely those of the individual author(s) and contributor(s) and not of MDPI and/or the editor(s). MDPI and/or the editor(s) disclaim responsibility for any injury to people or property resulting from any ideas, methods, instructions or products referred to in the content.

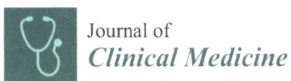

Article

Epidemiology, Ventilation Management and Outcomes of COPD Patients Receiving Invasive Ventilation for COVID-19—Insights from PRoVENT-COVID

Athiwat Tripipitsiriwat [1], Orawan Suppapueng [2], David M. P. van Meenen [3,4,*], Frederique Paulus [3,5], Markus W. Hollmann [4], Chaisith Sivakorn [6] and Marcus J. Schultz [3,7,8,9,†] on behalf of the PRoVENT-COVID Investigators

[1] Division of Respiratory Disease and Tuberculosis, Department of Medicine, Faculty of Medicine Siriraj Hospital, Mahidol University, Bangkok 10400, Thailand; athiwattri@gmail.com
[2] Division of Clinical Epidemiology, Department of Research, Faculty of Medicine Siriraj Hospital, Mahidol University, Bangkok 10400, Thailand; aorstat@gmail.com
[3] Department of Intensive Care, Amsterdam UMC, Location AMC, 1105 AZ Amsterdam, The Netherlands; f.paulus@amsterdamumc.nl (F.P.); marcus.j.schultz@gmail.com (M.J.S.)
[4] Department of Anesthesiology, Amsterdam UMC, Location AMC, 1105 AZ Amsterdam, The Netherlands; m.w.hollmann@amsterdamumc.nl
[5] Center of Expertise Urban Vitality, Faculty of Health, Amsterdam University of Applied Sciences, 1101 CD Amsterdam, The Netherlands
[6] Intensive Care Unit, University College London Hospital, London NW1 2BU, UK; chaisith.sivakorn@nhs.net
[7] Mahidol–Oxford Tropical Medicine Research Unit (MORU), Mahidol University, Bangkok 10400, Thailand
[8] Nuffield Department of Medicine, University of Oxford, Oxford OX3 7BN, UK
[9] Department of Anesthesia, General Intensive Care and Pain Management, Division of Cardiothoracic and Vascular Anesthesia & Critical Care Medicine, Medical University of Vienna, 1090 Vienna, Austria
* Correspondence: d.m.vanmeenen@amsterdamumc.nl
† The list of investigators is provided in Appendix A.

Abstract: Chronic obstructive pulmonary disease (COPD) is a risk factor for death in patients admitted to intensive care units (ICUs) for respiratory support. Previous reports suggested higher mortality in COPD patients with COVID-19. It is yet unknown whether patients with COPD were treated differently compared to non-COPD patients. We compared the ventilation management and outcomes of invasive ventilation for COVID-19 in COPD patients versus non-COPD patients. This was a post hoc analysis of a nation-wide, observational study in the Netherlands. COPD patients were compared to non-COPD patients with respect to key ventilation parameters. The secondary endpoints included adjunctive treatments for refractory hypoxemia, and 28-day mortality. Of a total of 1090 patients, 88 (8.1%) were classified as having COPD. The ventilation parameters were not different between COPD patients and non-COPD patients, except for FiO_2, which was higher in COPD patients. Prone positioning was applied more often in COPD patients. COPD patients had higher 28-day mortality than non-COPD patients. COPD had an independent association with 28-day mortality. In this cohort of patients who received invasive ventilation for COVID-19, only FiO_2 settings and the use of prone positioning were different between COPD patients and non-COPD patients. COPD patients had higher mortality than non-COPD patients.

Keywords: COPD; ARDS; COVID-19; invasive ventilation; ventilation management; outcome

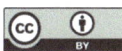

1. Introduction

Chronic obstructive pulmonary disease (COPD) is a common airway condition that affects around 10% of the world's population and causes approximately 3,000,000 deaths each year [1]. COPD has been linked to a higher risk of mortality in a variety of respiratory tract infections, including bacterial [2] and viral pneumonia [3]. COPD is also considered a risk factor for death in patients who need admission to an intensive care unit (ICU) for respiratory support [4,5], though mortality in these patients mainly depends on the cause of respiratory failure.

The coronavirus disease 2019 (COVID-19) pandemic unavoidably afflicted this large group of patients. Previous reports suggested a higher mortality rate in COPD patients with COVID-19 [6]. It is yet unknown whether patients with a history of COPD were treated differently compared to non-COPD patients. In particular, the ways in which invasive ventilation was applied might have been different. There may also have been differences in how refractory hypoxemia was treated. Such differences, if any, could have affected patient outcomes.

We conducted a post hoc analysis of a conveniently sized multicenter observational study, named 'Practice of Ventilation in COVID-19' (PRoVENT-COVID) [7]. Herein, we determined and compared ventilator settings and ventilation parameters, supportive treatments for refractory hypoxemia and outcomes in COPD patients versus non-COPD patients. We hypothesized that ventilation management in COPD patients would be different from that in non-COPD patients. We also determined which factors had an independent association with outcomes.

2. Materials and Methods

2.1. Study Design

This is a post hoc analysis of PRoVENT-COVID, a nation-wide, multicenter, observational cohort study [7]. PRoVENT-COVID included patients in 22 ICUs in the Netherlands. The study protocol was approved by the Institutional Review Board of the Amsterdam University Medical Centers, 'AMC' location. Members of the PRoVENT-COVID steering committee were responsible for the recruitment of study sites; local investigators and data collectors sought approval from their respective Institutional Review Boards or Research Ethics Committees. The study protocol was prepublished [8], and the study was registered at ClinicalTrials.gov (NCT04346342). The need for individual informed consent was waived due to the observational nature of this investigation. The study coordinators and trained data collectors assisted local doctors and monitored the study according to the International Conference on Harmonization's Good Clinical Practice Guideline, ensuring the integrity and timely completion of data collection.

2.2. Patients

Patients were eligible for participation if: (1) they were aged 18 years or older; (2) they had been admitted to one of the participating ICUs in the first wave of the national outbreak; (3) had acute respiratory failure related to COVID-19; and (4) required invasive ventilation. COVID-19 was confirmed via RT–PCR in all patients. Patients who received noninvasive ventilation, and patients who were transferred to a non-participating ICU within 1 h after intubation and underwent invasive ventilation, were excluded. For the current analysis, we pragmatically excluded patients under the age of 40 years, to improve the accuracy of the history of COPD.

2.3. Patient Classification

Patients with a known history of COPD were classified as COPD patients; patients without a known history of COPD were classified as non-COPD patients. History of COPD was based on information recorded in the medical records, which was collected for PRoVENT-COVID.

2.4. Collected Data

Demographic data, the severity of illness scores expressed in Acute Physiology and Chronic Health Evaluation (APACHE) scores II or IV, Simplified Acute Physiology Score (SAPS) II or the Sequential Organ Failure Assessment (SOFA) score were collected at baseline. Trained data collectors scored chest imaging performed to determine the extent of lung involvement; chest X-rays were scored as having opacities in one, two, three or four quadrants; chest computed tomography (CT) scans were scored as having 0%, 25%, 50%, 75% or 100% involvement. ARDS severity was categorized using the current Berlin definition of ARDS [9]. Laboratory tests, including arterial blood gas, lactate and serum creatinine, were collected at baseline.

Ventilator settings and parameters were collected after the first hour of invasive ventilation, and thereafter at fixed time points (08:00 a.m., 4:00 p.m. and 12:00 p.m.) over the first four calendar days of ventilation. The first day a patient received invasive ventilation in a participating ICU was named 'day 0'. Adjunctive treatments of refractory hypoxemia were also recorded during those four days, including the use of recruitment maneuvers, prone positioning and neuromuscular blocking agents. Typical ICU events and complications, including pneumothorax, thromboembolic complications, extubation and re-intubation, tracheostomy and acute kidney injury were collected up to day 28. At day 90, the intubation status, day of discharge from the ICU and hospital, and day of death in non-survivors were recorded.

2.5. Calculations

The driving pressure (ΔP) was calculated by subtracting the positive end-expiratory pressure (PEEP) from the plateau pressure (P_{plat}) during volume-controlled ventilation, or from the maximum airway pressure (P_{max}) during pressure-controlled ventilation, and only at timepoints with evidence of the absence of spontaneous breathing. The dead space fraction was calculated by subtracting the end-tidal carbon dioxide (et-CO_2) from the arterial carbon dioxide pressure ($PaCO_2$) and dividing by $PaCO_2$. Respiratory system compliance (C_{RS}) was calculated by dividing the tidal volume (V_T) by ΔP. The mechanical power of ventilation (MP) was calculated from V_T, respiratory rate (RR), peak pressure (P_{peak}) and ΔP ($0.098 \times 2217 V_T \times RR \times [P_{peak} - 0.5 \times \Delta P]$); if P_{peak} was not available, we used P_{plat} ($0.098 \times V_T \times RR \times [P_{plat} - 0.5 \times \Delta P]$). The number of days free from the ventilator at day 28 (VFD–28) was defined as the number of days a patient was not connected to a ventilator in the first 28 days after the start of ventilation, wherein patients who died before day 28 days received zero free days, even if weaned from ventilation within this timeframe.

2.6. Endpoints

The primary endpoint was marked by the collection of key ventilator settings and ventilation parameters over the first four calendar days of invasive ventilation, including V_T, PEEP, ΔP and C_{RS}. The secondary endpoints included other settings and parameters, including the mode of ventilation, alveolar minute ventilation (AMV), P_{peak}, RR, fraction of inspired oxygen (FiO_2), MP, dead space fraction and arterial blood gas analysis results, and et-CO_2. The other secondary endpoints were the use of adjunctive therapies, typical ICU events and complications, the duration of ventilation, the length of ICU and hospital stays, the number of VFD–28 and 28-day mortality.

2.7. Power Calculation

We did not perform a formal power calculation; instead, the sample size was based on the number of patients included in the original study.

2.8. Statistical Analysis

Quantitative data are presented as mean ± standard deviation or median with interquartile ranges were appropriate. Categorical data are presented as numbers and proportions. A Chi-square test or Fisher's exact test were used to compare categorical variables. An independent *t*-test or Mann–Whitney U test was used to compare continuous data. Cumulative distribution plots were created for the ventilator settings and parameters to visualize differences between COPD and non-COPD patients.

To assess the mortality impact of COPD, hazard ratios were calculated using shared frailty adjusted Cox regression with the center set as frailty for mortality. The subdistribution hazard ratios were also calculated for ICU and hospital length of stay, and the duration of ventilation, using a Fine–Gray competing risk analysis with death as the competing risk. Forward stepwise selection was used, defined by $p < 0.2$ according to a univariable analysis of the two groups, which were added to a multivariable model to demonstrate the impact of COPD on 28-day mortality. These included age; sex; body mass index; dead space fraction; PaO_2/FiO_2; plasma creatinine; history of hypertension, heart failure, diabetes mellitus, chronic kidney disease and active malignancy; the use of angiotensin-converting enzyme inhibitors; the use of angiotensin II receptor blockers; the use of a vasopressor or inotropes; fluid balance; pH; mean arterial pressure; heart rate; and C_{RS}.

All analyses were performed in STATA statistics version 14 (StataCorp, College Station, TX, USA). A p-value of <0.05 was considered statistically significant.

3. Results

3.1. Patients

Between 1 March and 1 June 2020, 1122 patients were included in PRoVENT-COVID. The main reasons for exclusion were not having received invasive ventilation or having an alternative diagnosis for acute hypoxemic respiratory failure. Of the remaining 1090 patients, 88 (8.1%) were classified as COPD patients (Supplement Figure S1). COPD patients were older and used corticosteroids, angiotensin-converting enzyme inhibitors and angiotensin ll receptor blockers more often than non-COPD patients (Table 1). At baseline, COPD patients had lower PaO_2/FiO_2, lower et–CO_2 and a higher dead space fraction (Table 2). ARDS was classified as severe more often in COPD patients, but none of the severity of disease scores were different between the two groups.

Table 1. Patient demographics and baseline characteristics.

	COPD Patients N = 88	Non-COPD Patients N = 1002	p-Value
Demographics			
Age, year, median [IQR]	68 [62–72]	65 [58–72]	0.03
Male sex, n (%)	60 (68.2)	735 (73.4)	0.30
BMI, kg/m^2, median [IQR]	28 [26–30]	28 [25–31]	0.84
Severity of illness			
SAPS II, median [IQR]	35 [30–48]	36 [29–43]	0.32
APACHE II score, median [IQR]	15 [13–20]	16 [12–20]	0.41
APACHE IV score, median [IQR]	55 [49–71]	56 [45–69]	0.33
SOFA score, median [IQR]	8 [6–11]	7 [6–10]	0.73
Severity of ARDS, n (%)			0.01
No ARDS	2 (2.4)	16 (1.6)	
Mild	1 (1.2)	104 (10.7)	
Moderate	50 (59.5)	602 (61.7)	
Severe	31 (36.9)	254 (26.0)	
Co-existing disorders, n (%)			
Hypertension	28 (31.8)	351 (35.0)	0.54
Heart failure	3 (3.4)	45 (4.5)	1.00
Diabetes mellitus	13 (14.8)	236 (23.6)	0.06
Chronic kidney disease	5 (5.7)	41 (4.1)	0.41
Liver cirrhosis	0 (0.0)	3 (0.3)	1.00
Active hematological neoplasia	0 (0.0)	16 (1.6)	0.63
Active solid neoplasia	4 (4.5)	23 (2.3)	0.27
Neuromuscular disease	0 (0.0)	7 (0.7)	1.00
Immunosuppression	2 (2.3)	22 (2.2)	1.00
Current medication, n (%)			
Systemic steroids	7 (8.0)	31 (3.1)	0.03
Inhaled steroids	48 (54.5)	73 (7.3)	<0.001
Angiotensin-converting enzyme inhibitors	8 (9.1)	181 (18.1)	0.03

Table 1. Cont.

	COPD Patients N = 88	Non-COPD Patients N = 1002	p-Value
Angiotensin II receptor blockers	16 (18.2)	111 (11.1)	0.05
Beta-blockers	21 (23.9)	189 (18.9)	0.25
Insulin	3 (3.4)	75 (7.5)	0.16
Metformin	8 (9.1)	166 (16.6)	0.07
Statins	30 (34.1)	300 (29.9)	0.42
Calcium channel blockers	19 (21.6)	176 (17.6)	0.35
Chest imaging			
Chest CT scan performed, n (%)	25 (29.4)	321 (33.6)	0.43
Lung parenchyma affected at chest CT, n (%)			0.70
<25%	11 (44.0)	115 (35.8)	
50%	7 (28.0)	92 (28.7)	
75%	6 (24.0)	95 (29.6)	
100%	1 (4.0)	19 (5.9)	
Lung parenchyma affected at CXR, number of quadrants, n (%)			0.48
1	4 (8.0)	37 (7.0)	
2	14 (28.0)	118 (22.2)	
3	16 (32.0)	146 (27.5)	
4	16 (32.0)	230 (43.3)	
Laboratory tests			
Plasma lactate, mmol/L, median [IQR]	1.2 [0.9–1.4]	1.2 [0.9–1.5]	0.44
Plasma creatinine, μmol/L (median [IQR])	77 [60–101]	78 [63–98]	0.89

Abbreviations: BMI, body mass index; COPD, chronic obstructive pulmonary disease; APACHE, Acute Physiology and Chronic Health Evaluation; SOFA, Sequential Organ Failure Assessment; ARDS, acute respiratory distress syndrome; CT, computed tomography; CXR, chest X-ray.

Table 2. Mechanical ventilation use during the first day of mechanical ventilation.

	COPD Patients N = 88	Non-COPD Patients N = 1002	p-Value
Mode of mechanical ventilation, n (%)			0.12
Volume-controlled	18 (21)	143 (14)	
Pressure-controlled	41 (47)	561 (56)	
Pressure support	3 (3)	50 (5)	
SIMV	9 (10)	72 (7)	
APRV	5 (6)	27 (3)	
INTELLiVENT–ASV	5 (6)	36 (4)	
Other	6 (7)	109 (11)	
Ventilation Parameters			
Expiratory V_T, mL, median [IQR]	440 [387–498]	451 [408–502]	0.13
V_T per PBW, mL/kg, median [IQR]	6.2 [5.9–7.0]	6.4 [5.9–7.0]	0.67
PEEP, cmH$_2$O, median [IQR]	13 [12–15]	13 [11–15]	0.24
Total Respiratory rate, median [IQR]	22 [20–24]	22 [19–24]	0.84
FiO$_2$, median [IQR]	0.6 [0.5–0.7]	0.6 [0.5–0.7]	0.01
P_{peak}, cmH$_2$O, median [IQR]	27 [24–29]	27 [24–30]	0.78
Driving pressure, cmH$_2$O, median [IQR]	14 [12–16]	14 [12–16]	0.87
Compliance, cmH$_2$O/L, median [IQR]	32 [26.8–39]	33 [27–40]	0.70
Mechanical power, J/min, median [IQR]	18 [15–20]	19 [16–22]	0.07
Minute ventilation, L/min, median [IQR]	9 [8–10]	10 [8–11]	0.07
pH, median [IQR]	7.35 [7.29–7.39]	7.37 [7.31–7.41]	0.02
PaO$_2$, kPa, median [IQR]	10 [9–12]	11 [9–13]	0.08
PaO$_2$/FiO$_2$, mmHg, median [IQR]	114 [89–149]	128 [99–168]	0.01

Table 2. Cont.

	COPD Patients N = 88	Non-COPD Patients N = 1002	p-Value
$PaCO_2$, kPa, median [IQR]	6.1 [5.5–6.5]	5.9 [5.2–6.7]	0.25
End-tidal CO_2, kPa, median [IQR]	4.6 [4.1–5.3]	4.9 [4.4–5.6]	0.01
Dead space fraction, median [IQR]	0.24 [0.14–0.33]	0.16 [0.06–0.26]	<0.001

Abbreviations: APRV, airway pressure release ventilation; ASV, adaptive support ventilation; COPD, chronic obstructive pulmonary disease; FiO_2, fraction of inspired oxygen; IQR; interquartile range; J/min, joules per minute; kg, kilogram; kPa, kiloPascal; mL, milliliter; $PaCO_2$, arterial pressure of carbon dioxide; PaO_2, arterial pressure of oxygen; PBW, predicted body weight; PEEP, positive end-expiratory pressure; P_{peak}, peak airway pressure; SIMV, synchronized intermittent mandatory ventilation; V_T, tidal volume.

3.2. Ventilation Management

Ventilation management is detailed in Table 2 and Figure 1. V_T and PEEP were not different between COPD and non-COPD patients. There were also no differences between ΔP and C_{RS}. COPD patients were ventilated with higher FiO_2. COPD patients also had lower arterial pH, lower $etCO_2$ and higher dead space fractions.

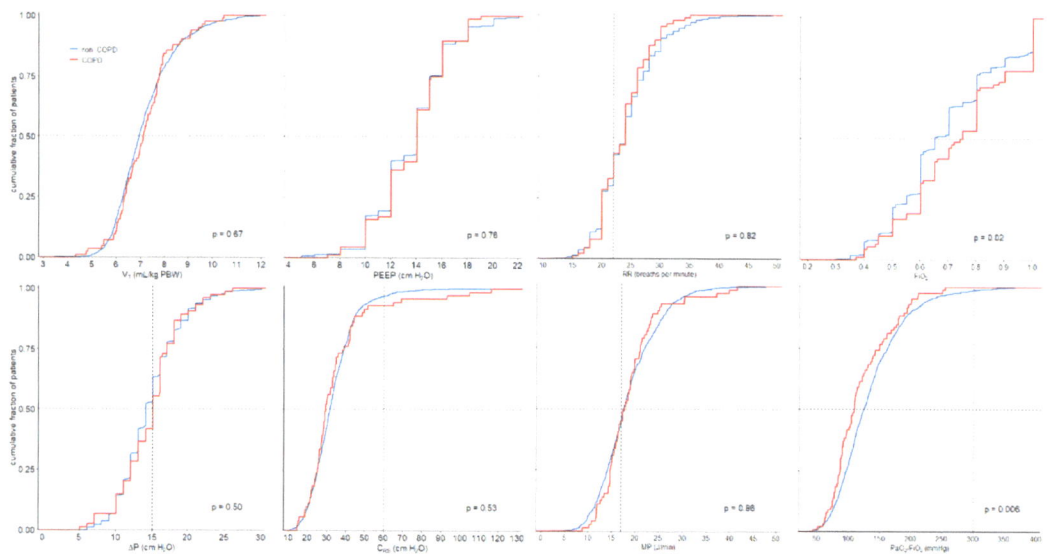

Figure 1. Cumulative distribution of ventilatory characteristics. The worst available value for each parameter was used.

Of the adjunctive treatments for refractory hypoxemia, prone positioning was used more often in COPD patients (Supplement Table S1). There were no differences in the use of recruitment maneuvers or neuromuscular blocking agents.

3.3. Outcomes

Air leaks, thromboembolic complications, acute kidney injury and re-intubations occurred as often in COPD patients as in non-COPD patients (Table 3). The duration of ventilation and the number of VFD–28 patients were not different between COPD and non-COPD patients (Figure 2). COPD patients had higher ICU and in-hospital mortality, and also higher 28-day and 90-day mortality.

In the multivariable analysis, COPD was an independent risk factor for 28-day mortality (Supplement Table S2). Fine–Gray competing risk analysis with death as the competing risk showed that the duration of ventilation, ICU length of stay and hospital length of stay were longer in COPD patients compared to non-COPD patients (Supplement Figure S2).

Table 3. Clinical outcomes and ICU complications.

	All N = 1090	COPD N = 88	Non-COPD N = 1002	*p*-Value
28-day mortality, n (%)	319 (29%)	36 (41%)	283 (28%)	0.02
90-day mortality, n (%)	369 (34%)	39 (44%)	330 (33%)	0.04
In-hospital mortality, n (%)	364 (37%)	39 (49%)	325 (36%)	0.02
ICU mortality, n (%)	354 (33%)	38 (45%)	316 (32%)	0.02
Length of hospital stay, days, median [IQR]	23 [14–37]	20 [11–31]	24 [14–37]	0.06
Length of ICU stay, days, median [IQR]	15 [9–26]	12 [8–24]	16 [9–26]	0.11
Ventilator-free days at day 28, days, median [IQR]	16 [10–28]	14 [10–30]	16 [10–28]	0.92
Duration of ventilation, days, median [IQR]	14 [8–23]	11 [8–20]	14 [8–23]	0.07
Tracheostomy, n (%)	187 (17%)	14 (16%)	173 (17%)	0.76
Pneumothorax, n (%)	41 (4%)	4 (5%)	37 (4%)	0.57
Thromboembolic complications, n (%)				
Pulmonary embolism	244 (22%)	20 (23%)	224 (22%)	0.94
Deep vein thrombosis	53 (5%)	5 (6%)	48 (5%)	0.61
Ischemic stroke	31 (3%)	3 (3%)	28 (3%)	0.73
Myocardial infarction	16 (1%)	0 (0%)	16 (2%)	0.63
Systemic arterial thrombosis	4 (0%)	1 (1%)	3 (0%)	0.29
Acute kidney injury, n (%)	488 (45%)	38 (43%)	450 (45%)	0.73
Re-intubation, n (%)	138 (13%)	8 (9%)	130 (13%)	0.30

Abbreviations: COPD, chronic obstructive pulmonary disease; ICU, intensive care unit; IQR, interquartile range.

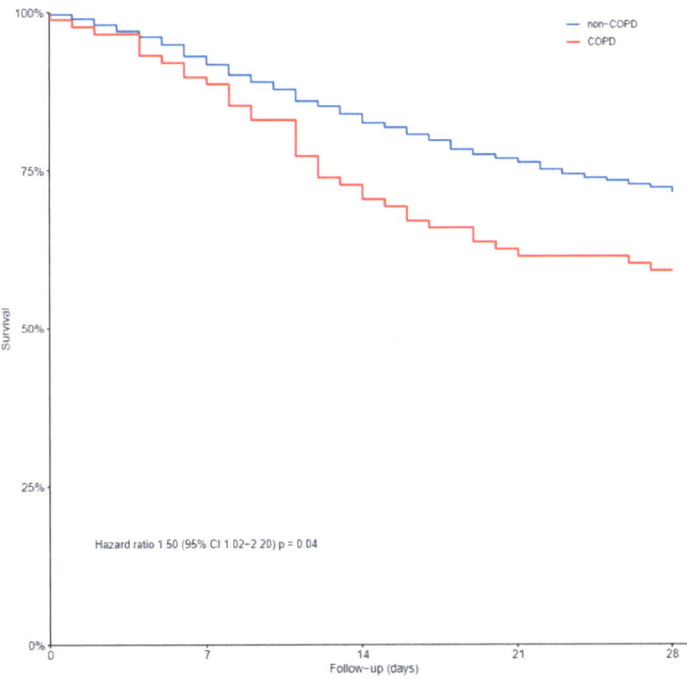

Figure 2. Kaplan–Meier graph showing mortality in COPD patients and non-COPD patients.

4. Discussion

The main findings of this post hoc analysis of a nation-wide, multicenter, observational study of invasively ventilated COVID-19 patients can be summarized as follows: (1) compared to non-COPD patients, COPD patients had more severe hypoxemia and ARDS; (2) the key ventilator settings and parameters were not different between COPD and non-COPD patients; (3) COPD patients were ventilated with higher FiO_2 and had lower PaO_2/FiO_2; (4) COPD patients had lower arterial pH and et–CO_2, and a higher dead space fraction; and (5) COPD patients received prone positioning more often. In addition, (6) COPD patients had higher mortality than non-COPD patients, and (7) COPD and a history of hypertension were independent risk factors for 28-day mortality.

Our study has several strengths. This analysis is one of the first to investigate ventilation management in COPD patients who received invasive ventilation for COVID-19. Trained investigators collected granular ventilation data over the first four days, increasing the robustness of the data. Patients were recruited in different types of hospitals, increasing the generalizability of our findings. The caregivers were not aware of the study at the time of data collection, minimizing the risk of observation bias. We had a sophisticated pre-defined statistical analysis plan in place, which was strictly followed.

The findings of this study extend our knowledge of ventilation practices in COPD patients with COVID-19. To the best of our knowledge, this study is the first to compare ventilation management between COPD and non-COPD patients in the context of COVID-19 in such great detail. The similarity in ventilator practices may not be unexpected given that both groups suffered from severe acute hypoxemic respiratory failure. The main difference between the groups was the severity of gas exchange abnormalities, resulting in the use of higher FiO_2 and more frequent use of prone positioning for refractory hypoxemia.

The best practice in invasive ventilation in COPD patients with ARDS remains uncertain. It is questionable whether low V_T ventilation should be used in COPD patients as strictly as has been advised for ARDS patients [10]. It is also uncertain whether PEEP titration should follow PEEP/FiO_2 tables as in ARDS patients [11], especially because COPD patients may be at increased risk of dynamic overinflation with deleterious consequences [11,12]. The findings of a previous study using electrical impedance tomography to determine the best PEEP in ARDS patients suggested that PEEP in COPD patients should be lower than that based on a PEEP/FiO_2 table [13]. In a study of adaptive support ventilation, PEEP was also lower in COPD patients than in patients with ARDS, but this study did not include patients with COPD with ARDS [14]. Notably, Practice of Ventilation was similar between COPD patients and non-COPD patients. There are several possible explanations for this finding. First, it is quite possible that during the firsts months of the pandemic, caregivers were not sure how to ventilate COVID-19 patients, let alone COVID-19 patients with COPD. It could also be that because of the severity of gas exchange impairment, it was not possible to apply different strategies. Lastly, it could be that patients with severe or exacerbated COPD were not admitted to the ICU during this time as there was a shortage of ICU beds, leading to COPD patients admitted to ICU being ventilated in a similar way to non-COPD patients.

We found a higher dead space fraction in COPD patients compared to non-COPD patients. This is, at least in part, in line with previous studies that showed a higher dead space fraction in ventilated COPD patients for reasons other than COVID-19 [15]. The higher dead space fraction in COPD patients in our cohort may, at least to some extent, be due to the application of a too high a level of PEEP [16,17]. However, there are no clinical trials that compare the effects of different levels of PEEP, either on the dead space fraction or on outcomes, in COPD patients with ARDS. Similarly, there are no clinical trials of prone positioning in this patient group, and such studies remain needed to determine the best ventilation practice in COPD patients with ARDS.

COPD is a risk factor for mortality in critically ill invasively ventilated patients [4,18]. Our findings extend this knowledge by showing that COPD is a risk factor for death in critically ill invasively ventilated COVID-19 patients, independent of age, sex, BMI, PaO_2/FiO_2, comorbidities and the use of antihypertensive drugs. COPD was also associated with a prolonged length of stay in the ICU and in hospitals as well as a prolonged duration of ventilation. Notably, the use of lower PEEP is suggested in patients with COPD [13]. In this study, COPD patients received a level of PEEP comparable to non-COPD patients, possibly adding to worse outcomes in the COPD patients.

The main limitation of our study is that presence of COPD was based on whether this was reported in the medical record. It could have been that clinicians also scored COPD in cases of asthma and other chronic airway diseases, thereby over-diagnosing COPD, or that patients with undiagnosed COPD were scored as not having COPD, or that COPD diagnosis was influenced mainly by smoking history, leading to under-reporting. This study also did not allow us to capture spirometry data. For these reasons, we restricted our analysis to patients aged older than 40 years [19]. Furthermore, data on the use of bronchodilating drugs were not collected, and whether or not patients received these drugs could have influenced their outcomes. We restricted the collection of data on ventilation characteristics and adjunctive therapy to the first four days of invasive ventilation. After these days, ventilation may have been different between the two patient groups, and we cannot exclude the possibility that ventilator management after the first four days of ventilation affects outcomes. Finally, as this is an analysis of an observational study, no causality can be claimed and the results should be seen as exploratory.

5. Conclusions

In this cohort of critically ill patients who received invasive ventilation for acute hypoxemic respiratory failure due to COVID-19, ventilation management was not different between COPD and non-COPD patients, except for FiO_2 settings and the use of prone positioning. COPD had independent associations with 28-day mortality.

Supplementary Materials: The following supporting information can be downloaded at: https://www.mdpi.com/article/10.3390/jcm12185783/s1, Supplementary Table S1: Rescue therapies for refractory hypoxemia, and other therapies during the first four days of mechanical ventilation; Supplementary Table S2: Multivariable analysis of factors in 28-day mortality; Supplementary Figure S1: CONSORT diagram; Supplementary Figure S2: Competing risk analysis for ICU length of stay, hospital length of stay and duration of ventilation with death as the competing risk.

Author Contributions: Conceptualization, A.T., D.M.P.v.M., F.P., C.S. and M.J.S.; methodology, A.T., O.S. and D.M.P.v.M.; formal analysis, O.S., A.T. and D.M.P.v.M.; writing—original draft preparation, A.T., D.M.P.v.M. and M.J.S.; writing—review and editing, D.M.P.v.M., M.W.H., M.J.S. and F.P.; visualization, A.T., D.M.P.v.M. and C.S.; supervision, M.J.S., F.P. and D.M.P.v.M.; funding acquisition, D.M.P.v.M., M.W.H., M.J.S. and F.P. All authors have read and agreed to the published version of the manuscript.

Funding: This research did not receive any specific grants from funding agencies in the public, commercial or not-for-profit sectors.

Institutional Review Board Statement: This study was conducted in accordance with the Declaration of Helsinki, and approved by the local Institutional Review Board of the Amsterdam University Medical Centers. All handling of personal data complies with the EU General Data Protection Regulation (GDPR).

Informed Consent Statement: The need for patients' individual written informed consent was waived due to the observational nature of the study.

Data Availability Statement: The data used in this study are available upon request to the steering committee of the PRoVENT-COVID study.

Conflicts of Interest: The authors declare no conflict of interest. The funders had no role in the design of the study; in the collection, analyses or interpretation of the data; in the writing of the manuscript; or in the decision to publish the results.

Registration: PRoVENT-COVID is registered at ClinicalTrials.gov (NCT04346342).

Appendix A

PRoVENT-COVID Investigators: PRoVENT-COVID stands for the Practice of Ventilation in COVID-19 Patients study. Investigator list in alphabetical order: S. Ahuja; J.P. van Akkeren; A.G. Algera; C.K. Algoe; R.B. van Amstel; P. van de Berg; D.C. Bergmans; D.I. van den Bersselaar; F.A. Bertens; A.J. Bindels; J.S. Breel; C.L. Bruna; M.M. de Boer; S. den Boer; L.S. Boers; M. Bogerd; L.D. Bos; M. Botta; O.L. Baur; H. de Bruin; L.A. Buiteman–Kruizinga; O. Cremer; R.M. Determann; W. Dieperink; J. v. Dijk; D.A. Dongelmans; M.J. de Graaff; M.S. Galekaldridge; L.A. Hagens; J.J. Haringman; S.T. van der Heide; P.L. van der Heiden; L.L. Hoeijmakers; L. Hol; M. W. Hollmann; J. Horn; R. van der Horst; E.L. Ie; D. Ivanov; N.P. Juffermans; E. Kho; E.S. de Klerk; A.W. Koopman; M. Koopmans; S. Kucukcelebi; M.A. Kuiper; D.W. de Lange; I. Martin–Loeches; G. Mazzinari; D.M. van Meenen; N. van Mourik; S.G. Nijbroek; E.A. Oostdijk; F. Paulus; C. J. Pennartz; J. Pillay; I.M. Purmer; T.C. Rettig; O. Roca; J.P. Roozeman; M.J. Schultz; A. Serpa Neto; G.S. Shrestha; M.E. Sleeswijk; P.E. Spronk; A.C. Strang; W. Stilma; P. Swart; A.M. Tsonas; C.M.A. Valk; A.P. Vlaar; L.I. Veldhuis; W.H. van der Ven; P. van Velzen; P. van Vliet; P. van der Voort; L. van Welie; B. van Wijk; T. Winters; W.Y. Wong; A.R. van Zanten.

References

1. Venkatesan, P. GOLD report: 2022 update. *Lancet Respir. Med.* **2022**, *10*, e20. [CrossRef] [PubMed]
2. Torres, A.; Menendez, R. Mortality in COPD patients with community-acquired pneumonia: Who is the third partner? *Eur. Respir. J.* **2006**, *28*, 262–263. [CrossRef] [PubMed]
3. Kalil, A.C.; Thomas, P.G. Influenza virus-related critical illness: Pathophysiology and epidemiology. *Crit. Care* **2019**, *23*, 258. [CrossRef] [PubMed]
4. Funk, G.-C.; Bauer, P.; Burghuber, O.C.; Fazekas, A.; Hartl, S.; Hochrieser, H.; Schmutz, R.; Metnitz, P. Prevalence and prognosis of COPD in critically ill patients between 1998 and 2008. *Eur. Respir. J.* **2013**, *41*, 792–799. [CrossRef] [PubMed]
5. Nevins, M.L.; Epstein, S.K. Predictors of outcome for patients with COPD requiring invasive mechanical ventilation. *Chest* **2001**, *119*, 1840–1849. [CrossRef] [PubMed]
6. Gerayeli, F.V.; Milne, S.; Cheung, C.; Li, X.; Yang, C.W.T.; Tam, A.; Choi, L.H.; Bae, A.; Sin, D.D. COPD and the risk of poor outcomes in COVID-19: A systematic review and meta-analysis. *eClinicalMedicine* **2021**, *33*, 100789. [CrossRef] [PubMed]
7. Botta, M.; Tsonas, A.M.; Pillay, J.; Boers, L.S.; Algera, A.G.; Bos, L.D.; Dongelmans, D.A.; Hollmann, M.W.; Horn, J.; Vlaar, A.P.J.; et al. Ventilation management and clinical outcomes in invasively ventilated patients with COVID-19 (PRoVENT-COVID): A national, multicentre, observational cohort study. *Lancet Respir. Med.* **2021**, *9*, 139–148. [CrossRef] [PubMed]
8. Boers, N.S.; Botta, M.; Tsonas, A.M.; Algera, A.G.; Pillay, J.; Dongelmans, D.A.; Horn, J.; Vlaar, A.P.J.; Hollmann, M.W.; Bos, L.D.J.; et al. PRactice of VENTilation in Patients with Novel Coronavirus Disease (PRoVENT-COVID): Rationale and protocol for a national multicenter observational study in The Netherlands. *Ann. Transl. Med.* **2020**, *8*, 1251. [CrossRef] [PubMed]
9. Ranieri, V.M.; Rubenfeld, G.D.; Thompson, B.T.; Ferguson, N.D.; Caldwell, E.; Fan, E.; Camporota, L.; Slutsky, A.S. Acute respiratory distress syndrome: The Berlin Definition. *JAMA* **2012**, *307*, 2526–2533. [PubMed]
10. Mowery, N.T. Ventilator Strategies for Chronic Obstructive Pulmonary Disease and Acute Respiratory Distress Syndrome. *Surg. Clin. N. Am.* **2017**, *97*, 1381–1397. [CrossRef] [PubMed]
11. Gattinoni, L.; Carlesso, E.; Cressoni, M. Selecting the 'right' positive end-expiratory pressure level. *Curr. Opin. Crit. Care* **2015**, *21*, 50–57. [CrossRef] [PubMed]
12. Karagiannidis, C.; Waldmann, A.D.; Róka, P.L.; Schreiber, T.; Strassmann, S.; Windisch, W.; Böhm, S.H. Regional expiratory time constants in severe respiratory failure estimated by electrical impedance tomography: A feasibility study. *Crit. Care* **2018**, *22*, 221. [CrossRef] [PubMed]
13. Liu, X.; Liu, X.; Meng, J.; Liu, D.; Huang, Y.; Sang, L.; Xu, Y.; Xu, Z.; He, W.; Chen, S.; et al. Electrical impedance tomography for titration of positive end-expiratory pressure in acute respiratory distress syndrome patients with chronic obstructive pulmonary disease. *Crit. Care* **2022**, *26*, 339. [CrossRef] [PubMed]
14. Arnal, J.M.; Garnero, A.; Novonti, D.; Demory, D.; Ducros, L.; Berric, A.; Donati, S.Y.; Corno, G.; Jaber, S.; Durand-Gasselin, J. Feasibility study on full closed-loop control ventilation (IntelliVent-ASV™) in ICU patients with acute respiratory failure: A prospective observational comparative study. *Crit. Care* **2013**, *17*, R196. [CrossRef] [PubMed]
15. Chuang, M.-L. Combining Dynamic Hyperinflation with Dead Space Volume during Maximal Exercise in Patients with Chronic Obstructive Pulmonary Disease. *J. Clin. Med.* **2020**, *9*, 1127. [CrossRef] [PubMed]
16. Tusman, G.; Gogniat, E.; Madorno, M.; Otero, P.; Dianti, J.; Ceballos, I.F.; Ceballos, M.; Verdier, N.; Böhm, S.H.; Rodriguez, P.O.; et al. Effect of PEEP on Dead Space in an Experimental Model of ARDS. *Respir. Care* **2020**, *65*, 11–20. [CrossRef] [PubMed]
17. Ferluga, M.; Lucangelo, U.; Blanch, L. Dead space in acute respiratory distress syndrome. *Ann. Transl. Med.* **2018**, *6*, 388. [CrossRef] [PubMed]

18. Rello, J.; Rodriguez, A.; Torres, A.; Roig, J.; Sole-Violan, J.; Garnacho-Montero, J.; de la Torre, M.V.; Sirvent, J.M.; Bodi, M. Implications of COPD in patients admitted to the intensive care unit by community-acquired pneumonia. *Eur. Respir. J.* **2006**, *27*, 1210–1216. [CrossRef] [PubMed]
19. Torén, K.; Murgia, N.; Olin, A.-C.; Hedner, J.; Brandberg, J.; Rosengren, A.; Bergström, G. Validity of physician-diagnosed COPD in relation to spirometric definitions of COPD in a general population aged 50–64 years—The SCAPIS pilot study. *Int. J. Chron. Obstruct. Pulmon. Dis.* **2017**, *12*, 2269–2275. [CrossRef] [PubMed]

Disclaimer/Publisher's Note: The statements, opinions and data contained in all publications are solely those of the individual author(s) and contributor(s) and not of MDPI and/or the editor(s). MDPI and/or the editor(s) disclaim responsibility for any injury to people or property resulting from any ideas, methods, instructions or products referred to in the content.

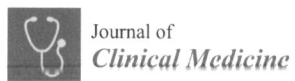

Article

The Outcome Relevance of Pre-ECMO Liver Impairment in Adults with Acute Respiratory Distress Syndrome

Stany Sandrio *, Manfred Thiel and Joerg Krebs

Department of Anesthesiology and Critical Care Medicine, University Medical Centre Mannheim, Medical Faculty Mannheim, University of Heidelberg, Theodor-Kutzer-Ufer 1-3, 68165 Mannheim, Germany; manfred.thiel@medma.uni-heidelberg.de (M.T.); joerg.krebs@umm.de (J.K.)
* Correspondence: stany.sandrio@umm.de

Abstract: We hypothesize that (1) a significant pre-ECMO liver impairment, which is evident in the presence of pre-ECMO acute liver injury and a higher pre-ECMO MELD (model for end-stage liver disease) score, is associated with increased mortality; and (2) the requirement of veno-veno-arterial (V-VA) ECMO support is linked to a higher prevalence of pre-ECMO acute liver injury, a higher pre-ECMO MELD score, and increased mortality. We analyze 187 ECMO runs (42 V-VA and 145 veno-venous (V-V) ECMO) between January 2017 and December 2020. The SAPS II score is calculated at ICU admission; hepatic function and MELD score are assessed at ECMO initiation (pre-ECMO) and during the first five days on ECMO. SOFA, PRESERVE and RESP scores are calculated at ECMO initiation. Pre-ECMO cardiac failure, acute liver injury, ECMO type, SAPS II and MELD, SOFA, PRESERVE, and RESP scores are associated with mortality. However, only the pre-ECMO MELD score independently predicts mortality (p = 0.04). In patients with a pre-ECMO MELD score > 16, V-VA ECMO is associated with a higher mortality risk (p = 0.0003). The requirement of V-VA ECMO is associated with the development of acute liver injury during ECMO support, a higher pre-ECMO MELD score, and increased mortality.

Keywords: ARDS; ECMO; liver injury; MELD score

1. Introduction

Extrapulmonary organ dysfunction has been associated with poor outcomes in patients with acute respiratory distress syndrome (ARDS) managed with extracorporeal membrane oxygenation (ECMO). A meta-analysis of two randomized controlled trials (conventional ventilator support versus extracorporeal membrane oxygenation for severe acute respiratory failure "CESAR" and ECMO to rescue lung injury in severe ARDS "EOLIA") suggested that veno-venous (V-V) ECMO lacks the ability to improve the outcome of ARDS patients with more than two organ failures [1] and that mortality in patients receiving ECMO for respiratory failure is correlated with the amount and the extent of extrapulmonary organ dysfunction at the time of ECMO initiation [2]. In these patients, cardiovascular failure due to shock and sepsis contributes disproportionately to mortality [3–6]. Additionally, hepatic dysfunction, which is known to be an independent factor contributing to mortality in ARDS [7], might play a role in determining the outcome of respiratory ECMO [8,9]. To date, studies assessing the outcome relevance of liver dysfunction and injury before the initiation of ECMO support have centered on patients supported by veno-arterial ECMO for cardiogenic shock [10,11]. Given the limited literature, evaluation of the relevance of liver injury and dysfunction before and after the initiation of ECMO therapy in relation to the outcomes of ARDS patients supported with ECMO is warranted.

Liver dysfunction refers to impaired clearance and synthetic hepatic function with increased bilirubin and international normalized ratio (INR) [12]. Both values are incorporated in the Model for End-Stage Liver Disease (MELD) score, which has been proposed as a predictor of hepatic, cardiac, and renal dysfunction [13]. Among patients with liver failure, the MELD score has been shown to predict mortality [14]. The MELD score has been also reported as an outcome predictor in patients with respiratory or cardiocirculatory failure managed with V-V and veno-arterial ECMO [8,15].

Acute liver injury, also known as hypoxic liver injury, is diagnosed based on clinical criteria: (1) a massive, rapid, and often transient increase in serum transaminases, (2) the presence of a respiratory or cardiocirculatory failure with reduced hepatic oxygen delivery or utilization, and (3) the exclusion of other causes of liver injury, particularly drug- or viral-induced hepatitis [16,17]. Transaminases level at 2.5 to 20 times the normal upper limit has been used to define acute/hypoxic liver injury [17]. Henrion et al. reported that cardiac failure, particularly in conjunction with congestive heart failure, as well as respiratory failure and septic shock frequently causes acute liver injury [16]. Hence, ARDS patients with acute cor pulmonale due to elevated pulmonary artery pressure [18] or septic-induced vasoplegia that is unresponsive to catecholamines [19,20] might be especially vulnerable to acute liver injury due to systemic hypoxia, hepatic congestion, and diminished hepatic blood flow.

In ARDS with concomitant right ventricular failure due to acute cor pulmonale or septic cardiomyopathy, veno-veno-arterial (V-VA) ECMO might be indicated [3,21]. In this cannulation approach, the arterial outflow is bifurcated, with one portion directed retrograde towards the aorta and the other towards the right atrium [3,21–23]. This hybrid configuration combines the benefits and distinctive features of both V-V and veno-arterial ECMO, enabling concurrent and robust respiratory and circulatory support [21,22].

In this study, we hypothesize that in patients with primary respiratory failure:

1. A significant liver impairment before ECMO initiation (pre-ECMO), indicated by the presence of acute liver injury or a higher MELD score, is associated with increased mortality;
2. The requirement of V-VA ECMO support due to an acute cor pulmonale or catecholamine refractory shock is associated with (a) a higher prevalence of pre-ECMO acute liver injury and (b) a higher pre-ECMO MELD score and, therefore, (c) an increased mortality.

2. Materials and Methods

2.1. Data Acquisition, Inclusion, and Exclusion Criteria

After institutional ethics committee approval (Medizinische Ethikkommission II, University Medical Centre Mannheim, Medical Faculty Mannheim of the University of Heidelberg, study registration number 2021-881), and registration in the German Clinical Trials Register (DRKS00028509), a retrospective review of electronic medical records was performed to identify patients with V-V and V-VA ECMO support between January 2017 and December 2020 at the Department of Anesthesiology and Critical Care Medicine, University Medical Centre Mannheim, Germany.

We performed a comprehensive data collection for each eligible patient. We include all ARDS patients receiving V-V and V-VA ECMO due to primary respiratory failure. Patients who required ECMO support for other reasons (e.g., ECMO as intraprocedural support during aortic surgery, extracorporeal cardiopulmonary resuscitation) are excluded from the analysis. In these patients, we aggregate age, sex, body-mass index, diagnosis, duration of mechanical ventilation before ECMO initiation, the parameter of mechanical ventilation, the length and type of ECMO support, the length of ICU stay, the presence of chronic kidney or liver disease, the need of renal replacement therapy, history of pre-ECMO cardiac arrest, cardiac failure, septic shock, and central nervous system injury. We further collected laboratory data including the daily serum levels of total bilirubin, international normalized ratio (INR), aspartate aminotransferase (AST), and alanine aminotransferase (ALT). These comprehensive data points provide a detailed overview of the patients' clinical profiles for further analysis.

2.2. ECMO Management

Our clinical workflow and management strategy for patients on ECMO support due to respiratory failure are detailed previously [3]. Briefly, in accordance with the EOLIA trial [5] and recent guidelines [24], V-V ECMO is initiated in severe hypoxic ($PaO_2/FiO_2 < 80$ for longer than six hours or $PaO_2/FiO_2 < 50$ for longer than three hours) or hypercapnic (arterial pH < 7.25 and $PaCO_2 > 60$ mmHg for longer than six hours) ARDS patients [3,5,24]. V-VA ECMO is applied in patients with severe respiratory failure and concomitant hemodynamic instability with tissue hypoperfusion, a systolic blood pressure less than 90 mmHg, and a cardiac index less than 2.0 L/min/m^2 despite preload optimization and the continuous infusion of catecholamines [3]. These patients commonly show primary respiratory failure accompanied by acute cor pulmonale or catecholamine-refractory septic shock.

Per the standard of our unit, we insert a 29 French multistage drainage cannula through the right femoral vein and a 23 French venous return cannula through the jugular vein [3]. In the case of V-VA ECMO, an additional 17 French arterial cannula and a 7 French antegrade perfusion cannula are inserted into the left femoral artery [3].

2.3. Definitions and Scores Calculation

In this study, acute liver injury is defined as the presence of increased serum aspartate transaminase greater than 350 U/L and alanine transaminase greater than 400 U/L, which indicated transaminase levels greater than 10 times the upper limit of normal [16,17]. Daily serum levels of transaminases, bilirubin, and creatinine and international normalized ratio (INR), and MELD score are assessed immediately prior to ECMO initiation (pre-ECMO) and during the first five days on ECMO support.

The MELD score is calculated according to the current Organ Procurement and Transplantation Network (OPTN) policies [25] and as recommended by the United Network for Organ Sharing [26,27].

$$\text{MELD} = \left(0.957 \times \ln\left(\text{creatinine}\frac{\text{mg}}{\text{dL}}\right) + 0.378 \times \ln\left(\text{bilirubin}\frac{\text{mg}}{\text{dL}}\right) + 1.120 \times \ln(\text{INR}) + 0.643\right) \times 10$$

In patients with serum creatinine above 4.0 mg/dL, as well as in patients who require a minimum of two dialyses or 24 h of continuous renal replacement therapy within the last seven days, the value for serum creatinine used in the calculation is set to 4.0 mg/dL [25]. For bilirubin or creatinine value less than 1 mg/dL, a value of 1 mg/dL is used in the calculation [25]. The MELD score is then rounded to the nearest integer and assessed at ICU admission, just before ECMO initiation (pre-ECMO) and during the first five days on ECMO support.

In this study, we analyze a patient cohort under V-V and V-VA ECMO for primary respiratory failure. Most of the patients presented with hypernatremia and, thus, the sodium value is set to 137 in the MELD-Na calculation [25]. This calculation resulted in identical MELD and MELD-Na values. Therefore, we use the MELD score in this study (not MELD-Na).

To further characterize the study population SAPS II (simplified acute physiology score II), SOFA (sequential organ failure assessment), RESP (respiratory ECMO survival prediction), and PRESERVE (predicting death for severe ARDS on V-V ECMO) scores are calculated. The SAPS II score is calculated as previously described by Le Gall et al. with physiological variables, which are collected within the first 24 h of treatment in the ICU [28]. SOFA, RESP, and PRESERVE scores are calculated at ECMO initiation, as described by Vincent et al. and Schmidt et al., respectively [29–31].

2.4. Statistical Analysis

Statistical analysis is performed with JMP® Version 15 from SAS (SAS, Cary, NC, USA). Categorical variables are presented as frequencies of observation (%) and analyzed using a two-tailed Fisher's exact test. Continuous variables are reported as medians with corresponding 25–75% interquartile ranges and comparisons are made using the Wilcoxon nonparametric test. For data that are measured multiple times, a repeated measures ANOVA and F-test are employed for analysis.

The following risk factors are included in our analysis: age, sex, body-mass index, ECMO type (V-V or V-VA), relevant comorbidities (pre-ECMO cardiac failure, septic shock, preexisting chronic liver and renal diseases, as well as the presence of acute liver injury), SAPS II at ICU admission, as well as pre-ECMO MELD, SOFA, PRESERVE, and RESP scores. The ability of a risk factor to predict mortality is assessed with logistic regression. The cut-off values of a risk factor for predicting mortality are correspondingly determined through a ROC curve analysis.

As we aimed to evaluate the impact of extrapulmonary organ function at the time of ECMO initiation on mortality, univariate and multivariable analyses are based on values at ECMO initiation (pre-ECMO). The multivariable analysis includes all factors with a $p \leq 0.05$ at the univariate analysis. To avoid redundancy, single laboratory values (i.e., bilirubin, creatinine, INR, aspartate, and alanine transaminase) are excluded from the analysis.

The links between the requirement of V-VA ECMO support and (1) a higher prevalence of pre-ECMO acute liver injury, (2) a higher pre-ECMO MELD score, and (3) increased mortality are evaluated with logistic regression.

Survival estimates are completed with Kaplan–Meier and Cox proportional hazards analyses. Patients who were discharged alive from ICU are censored at the time of their discharge date.

3. Results

Between January 2017 and December 2020, we identified 187 ECMO runs (42 V-VA and 145 V-V ECMO) on 177 patients. Eight patients required two ECMO runs and one patient required three ECMO runs due to recurring respiratory failure.

3.1. Patient's Demographics and Characteristics

The patients' demographics and characteristics are presented in Table 1. Survivors have significantly lower SAPS II (69 (59–80) vs. 78 (64–90), $p = 0.002$), a lower incidence of cardiac failure (19% vs. 43%, $p = 0.0005$), and require significantly less V-VA ECMO support (12% vs. 34%, $p = 0.0004$). There is no significant difference in the pre-ECMO prevalence of septic shock and preexisting chronic liver or renal diseases between survivors and nonsurvivors. However, survivors show a lower pre-ECMO prevalence of acute liver injury ($p = 0.03$) and have a lower MELD score (12 (8–20) vs. 19 (11–23), $p = 0.0004$), SOFA score (13 (11–16) vs. 15 (13–17.7), $p = 0.001$), PRESERVE score (3 (2–5) vs. 4 (3–6), $p = 0.005$), and RESP score (1 (2–3) vs. 0 (−2–2), $p = 0.04$).

Table 1. Pre-ECMO patient's demographics and characteristics (survivor vs. nonsurvivor).

	Survivors n = 95	Nonsurvivors n = 92	p Values
Age (years)	55 (42–61)	57 (49–64)	0.07
Sex	female n = 29 (31%) male n = 66 (69%)	female n = 30 (33%) male n = 62 (67%)	0.87
Body-mass index (kg/m^2)	29 (25–35)	27 (25–31)	0.08
ICU length of stay (days)	21 (14–33)	11.5 (6–24)	<0.0001
ECMO strategies • V-V ECMO • V-VA ECMO	 n = 84 (88%) n = 11 (12%)	 n = 61 (66%) n = 31 (34%)	 0.0004

Table 1. Cont.

	Survivors n = 95	Nonsurvivors n = 92	p Values
Duration of ECMO support (days)	12 (8–16)	9.5 (4–19)	0.08
Clinical presentation prior to ECMO initiation other than respiratory failure:			
• chronic liver disease	n = 1 (1%)	n = 4 (4%)	0.2
• chronic renal disease	n = 3 (3%)	n = 9 (4.5%)	0.08
• cardiac failure	n = 18 (19%)	n = 40 (43%)	0.0005
• septic shock	n = 53 (56%)	n = 62 (67%)	0.13
• acute liver injury	n = 3 (3%)	n = 11 (12%)	0.03
Bilirubin	0.6 (0.3–1.2)	0.9 (0.5–1.8)	0.01
Aspartate transaminase	77 (38.2–146.5)	143 (58.2–414)	0.0002
Alanine transaminase	39 (28–70.2)	53 (30–159)	0.02
Creatinine	1.4 (0.7–2.4)	1.8 (1.1–2.9)	0.01
INR	1.1 (1.0–1.2)	1.2 (1.1–1.5)	<0.0001
MELD score	12 (8–20)	19 (11–23)	0.0004
SOFA score	13 (11–16)	15 (13–17.7)	0.001
PRESERVE score	3 (2–5)	4 (3–6)	0.005
RESP score	1 (−2–3)	0 (−2–2)	0.04
SAPS II score at ICU admission	69 (59–80)	78 (64–90)	0.002
Predicted mortality based on median SAPS II score	82.6%	91.2%	

ICU: intensive care unit; ECMO: extracorporeal membrane oxygenation; V-V: veno-venous; V-VA: veno-venoarterial; INR: International Normalized Ratio; MELD: Model for End-Stage Liver Disease; SOFA: Sequential Organ Failure Assessment; PRESERVE: PRedicting dEath for SEvere ARDS on V-V ECMO; RESP: Respiratory ECMO Survival Prediction; SAPS II: Simplified Acute Physiology Score II.

Survivors also show a significant lower pre-ECMO bilirubin (0.6 (0.3–1.2) vs. 0.9 (0.5–1.8), $p = 0.01$), creatinine (1.4 (0.7–2.4) vs. 1.8 (1.1–2.9), $p = 0.01$), INR (1.1 (1.0–1.2) vs. 1.2 (1.1–1.5), $p < 0.0001$), aspartate (77 (38.2–146.5) vs. 143 (58.2–414), $p = 0.0002$), and alanine transaminases (39 (28–70.2) vs. 53 (30–159), $p = 0.02$), Table 1.

3.2. The Development of Acute Liver Injury

Pre-ECMO acute liver injury is observed in 8 out of 145 V-V ECMO and 6 out of 42 V-VA ECMO cases ($p = 0.09$), Figure 1. Within the first five days after ECMO initiation, acute liver injury is identified in six additional patients on V-V ECMO and ten additional patients on V-VA ECMO ($p < 0.0001$), Figure 1.

3.3. The Course of MELD Score

Prior to ECMO initiation and during the first five days on ECMO, the repeated measures analyses show a significant increase of MELD score in both V-V ECMO (F test $p < 0.0001$) and V-VA ECMO (F test $p = 0.005$) groups, Figure 2. These are associated with increased total bilirubin and creatinine within individuals over time (F-test $p < 0.0001$ for both bilirubin and creatine). The increase in creatinine is contributed to the application of continuous renal replacement therapy and, thus, the creatinine value in the MELD score calculation is set to 4.0 mg/dL.

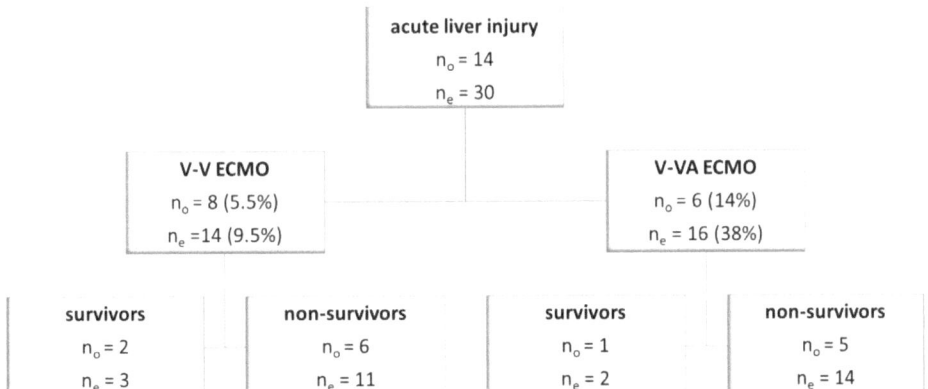

Figure 1. The prevalence of acute/hypoxic liver injury prior to ECMO initiation (n_o) and within the first five days on ECMO support (n_e).

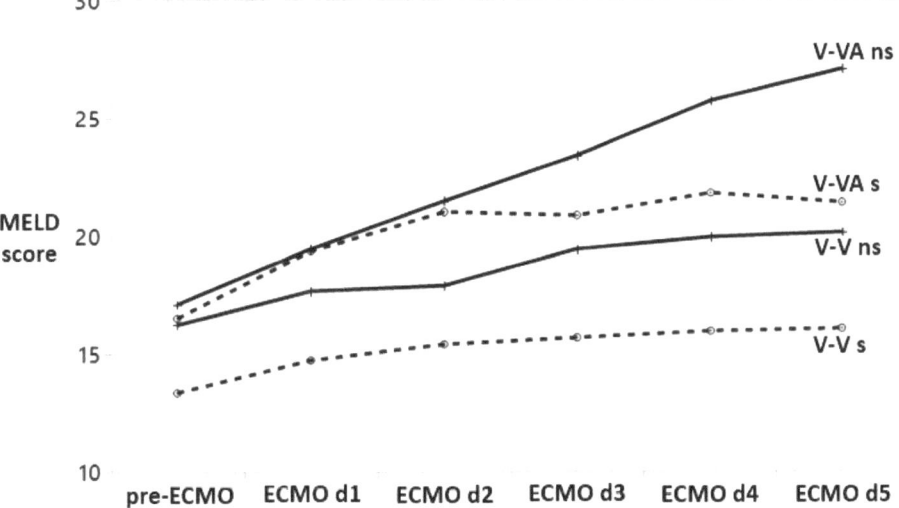

Figure 2. Repeated measures analyses of MELD scores at various assessment points. MELD values are displayed as means. Within individuals, MELD scores increase significantly over time both in V-VA ECMO (F-test $p = 0.005$) and in V-V ECMO groups (F-test $p < 0.0001$). However, in both V-V and V-VA groups, this increased MELD score does not significantly change the mortality rate over time (F-test $p = 0.2$ and $p = 0.3$, respectively). Dotted lines indicate survivors (V-V s and V-VA s); solid lines indicate nonsurvivors (V-V ns and V-VA ns).

In the V-V ECMO but not the V-VA ECMO group, there is a significant difference in pre-ECMO MELD values between nonsurvivors and survivors ($p = 0.01$). However, there is a striking increase in MELD score in V-VA ECMO nonsurvivors as compared to the V-VA ECMO survivors.

3.4. Outcome Predictors

Table 2 outlines the ability of pre-ECMO risk factors (age, sex, body-mass index, pre-ECMO cardiac failure, septic shock, chronic liver and kidney diseases, acute liver injury, levels of bilirubin, creatinine, INR, and both transaminase enzymes, as well as SAPS II at ICU admission, MELD score, and ECMO type) to predict mortality.

Table 2. The ability of pre-ECMO risk factors in predicting ICU mortality. SAPS II is calculated at ICU admission; pre-ECMO values are assessed just before ECMO initiation.

Risk Factors	Cut-Off Values	p-Values (Univariate)	AUROC	p-Values (Multivariable)
Age	60	0.06	0.58	
Male sex		0.9		
Body-Mass Index	27.7	0.4	0.60	
ECMO type (V-V or V-VA)		0.0003		0.2
Cardiac failure		0.0003		0.4
Septic shock		0.1		
Chronic liver disease		0.2		
Chronic renal disease		0.06		
Acute liver injury		0.03		0.2
Bilirubin	0.63	0.03	0.60	
Aspartate transaminase	112	0.0008	0.66	
Alanine transaminase	109	0.02	0.6	
Creatinine	1.6	0.23	0.60	
INR	1.15	<0.0001	0.69	
MELD score	16	0.0001	0.65	0.04
SOFA score	13	0.001	0.64	0.6
PRESERVE score	4	0.009	0.61	0.06
RESP score	2	0.05	0.58	0.7
SAPS II at admission	75	0.002	0.63	0.09

AUROC: Area Under the Receiver Operating Characteristic Curve; INR: International Normalized Ratio; ECMO: extracorporeal membrane oxygenation; MELD: Model for End-Stage Liver Disease; V-V: veno-venous; V-VA: veno-veno-arterial; SAPS II: Simplified Acute Physiology Score II; SOFA: Sequential Organ Failure Assessment; PRESERVE: PRedicting dEath for SEvere ARDS on V-V ECMO; RESP: Respiratory ECMO Survival Prediction.

In the univariate analysis, pre-ECMO cardiac failure, acute liver injury, bilirubin, transaminase enzymes, INR, pre-ECMO MELD, SOFA, PRESERVE and RESP scores, ECMO type, and SAPS II are related to ICU mortality. In the multivariable analysis, single laboratory values (i.e., bilirubin, creatinine, INR, aspartate, and alanine transaminase) are excluded from the analysis to avert redundancy. Here, only the pre-ECMO MELD score independently predicts ICU mortality ($p = 0.04$). The analysis shows a higher mortality in patients with a pre-ECMO MELD score greater than 16. Factors related to the pre-ECMO MELD score are summarized in Appendix A, Table A1.

3.5. The Impact of Liver Injury and a High Pre-ECMO MELD and SAPS II Scores on Outcome

According to the Cox proportional hazard model, acute liver injury occurring both before and after ECMO initiation is significantly associated with a 4.5-fold and 4.7-fold higher risk of mortality, respectively ($p < 0.0001$), Table 3. Additionally, the Cox model estimates a 1.9-fold and 2.3-fold higher mortality risk in patients with a pre-ECMO MELD score > 16 ($p = 0.002$) and SAPS II > 75 ($p = 0.0001$), Table 3.

Kaplan–Meier analyses reveal a notably higher survival probability within two months of ECMO initiation for patients who did not have pre-ECMO or developed acute liver injury during ECMO (Log-Rank $p < 0.0001$), Appendix A, Figures A1 and A2.

Table 3. Cox proportional hazard analyses of risk factors associated with ICU mortality. * during the first five days on ECMO support.

Risk Factors	Hazard Ratios (95% CI)	p Values
Pre-ECMO acute liver injury		
• all patients	4.5 (2.3–8.5)	<0.0001
• V-V ECMO	5.4 (2.3–12.9)	0.0001
• V-VA ECMO	2.4 (0.9–6.3)	0.07
Acute liver injury during ECMO *		
• all patients	4.7 (2.9–7.6)	<0.0001
• V-V ECMO	5.7 (2.9–11.2)	<0.0001
• V-VA ECMO	2.7 (1.3–5.8)	0.01
Pre-ECMO MELD score > 16		
• all patients	1.9 (1.3–3.0)	0.002
• V-V ECMO	1.7 (1.0–2.8)	0.04
• V-VA ECMO	2.6 (1.2–5.6)	0.01
SAPS II > 75		
• all patients	2.3 (1.5–3.5)	0.0001
• V-V ECMO	1.9 (1.1–3.1)	0.01
• V-VA ECMO	4 (1.8–8.6)	0.0004

V-V: veno-venous; V-VA: veno-veno-arterial; ECMO: extracorporeal membrane oxygenation; CI: confidence interval.

Irrespectively of the ECMO strategies, the Kaplan–Meier analysis shows a worse 30 days survival probability for patients with an acute liver injury, both prior to ECMO initiation (log-rank $p < 0.0001$), Figure 3 and within the first five days of ECMO support (log-rank $p < 0.0001$), Appendix A, Figure A3.

In the Cox proportional hazard model, pre-ECMO acute liver injury is associated with a 5.4 higher mortality risk in the V-V ECMO group ($p = 0.0001$); while the higher mortality risk in V-VA ECMO groups is statistically nonsignificant ($p = 0.07$), Table 3. Among patients with pre-ECMO acute liver injury, both the V-V and V-VA ECMO groups show a similar mortality risk (95% CI 0.3–3.3, $p = 1.0$).

The incidence of acute liver injury within the initial five days of V-V and V-VA ECMO correlates with a 5.7-fold and 2.7-fold increase in mortality ($p < 0.0001$ and $p = 0.01$), respectively, Table 3. Among patients with acute liver injury during ECMO, the V-V ECMO group shows a higher mortality risk than the V-VA-ECMO group; however, this difference is statistically nonsignificant (95% CI 0.5–2.6, $p = 0.7$).

The pre-ECMO MELD score is significantly lower in the V-V ECMO group than in the V-VA ECMO group (13 (8–21) vs. 17 (13.5–25), $p = 0.007$). The Kaplan–Meier analysis shows a worse 30 days survival probability for patients with a pre-ECMO MELD score greater than 16 in both V-V and V-VA ECMO groups, Figure 4.

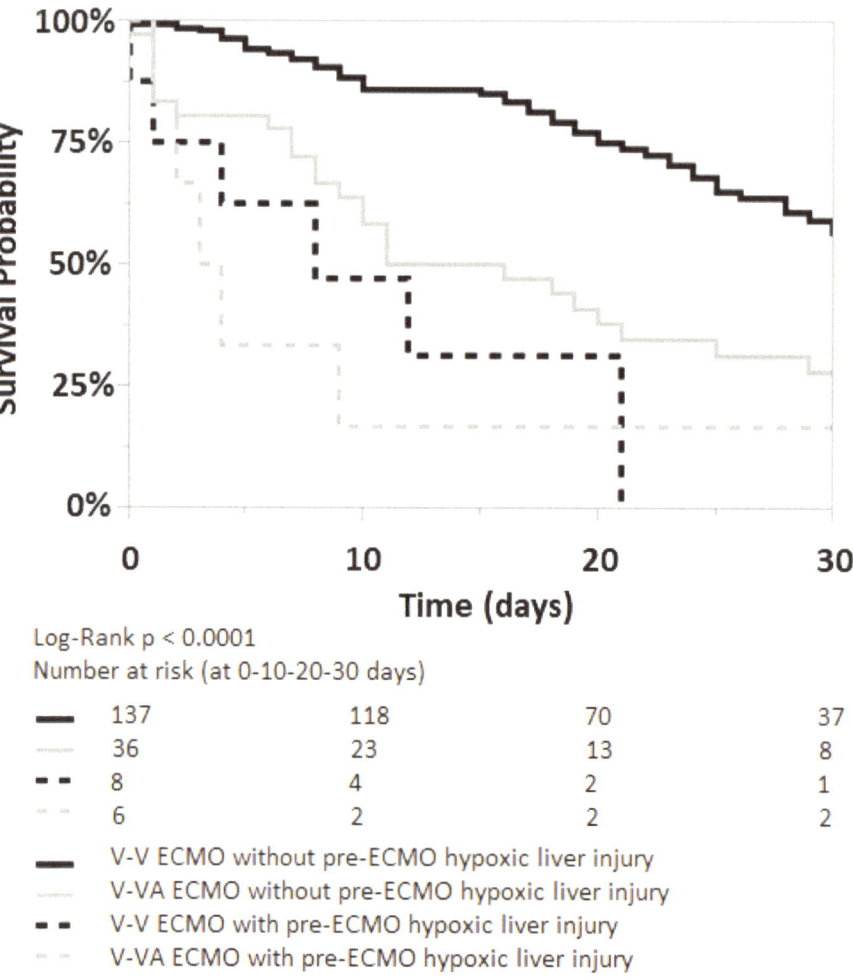

Figure 3. Kaplan–Meier curve for patients without (solid lines) and with (dotted lines) pre-ECMO acute/hypoxic liver injury; both in V-V and V-VA ECMO groups (black and grey lines, respectively). Log-Rank $p < 0.0001$.

Among patients with a pre-ECMO MELD score > 16, mortality increases by 1.7 and 2.6 times in those receiving V-V and V-VA ECMO support, respectively ($p = 0.04$ and $p = 0.0019$, Table 3. When comparing the two ECMO strategies in patients with a pre-ECMO MELD score > 16, V-VA ECMO is associated with a 2.7 times higher mortality risk compared to V-V ECMO support (95% CI 1.6–4.7, $p = 0.0003$).

In patients with a pre-ECMO SAPS II > 75, mortality increases by 1.9 times for those on V-V ECMO support ($p = 0.01$) and 4 times for those on V-VA ECMO support ($p = 0.0004$), Table 3. Here, the V-VA ECMO group demonstrates a 3.2 times higher mortality risk than the V-V ECMO group (95% CI 1.9–5.6, $p < 0.0001$).

The univariate analyses show that the requirement of V-VA ECMO support is associated with the development of acute liver injury during ECMO support ($p < 0.0001$), a higher pre-ECMO MELD score ($p = 0.01$), and a higher ICU mortality ($p = 0.0004$). However, it is not linked to a higher prevalence of pre-ECMO acute liver injury ($p = 0.09$).

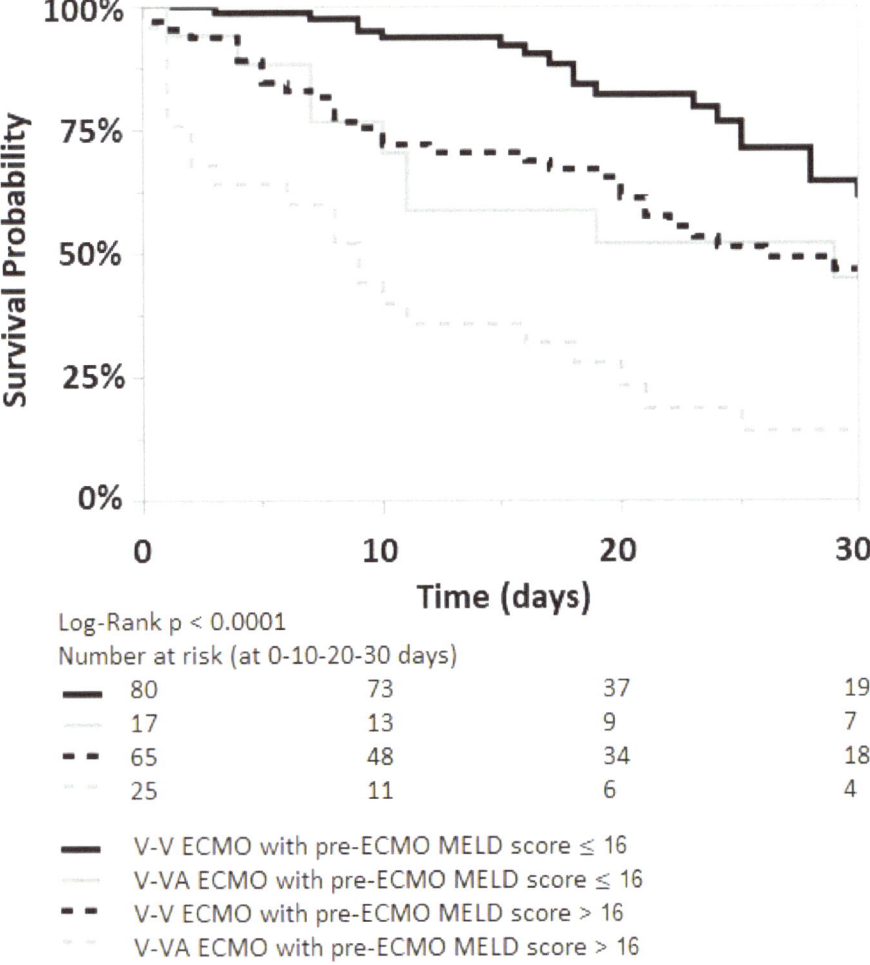

Figure 4. Kaplan–Meier curve for patients with pre-ECMO MELD score ≤ 16 (solid lines) and pre-ECMO MELD score > 16 (dotted lines); both in V-V and V-VA ECMO groups (black and grey lines, respectively). Log-Rank $p < 0.0001$.

4. Discussion

This study's main findings could be summarized as follows: (1) a significant pre-ECMO liver impairment, which is evident in the presence of pre-ECMO acute liver injury and a high pre-ECMO MELD score, is associated with increased mortality; (2) a pre-ECMO MELD score greater than 16 is an independent predictor of mortality in patients under ECMO support due to a primary respiratory failure; and (3) the requirement of V-VA ECMO support is associated with a higher pre-ECMO MELD score and increased mortality.

4.1. Acute Liver Injury

Our Cox analysis shows that the presence of pre-ECMO acute liver injury substantially increases the risk of ICU mortality. Hypoxic liver injury, also known as acute or ischemic liver injury, is characterized by a massive transaminases elevation resulting from reduced hepatic oxygen delivery or utilization [17]. Four mechanisms are potentially involved: (1) hypoxia, (2) ischemia due to hypoperfusion or hypotension, (3) hepatic venous congestion, and (4) the liver's inability to extract and utilize oxygen [16,32]. Moreover, Seeto et al. suggested that liver hypoxia and ischemia resulting from low cardiac output are not alone sufficient to cause typical hypoxic hepatitis [33]. In their analysis, 94% of patients with acute liver injury had a right ventricular dysfunction and the accompanying hepatic venous congestion [33]. All mechanisms are commonly present in patients with ARDS and the associated septic shock or acute cor pulmonale, which reflects our patient cohort under V-V and V-VA ECMO support in this study.

In our institution, V-VA ECMO is typically initiated in ARDS with either acute cor pulmonale or catecholamine-refractory septic shock [3]. Prior to ECMO cannulation, these patients show a high illness severity and already exhibit multiorgan failure. As expected, the V-VA ECMO group shows a higher prevalence of acute liver injury prior to ECMO initiation (14%) and within the first five days on ECMO support (38%), as compared to the V-V ECMO group (5.5% and 9.5%, respectively), Figure 1. Hypoxia, hypotension, and venous congestion might be addressed with V-VA ECMO. However, V-VA ECMO cannot alleviate the liver's inability to extract and utilize oxygen, which might occur in septic shock [16].

According to the findings presented in Table 3, pre-ECMO acute liver injury is associated with a significantly higher mortality risk in the V-V ECMO group. In the V-VA ECMO group, however, although the pre-ECMO transaminase levels are higher compared to the V-V group, the association between pre-ECMO acute liver injury and mortality does not reach statistical significance. This observation can be attributed to the profound hemodynamic instability in conjunction with hypoxemia prior to V-VA ECMO initiation, which contributes to mortality in V-VA patients irrespective of the presence or absence of pre-ECMO liver injury. As a result, the prognosis of patients receiving V-VA support is predominantly influenced by the severity of hemodynamic disturbance and the effectiveness of V-VA ECMO in rapidly stabilizing the cardio–circulatory system.

In this study, acute liver injury is defined as the presence of elevated serum aspartate transaminase levels exceeding 350 U/L and alanine transaminase levels surpassing 400 U/L. These thresholds, as suggested by Henrion et al., indicate transaminase levels that are more than 10 times higher than the upper limit of normal [16]. Both transaminase enzymes reach their peak levels within 24 h after a severe hemodynamic disturbance [17]. Given that the most severe hemodynamic disturbances typically occur during V-VA ECMO initiation [3], it is expected that both transaminase enzymes will reach their peak levels on the day following V-VA ECMO initiation.

Our results show that V-VA ECMO is linked to the occurrence of acute liver injury within the first five days of support (Table 3). However, among patients who develop an acute liver injury during ECMO, the V-VA ECMO group exhibits a lower mortality risk compared to the V-V ECMO group (Table 3). While this difference could be partially attributed to the ability of V-VA ECMO to stabilize hemodynamics, ensure adequate oxygen supply, and mitigate additional end-organ damage, the difference does not reach statistical significance (Table 3). Of note, our analyses include a relatively small sample size with only 42 V-VA ECMO runs. Consequently, the limited number of cases might not provide enough statistical power to establish a significant finding.

4.2. MELD Score as an Independent Outcome Predictor

MELD score is an objective metric and quickly assesses hepatic function [26]. It has a predictive value in acute liver failure [14] and has also been used widely to allocate livers for transplantation [26]. Wiesner et al. reported that without liver transplantation, patients with a MELD score < 9 experienced a 1.9% mortality at three months, whereas patients with a MELD score $\geq$ 40 had a mortality rate of 71.3% [34].

Outside of liver cirrhosis and transplants allocation, the MELD score has been proposed as a predictor of renal, hepatic, and cardiac dysfunction [13]. As the outcome of respiratory ECMO, it is associated with nonpulmonary organ dysfunction at the time of ECMO initiation [2]; our results that demonstrate the pre-ECMO MELD score as an independent outcome predictor are in line with the findings from the CESAR and EOLIA trial [1]. In our analysis, the MELD score has a superior predictive performance for mortality compared to the SOFA, PRESERVE, RESP, and SAPS II scores (Table 2). In addition, the MELD score has been shown to have prognostic value in patients with respiratory failure supported by V-V ECMO and in patients with cardiac failure who required left ventricular assist devices [8,13]. As the MELD score calculation is based solely on three readily available, routinely collected, and reproducible laboratory values (creatinine, total bilirubin, and INR), it is easy to implement in a clinical setting and independent of subjective values [25].

Watanabe reported that a MELD score greater than 12 is an independent predictor of mortality in 71 patients with respiratory failure supported with V-V ECMO [8]. Our analysis of 42 V-VA and 145 V-V ECMO cases for primary respiratory failure also shows that the pre-ECMO MELD score is associated with mortality in both univariate ($p = 0.0001$) and multivariable ($p = 0.04$) analyses. The calculated cut-off value of 16 is slightly higher than previously reported by Watanabe et al.

A Cox proportional hazard analysis shows that a pre-ECMO MELD score greater than 16 increases the hazard ratio for ICU mortality by a factor of 1.9, Table 3. Severe ARDS is commonly associated with the progressive deterioration of nonpulmonary organ functions. This nonpulmonary organ dysfunctions, such as acute liver injury and dysfunction, coagulopathy, right heart dysfunction, catecholamine-refractory septic vasoplegia, or acute kidney failure, is reflected in the higher pre-ECMO MELD score and, therefore, might explain the value of the MELD score as an independent outcome predictor in patients with severe ARDS managed with ECMO.

In line with our findings, Matthews et al. reported the association between the MELD score prior to the implantation of ventricular assist devices and the postoperative right ventricular failure, renal failure, and mortality [13]. They reported that a preoperative MELD score greater than 17 is associated with a three-fold increased odds of perioperative mortality [13].

In contrast, Sern Lim reported a reduced predictive performance of the pre-ECMO MELD excluding the INR (MELD-XI) score in patients with acute decompensated chronic left heart failure bridged with veno-arterial ECMO [35]. These patients typically exhibit cardiac congestion and sympathetic and neurohormonal activation resulting in various degrees of hepatorenal impairment [35]. The author claims that the progressive multiorgan deterioration "homogenizes" his patient cohort and might thereby reduce the discriminatory value of the pre-ECMO MELD score [35]. In our study, however, we analyzed a rather homogenous patient cohort with severe ARDS and various degrees of extrapulmonary organ dysfunction. In this population, survival depends on the extent of extrapulmonary organ dysfunction at ECMO initiation [2], which is reflected by the pre-ECMO MELD score.

As a higher MELD score reflects a higher severity of illness with established organ dysfunction, our analysis shows a significantly higher pre-ECMO MELD score in the V-VA ECMO group than in the V-V ECMO group. V-VA ECMO is used to maintain hemodynamic stability in patients with respiratory failure and a concomitant acute right heart failure or catecholamine-refractory septic shock. As patients who are supported with V-VA ECMO already had a minimum of two failing organs (pulmonary and cardiovascular) prior to ECMO initiation, hepatorenal dysfunction, which is reflected in a higher pre-ECMO MELD score, further increases the mortality risk. The Cox model estimates that, among patients with a pre-ECMO MELD score greater than 16, V-VA ECMO support has a 2.7 times higher hazard ratio of ICU mortality, as compared to the V-V ECMO.

4.3. Limitations

Our analysis is subject to the limitations inherent in a retrospective study conducted at a single center, which includes the possibility of selection bias. The relatively small sample size, especially in the V-VA ECMO group, poses challenges in achieving robust comparability for statistical analysis. It is important to acknowledge these limitations when interpreting the findings and recognizing the potential impact they may have on the generalizability of the results.

5. Conclusions

A MELD score numerically operationalizes multiorgan dysfunction. A Pre-ECMO MELD score, both as continuous and as a dichotomous variable, is an independent outcome predictor in patients with primary respiratory failure supported with V-V or V-VA ECMO. Additionally, in our analysis, the MELD score has a superior predictive performance for mortality compared to the SOFA, PRESERVE, RESP, and SAPS II scores.

Immediately prior to V-VA ECMO initiation, patients are severely debilitated, experiencing multiorgan failure involving the lungs, heart, and vasomotor system. This condition typically arises due to acute cor pulmonale or catecholamine-refractory shock. The need for V-VA ECMO support to stabilize the pulmonary and cardio–circulatory systems is linked to a higher pre-ECMO MELD score and an elevated risk of mortality.

Author Contributions: Conceptualization, S.S. and J.K.; methodology, S.S.; software, S.S.; validation, S.S. and J.K.; formal analysis, S.S. and J.K.; data curation, S.S.; writing—original draft preparation, S.S.; writing—review and editing, M.T. and J.K.; visualization, S.S.; supervision, M.T. and J.K. All authors have read and agreed to the published version of the manuscript.

Funding: This research received no external funding.

Institutional Review Board Statement: The study was conducted in accordance with the Declaration of Helsinki and approved by the Institutional Review Board (Medizinische Ethikkommission II, University Medical Centre Mannheim, Medical Faculty Mannheim of the University of Heidelberg, study registration number 2021-881, date of approval 21 September 2021) for studies involving humans.

Informed Consent Statement: Informed consent was obtained from all subjects involved in the study.

Data Availability Statement: The analyzed datasets for this study are available from the corresponding author upon reasonable request.

Conflicts of Interest: The authors declare no conflict of interest.

Appendix A. Model for End-Stage Liver Disease (MELD) Score

Appendix A.1. Factors Related to Pre-ECMO MELD Score

Table A1 summarizes factors affecting the pre-ECMO MELD score as a continued variable. In univariate analysis, age older than 60 years, male sex, SAPS II greater than 75 as well as pre-ECMO cardiac failure, septic shock, and acute liver injury are associated with pre-ECMO high MELD score. However, only male sex, SAPS II greater than 75 along with pre-ECMO septic shock and acute liver injury are linked to high pre-ECMO MELD score (p = 0.01, <0.0001, 0.0005 and 0.0005, respectively).

Table A1. Factors linked to pre-ECMO MELD score. As both creatinine and bilirubin are included in the MELD score calculation, the SOFA score, which also includes creatinine and bilirubin, is not included in the multivariable analysis. MELD: Model for End-Stage Liver Disease; SOFA: Sequential Organ Failure Assessment; PRESERVE: PRedicting dEath for SEvere ARDS on V-V ECMO; RESP: Respiratory ECMO Survival Prediction; SAPS II: Simplified Acute Physiology Score II.

Factors Affecting Pre-ECMO MELD Score	p-Values (Univariate)	p-Values (Multivariable)
Age > 60 years	0.01	0.2
Male sex	0.03	0.05
Body-Mass Index	0.4	
chronic liver disease	0.1	
chronic renal disease	0.1	
cardiac failure	0.009	0.9
septic shock	<0.0001	0.1

Table A1. Cont.

Factors Affecting Pre-ECMO MELD Score	p-Values (Univariate)	p-Values (Multivariable)
acute liver injury	<0.0001	0.005
SOFA score > 13	<0.0001	
PRESERVE score > 4	0.04	0.1
RESP score < 2	0.6	0.8
SAPS II > 75	<0.0001	<0.0001

High pre-ECMO MELD score is also associated with the development of (1) acute liver injury during the first five days on ECMO (MELD cut-off value 21, $p < 0.0001$, AUROC 0.80) and (2) acute kidney failure which required continuous renal replacement therapy (MELD cut-off value 10, $p < 0.0001$, AUROC 0.77).

Appendix A.2. The Impact of Pre-ECMO Acute/Hypoxic Liver Injury

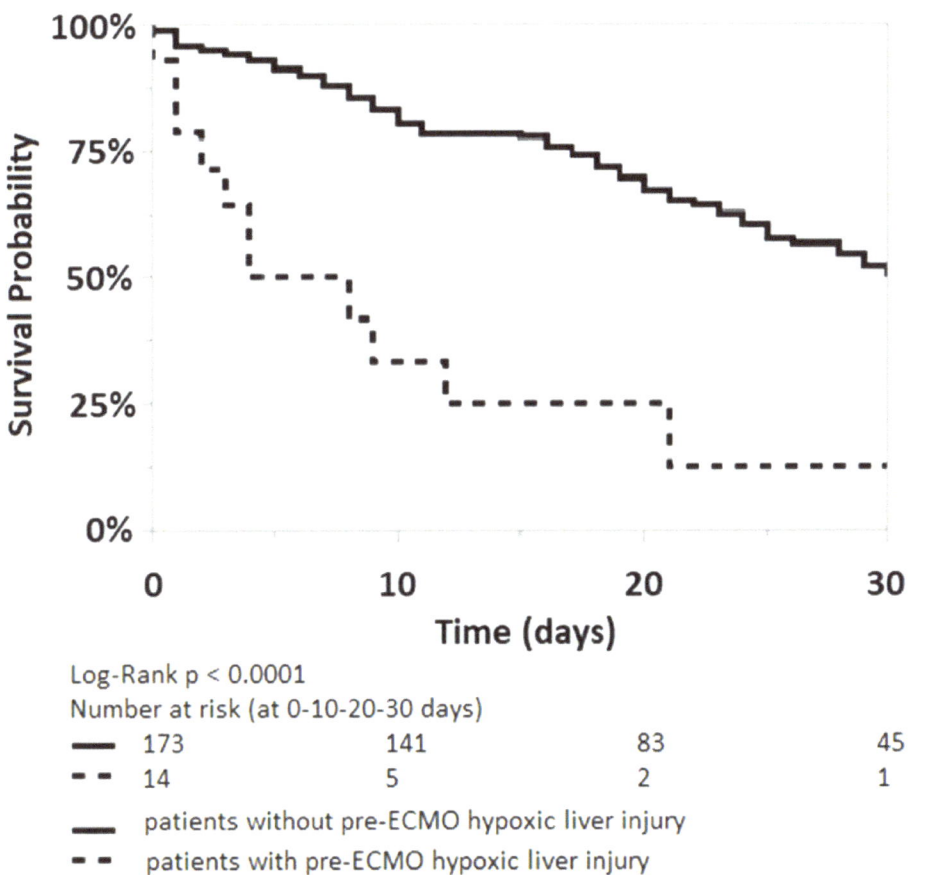

Figure A1. Kaplan–Meier curve for patients without (solid lines) and with (dotted lines) pre-ECMO acute/hypoxic liver injury.

Appendix A.3. The Impact of Acute/Hypoxic Liver Injury during the First Five Days on ECMO

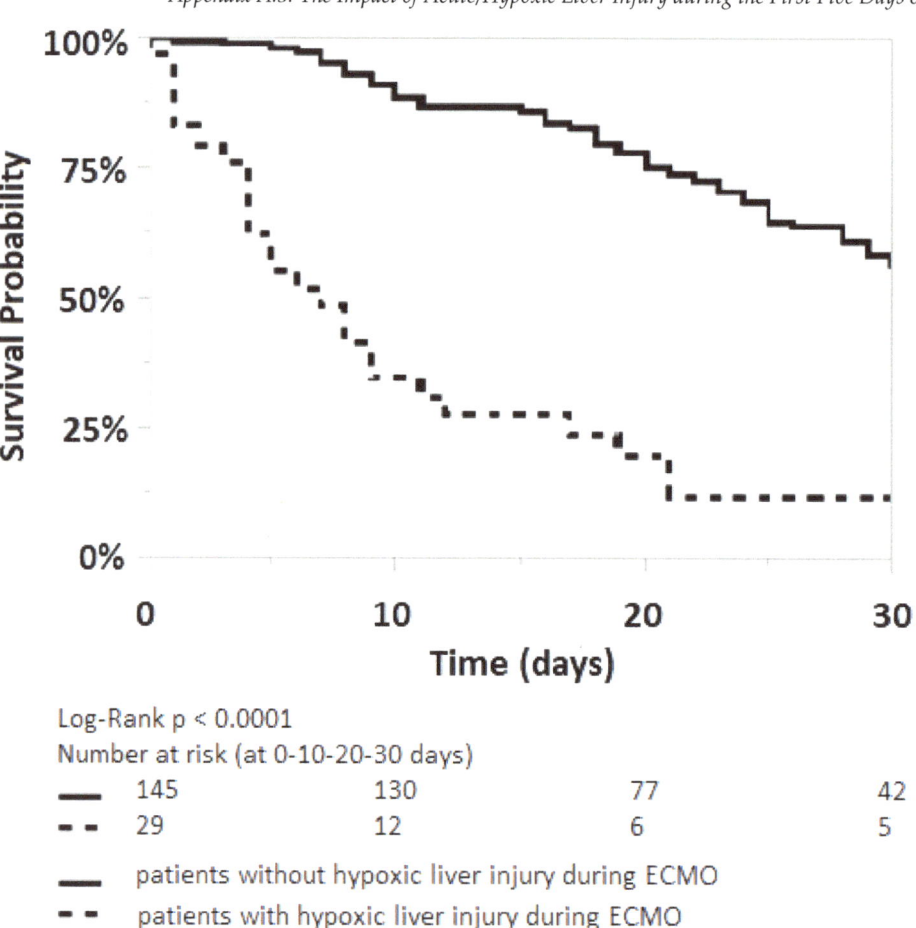

Figure A2. Kaplan–Meier curve for patients without (solid lines) and with (dotted lines) acute/hypoxic liver injury during the first five days on ECMO.

Appendix A.4. The Impact of V-V and V-VA ECMO Strategies in Patients with Acute Liver Injury

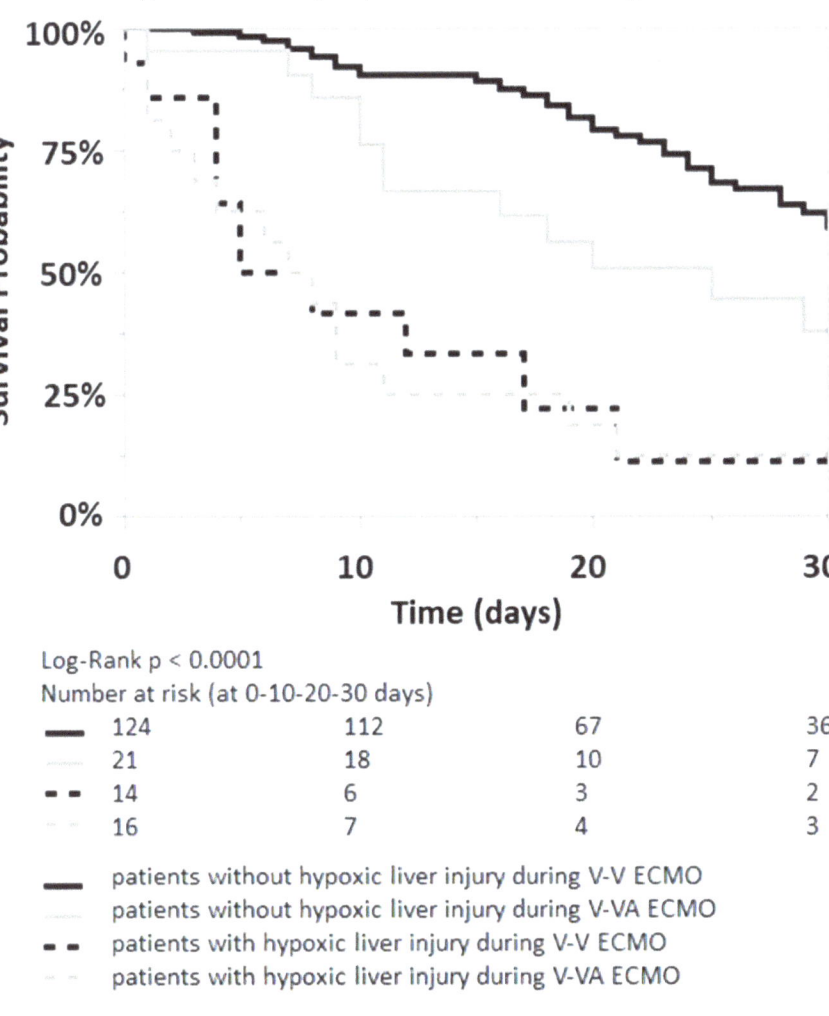

Figure A3. Kaplan–Meier curve for patients who did not develop (solid lines) and who developed (dotted lines) acute/hypoxic liver injury within the first five days on ECMO; both in V-V and V-VA ECMO groups (black and grey lines, respectively). Log-Rank $p < 0.0001$.

References

1. Combes, A.; Peek, G.J.; Hajage, D.; Hardy, P.; Abrams, D.; Schmidt, M.; Dechartres, A.; Elbourne, D. ECMO for severe ARDS: Systematic review and individual patient data meta-analysis. *Intensive Care Med.* **2020**, *46*, 2048–2057. [CrossRef]
2. Pappalardo, F.; Pieri, M.; Greco, T.; Patroniti, N.; Pesenti, A.; Arcadipane, A.; Ranieri, V.M.; Gattinoni, L.; Landoni, G.; Holzgraefe, B.; et al. Predicting mortality risk in patients undergoing venovenous ECMO for ARDS due to influenza A (H_1N_1) pneumonia: The ECMOnet score. *Intensive Care Med.* **2013**, *39*, 275–281. [CrossRef]
3. Sandrio, S.; Krebs, J.; Leonardy, E.; Thiel, M.; Schoettler, J.J. Vasoactive Inotropic Score as a Prognostic Factor during (Cardio-) Respiratory ECMO. *J. Clin. Med.* **2022**, *11*, 2390. [CrossRef]
4. Guerin, C.; Reignier, J.; Richard, J.C.; Beuret, P.; Gacouin, A.; Boulain, T.; Mercier, E.; Badet, M.; Mercat, A.; Baudin, O.; et al. Prone positioning in severe acute respiratory distress syndrome. *N. Engl. J. Med.* **2013**, *368*, 2159–2168. [CrossRef]
5. Combes, A.; Hajage, D.; Capellier, G.; Demoule, A.; Lavoue, S.; Guervilly, C.; Da Silva, D.; Zafrani, L.; Tirot, P.; Veber, B.; et al. Extracorporeal Membrane Oxygenation for Severe Acute Respiratory Distress Syndrome. *N. Engl. J. Med.* **2018**, *378*, 1965–1975. [CrossRef]

6. Peek, G.J.; Mugford, M.; Tiruvoipati, R.; Wilson, A.; Allen, E.; Thalanany, M.M.; Hibbert, C.L.; Truesdale, A.; Clemens, F.; Cooper, N.; et al. Efficacy and economic assessment of conventional ventilatory support versus extracorporeal membrane oxygenation for severe adult respiratory failure (CESAR): A multicentre randomised controlled trial. *Lancet* **2009**, *374*, 1351–1363. [CrossRef]
7. Kallet, R.H.; Lipnick, M.S.; Zhuo, H.; Pangilinan, L.P.; Gomez, A. Characteristics of Nonpulmonary Organ Dysfunction at Onset of ARDS Based on the Berlin Definition. *Respir. Care* **2019**, *64*, 493–501. [CrossRef] [PubMed]
8. Watanabe, S.; Kurihara, C.; Manerikar, A.; Thakkar, S.; Saine, M.; Bharat, A. MELD Score Predicts Outcomes in Patients Undergoing Venovenous Extracorporeal Membrane Oxygenation. *ASAIO J.* **2020**, *67*, 871–877. [CrossRef]
9. Lazzeri, C.; Bonizzoli, M.; Cianchi, G.; Batacchi, S.; Chiostri, M.; Fulceri, G.E.; Buoninsegni, L.T.; Peris, A. Bilirubin in the early course of venovenous extracorporeal membrane oxygenation support for refractory ARDS. *J. Artif. Organs* **2018**, *21*, 61–67. [CrossRef]
10. Masha, L.; Peerbhai, S.; Boone, D.; Shobayo, F.; Ghotra, A.; Akkanti, B.; Zhao, Y.; Banjac, I.; Gregoric, I.D.; Kar, B. Yellow Means Caution: Correlations Between Liver Injury and Mortality with the Use of VA-ECMO. *ASAIO J.* **2019**, *65*, 812–818. [CrossRef]
11. Schmidt, M.; Burrell, A.; Roberts, L.; Bailey, M.; Sheldrake, J.; Rycus, P.T.; Hodgson, C.; Scheinkestel, C.; Cooper, D.J.; Thiagarajan, R.R.; et al. Predicting survival after ECMO for refractory cardiogenic shock: The survival after veno-arterial-ECMO (SAVE)-score. *Eur. Heart J.* **2015**, *36*, 2246–2256. [CrossRef]
12. Lescot, T.; Karvellas, C.; Beaussier, M.; Magder, S. Acquired liver injury in the intensive care unit. *Anesthesiology* **2012**, *117*, 898–904. [CrossRef]
13. Matthews, J.C.; Pagani, F.D.; Haft, J.W.; Koelling, T.M.; Naftel, D.C.; Aaronson, K.D. Model for end-stage liver disease score predicts left ventricular assist device operative transfusion requirements, morbidity, and mortality. *Circulation* **2010**, *121*, 214–220. [CrossRef]
14. Kamath, P.S.; Heimbach, J.; Wiesner, R.H. Acute Liver Failure Prognostic Scores: Is Good Enough Good Enough? *Clin. Gastroenterol. Hepatol.* **2016**, *14*, 621–623. [CrossRef]
15. Ayers, B.; Wood, K.; Melvin, A.; Prasad, S.; Gosev, I. MELD-XI is predictive of mortality in venoarterial extracorporeal membrane oxygenation. *J. Card Surg.* **2020**, *35*, 1275–1282. [CrossRef]
16. Henrion, J.; Schapira, M.; Luwaert, R.; Colin, L.; Delannoy, A.; Heller, F.R. Hypoxic hepatitis: Clinical and hemodynamic study in 142 consecutive cases. *Medicine* **2003**, *82*, 392–406. [CrossRef]
17. Waseem, N.; Chen, P.H. Hypoxic Hepatitis: A Review and Clinical Update. *J. Clin. Transl. Hepatol.* **2016**, *4*, 263–268. [CrossRef] [PubMed]
18. Mekontso Dessap, A.; Boissier, F.; Charron, C.; Begot, E.; Repesse, X.; Legras, A.; Brun-Buisson, C.; Vignon, P.; Vieillard-Baron, A. Acute cor pulmonale during protective ventilation for acute respiratory distress syndrome: Prevalence, predictors, and clinical impact. *Intensive Care Med.* **2016**, *42*, 862–870. [CrossRef] [PubMed]
19. Ling, R.R.; Ramanathan, K.; Poon, W.H.; Tan, C.S.; Brechot, N.; Brodie, D.; Combes, A.; MacLaren, G. Venoarterial extracorporeal membrane oxygenation as mechanical circulatory support in adult septic shock: A systematic review and meta-analysis with individual participant data meta-regression analysis. *Crit. Care* **2021**, *25*, 246. [CrossRef] [PubMed]
20. Kon, Z.N.; Bittle, G.J.; Pasrija, C.; Pham, S.M.; Mazzeffi, M.A.; Herr, D.L.; Sanchez, P.G.; Griffith, B.P. Venovenous Versus Venoarterial Extracorporeal Membrane Oxygenation for Adult Patients With Acute Respiratory Distress Syndrome Requiring Precannulation Hemodynamic Support: A Review of the ELSO Registry. *Ann. Thorac. Surg.* **2017**, *104*, 645–649. [CrossRef]
21. Vogel, D.J.; Murray, J.; Czapran, A.Z.; Camporota, L.; Ioannou, N.; Meadows, C.I.S.; Sherren, P.B.; Daly, K.; Gooby, N.; Barrett, N. Veno-arterio-venous ECMO for septic cardiomyopathy: A single-centre experience. *Perfusion* **2018**, *33*, 57–64. [CrossRef] [PubMed]
22. Ius, F.; Sommer, W.; Tudorache, I.; Avsar, M.; Siemeni, T.; Salman, J.; Puntigam, J.; Optenhoefel, J.; Greer, M.; Welte, T.; et al. Veno-veno-arterial extracorporeal membrane oxygenation for respiratory failure with severe haemodynamic impairment: Technique and early outcomes. *Interact. Cardiovasc. Thorac. Surg.* **2015**, *20*, 761–767. [CrossRef] [PubMed]
23. Stohr, F.; Emmert, M.Y.; Lachat, M.L.; Stocker, R.; Maggiorini, M.; Falk, V.; Wilhelm, M.J. Extracorporeal membrane oxygenation for acute respiratory distress syndrome: Is the configuration mode an important predictor for the outcome? *Interact. Cardiovasc. Thorac. Surg.* **2011**, *12*, 676–680. [CrossRef] [PubMed]
24. Grasselli, G.; Calfee, C.S.; Camporota, L.; Poole, D.; Amato, M.B.P.; Antonelli, M.; Arabi, Y.M.; Baroncelli, F.; Beitler, J.R.; Bellani, G.; et al. ESICM guidelines on acute respiratory distress syndrome: Definition, phenotyping and respiratory support strategies. *Intensive Care Med.* **2023**, *49*, 727–759. [CrossRef]
25. OPTN Policies. Available online: https://optn.transplant.hrsa.gov/media/eavh5bf3/optn_policies.pdf (accessed on 27 November 2022).
26. Organ Procurement and Transplantation Network, L.a.I.O.T.C. Clerical Changes for Implementation of Adding Serum Sodium to the MELD Score. Available online: https://optn.transplant.hrsa.gov/media/1575/policynotice_20151101.pdf (accessed on 27 November 2022).
27. Kamath, P.S. MELD Score (Model for End-Stage Liver Disease) (12 and Older). Available online: https://www.mdcalc.com/meld-score-model-end-stage-liver-disease-12-older (accessed on 1 November 2022).
28. Le Gall, J.R.; Lemeshow, S.; Saulnier, F. A new Simplified Acute Physiology Score (SAPS II) based on a European/North American multicenter study. *JAMA* **1993**, *270*, 2957–2963. [CrossRef]

29. Schmidt, M.; Bailey, M.; Sheldrake, J.; Hodgson, C.; Aubron, C.; Rycus, P.T.; Scheinkestel, C.; Cooper, D.J.; Brodie, D.; Pellegrino, V.; et al. Predicting survival after extracorporeal membrane oxygenation for severe acute respiratory failure. The Respiratory Extracorporeal Membrane Oxygenation Survival Prediction (RESP) score. *Am. J. Respir. Crit. Care Med.* **2014**, *189*, 1374–1382. [CrossRef]
30. Schmidt, M.; Zogheib, E.; Roze, H.; Repesse, X.; Lebreton, G.; Luyt, C.E.; Trouillet, J.L.; Brechot, N.; Nieszkowska, A.; Dupont, H.; et al. The PRESERVE mortality risk score and analysis of long-term outcomes after extracorporeal membrane oxygenation for severe acute respiratory distress syndrome. *Intensive Care Med.* **2013**, *39*, 1704–1713. [CrossRef]
31. Vincent, J.L.; Moreno, R.; Takala, J.; Willatts, S.; De Mendonca, A.; Bruining, H.; Reinhart, C.K.; Suter, P.M.; Thijs, L.G. The SOFA (Sepsis-related Organ Failure Assessment) score to describe organ dysfunction/failure. *Intensive Care Med.* **1996**, *22*, 707–710. [CrossRef]
32. Ucgun, I.; Ozakyol, A.; Metintas, M.; Moral, H.; Orman, A.; Bal, C.; Yildirim, H. Relationship between hypoxic hepatitis and cor pulmonale in patients treated in the respiratory ICU. *Int. J. Clin. Pract.* **2005**, *59*, 1295–1300. [CrossRef]
33. Seeto, R.K.; Fenn, B.; Rockey, D.C. Ischemic hepatitis: Clinical presentation and pathogenesis. *Am. J. Med.* **2000**, *109*, 109–113. [CrossRef]
34. Wiesner, R.; Edwards, E.; Freeman, R.; Harper, A.; Kim, R.; Kamath, P.; Kremers, W.; Lake, J.; Howard, T.; Merion, R.M.; et al. Model for end-stage liver disease (MELD) and allocation of donor livers. *Gastroenterology* **2003**, *124*, 91–96. [CrossRef] [PubMed]
35. Sern Lim, H. Baseline MELD-XI score and outcome from veno-arterial extracorporeal membrane oxygenation support for acute decompensated heart failure. *Eur. Heart J. Acute Cardiovasc. Care* **2016**, *5*, 82–88. [CrossRef] [PubMed]

Disclaimer/Publisher's Note: The statements, opinions and data contained in all publications are solely those of the individual author(s) and contributor(s) and not of MDPI and/or the editor(s). MDPI and/or the editor(s) disclaim responsibility for any injury to people or property resulting from any ideas, methods, instructions or products referred to in the content.

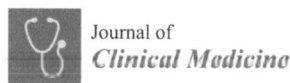

Article

Response to Prone Position in COVID-19 and Non-COVID-19 Patients with Severe ARDS Supported by vvECMO

Laura Textoris [1], Ines Gragueb-Chatti [1], Florence Daviet [1], Sabine Valera [1], Céline Sanz [1], Laurent Papazian [1,2], Jean-Marie Forel [1,3], Sami Hraiech [1,3], Antoine Roch [1,3] and Christophe Guervilly [1,3,*]

[1] Service de Médecine Intensive Réanimation, Hôpital Nord, Assistance Publique-Hôpitaux de Marseille, 13015 Marseille, France; laura.textoris@ap-hm.fr (L.T.); ines.gragueb-chatti@ap-hm.fr (I.G.-C.); florence.daviet@ap-hm.fr (F.D.); sabine.valera@ap-hm.fr (S.V.); celine.sanz@ap-hm.fr (C.S.); laurent.papazian.pro@gmail.com (L.P.); jean-marie.forel@ap-hm.fr (J.-M.F.); sami.hraiech@ap-hm.fr (S.H.); antoine.roch@ap-hm.fr (A.R.)

[2] Centre Hospitalier de Bastia, Service de Réanimation, 604 Chemin de Falconaja, 20600 Bastia, France

[3] Centre d'Études et de Recherches sur les Services de Santé et Qualité de vie EA 3279, Aix-Marseille Université, 13005 Marseille, France

* Correspondence: christophe.guervilly@ap-hm.fr; Tel.: +33-491-965-842; Fax: +33-491-965-837

Abstract: Background: For moderate to severe acute respiratory distress syndrome (ARDS), lung-protective ventilation combined with prolonged and repeated prone position (PP) is recommended. For the most severe patients for whom this strategy failed, venovenous extracorporeal membrane oxygenation (vv-ECMO) allows a reduction in ventilation-induced lung injury and improves survival. Some aggregated data have suggested a benefit regarding survival in pursuing PP during vv-ECMO. The combination of PP and vv-ECMO has been also documented in COVID-19 studies, although there is scarce evidence concerning respiratory mechanics and gas exchange response. The main objective was to compare the physiological response of the first PP during vv-ECMO in two cohorts of patients (COVID-19-related ARDS and non-COVID-19 ARDS) regarding respiratory system compliance (C_{RS}) and oxygenation changes. Methods: This was a single-center, retrospective, and ambispective cohort study in the ECMO center of Marseille, France. ECMO was indicated according to the EOLIA trial criteria. Results: A total of 85 patients were included, 60 in the non-COVID-19 ARDS group and 25 in the COVID-19-related ARDS group. Lung injuries of the COVID-19 cohort exhibited significantly higher severity with a lower C_{RS} at baseline. Concerning the main objective, the first PP during vv-ECMO was not associated with a change in C_{RS} or other variation in respiratory mechanic variables in both cohorts. By contrast, oxygenation was improved only in the non-COVID-19 ARDS group after a return to the supine position. Mean arterial pressure was higher during PP as compared with a return to the supine position in the COVID-19 group. Conclusion: We found distinct physiological responses to the first PP in vv-ECMO-supported ARDS patients according to the COVID-19 etiology. This could be due to higher severity at baseline or specificity of the disease. Further investigations are warranted.

Keywords: COVID-19; severe ARDS; venovenous ECMO; prone position; respiratory system compliance

Citation: Textoris, L.; Gragueb-Chatti, I.; Daviet, F.; Valera, S.; Sanz, C.; Papazian, L.; Forel, J.-M.; Hraiech, S.; Roch, A.; Guervilly, C. Response to Prone Position in COVID-19 and Non-COVID-19 Patients with Severe ARDS Supported by vvECMO. *J. Clin. Med.* **2023**, *12*, 3918. https://doi.org/10.3390/jcm12123918

Academic Editors: Paolo Pelosi and Denise Battaglini

Received: 23 May 2023
Revised: 2 June 2023
Accepted: 6 June 2023
Published: 8 June 2023

Copyright: © 2023 by the authors. Licensee MDPI, Basel, Switzerland. This article is an open access article distributed under the terms and conditions of the Creative Commons Attribution (CC BY) license (https://creativecommons.org/licenses/by/4.0/).

1. Introduction

Acute respiratory distress syndrome (ARDS) is an acute respiratory failure that is classified into three stages of severity according to the Berlin definition [1]. For moderate-to-severe ARDS, lung-protective ventilation which includes a low tidal volume (V_t)–low plateau pressure (P_{plat}) ventilation strategy combined with prolonged and repeated prone position (PP) is recommended [2].

Venovenous extracorporeal membrane oxygenation (vv-ECMO) allows decreasing V_t, airway inspiratory pressures, and the respiratory rate (RR), which all individually can induce or worsen ventilator-induced lung injuries (VILIs) [3,4]. For the most severe ARDS patients for whom the combination of lung-protective ventilation combined with PP failed, the early initiation of vv-ECMO increased survival [5].

In addition, retrospective aggregated data suggest a potential benefit of continuation or initiation of PP in vv-ECMO patients.

In December 2019, a new virus emerged in the region of Wuhan in China, the severe acute respiratory syndrome coronavirus 2 (SARS-CoV-2) which was responsible for the global pandemic of coronavirus disease 2019 (COVID-19) [6]. Although most patients infected by COVID-19 present mild or moderate symptoms, about 10% will need hospitalization and 1.5% will require intensive care unit (ICU) hospitalization. Among them, around 70% need respiratory support for acute respiratory failure. vv-ECMO has been increasingly used during the first wave of the pandemic and thereafter [7].

Interestingly, some observational cohorts report a very high rate of PP use (up to 70–90%) during vv-ECMO [8–10].

Therefore, the aim of the study was to compare the physiological response of PP between two cohorts of severe ARDS patients (COVID-19-related ARDS and non-COVID-19 ARDS) supported by vv-ECMO.

2. Materials and Methods

2.1. Study Design and Ethics Approval

We performed a single-center, retrospective, and ambispective cohort study. The study protocol was reviewed and approved by the Marseille Teaching Hospital Institutional Review Board (PADS21-89) and by the ethics committee of the French intensive care society (CE SRLF 21-47). According to French law, informed consent was not required due to the design of the study, and we only collected the non-opposition form from the patient or their surrogate.

2.2. Study Settings

All patients included were in a tertiary university hospital in Marseille, France. Patients were cannulated either directly in the department or in another ICU in the Provence-Alpes-Côtes-d'Azur region and immediately transferred by the vv-ECMO mobile retrieval team [11].

2.3. Population

The non-COVID-19 cohort was built from a previous study [12]. Only patients with available physiological data were included in the cohort. The ambispective cohort included consecutive COVID-19 patients hospitalized between 1 January 2021 and 31 December 2021 and supported by vv-ECMO. The first patient was included on 2 February 2021, and the last patient was included on 11 November 2021.

vv-ECMO was indicated according to the EOLIA trial criteria, either refractory hypoxemia defined by a ratio of partial pressure of arterial oxygen to fraction of inspired oxygen (PaO_2:FiO_2 ratio) < 50 mmHg for at least 3 h or a PaO_2:FiO_2 ratio < 80 mmHg for at least 6 h despite a $FiO_2 \geq 80\%$ and a positive end-expiratory pressure (PEEP) ≥ 10 cm H_2O, or respiratory acidosis with arterial blood pH < 7.25 with a partial pressure of arterial carbon dioxide (PaCO2) > 60 mmHg for > 6 h (with RR increased to 35 cycles/minute) resulting from mechanical ventilation settings adjusted to keep $P_{plat} \leq 32$ cm H_2O (first, V_t reduction by 1 mL/kg decrements to 4 mL/kg; then, PEEP reduction to a minimum of 8 cm H_2O) [5].

2.4. Primary and Secondary Endpoints

The primary endpoint was the change in the respiratory system compliance and oxygenation between the start and the end of the first PP session during vv-ECMO in the two cohorts (COVID-19 and non-COVID-19 patients).

Secondary endpoints were the changes in other respiratory mechanics variables, arterial blood gas and ECMO settings during the same time frame, safety assessment of the first PP, and clinical outcomes in the two cohorts.

2.5. vv-ECMO Management

All the patients were cannulated using a percutaneous approach. The oxygen fraction delivered by the membrane oxygenator (FmO_2, %) was set at 100. Then, the sweep gas flow was progressively increased to reach an arterial pH value above 7.30. The vv-ECMO blood flow was progressively increased to obtain a pulsed oxygen saturation (SpO_2) > 90% (or PaO_2 > 60 mmHg) and to reach at least 60 % of the actual cardiac output. Anticoagulation with intravenous unfractionated heparin was used to target an anti-Xa activity between 0.3 and 0.6 IU/mL. The triggering limit for transfusion was 8 g/dL for hemoglobin, 50 Giga/L for platelet, and 1.5 g/L for fibrinogen. Hemolysis was also investigated daily during the vv-ECMO run.

2.6. Mechanical Ventilation Protocol during vv-ECMO

Volume-controlled with constant flow mode was first used. V_t was set to obtain a maximum P_{plat} of 25 cm H_2O while PEEP was kept above 10 cm H_2O. RR was decreased between 10 and 15 cycles/min. Continuous perfusion of neuromuscular blockers was pursued for 48 h after cannulation.

In case of the early improvement of respiratory function or after 48 h, a switch to partial assisted pressure-controlled mode as airway pressure release ventilation (APRV) or bi-level positive airway pressure (Bi-PAP) was encouraged after interruption of neuromuscular blockers.

2.7. Prone Position Procedure

All included patients received at least one 16 h session of PP during the vv-ECMO run. The ICU team followed a written protocol for each maneuver including eye occlusion protection and protection of skin from all catheters and invasive devices (vv-ECMO cannulas, tubing, thoracic drain, and bladder probe). The intensivists in charge of the patient stood at the head to hold the intubation tube and jugular cannula in place. Two people stood on either side of the patient. A fifth person secured vv-ECMO tubing and prevented any dislodgment of vv-ECMO cannulas. Two specific air mattresses were then placed on the patient's head, thorax, and hips to prevent pressure sores.

2.8. Data Collection

Demographics (gender, age, weight, height, BMI, comorbidities) and severity scores were recorded at the inclusion.

Before vv-ECMO, data on duration of mechanical ventilation, worse PaO_2:FiO_2 ratio, use and number of PP sessions, administration of inhaled nitric oxide (iNO), and eventual renal replacement therapy were collected.

The date of cannulation, vv-ECMO configuration, and number of PP sessions on vv-ECMO were also recorded. We computed the duration of vv-ECMO, vv-ECMO weaning rate, and ICU and hospital mortality rates as outcomes.

Concerning respiratory mechanics variables, we recorded V_t (mL), RR (cycles/min), minute ventilation (V_M, L/min), PEEP (cm H_2O), peak inspiratory pressure (P_{peak}, cm H_2O), and FiO_2 (%) for each patient. At the same time, we measured P_{plat} (cm H_2O) by using an inspiratory pause (1 s) and calculated the compliance of the respiratory system (C_{RS}, mL/cm H_2O) by dividing V_t by the difference between P_{plat} and total PEEP, measured by using an expiratory pause (5 s), also called driving pressure ($\Delta P = P_{plat} - PEEP_{total}$, cm H_2O). Mechanical power (MP, J/min) was only available in COVID-19 patients and was calculated as follows:

$$MP = 0.098 \times Vt(L) \times RR(c/min) \times \left(Ppeak - \frac{\Delta P}{2}\right) (cm\ H_2O)$$

with 0.098 the conversion factor from L/cm H_2O to joules [13].

For the COVID-19 ambispective cohort, we collected additional data. One hour before (H-1 PP) and one hour after the PP (H+1 PP), and one hour before the supine position (H-1

SP) and one hour after (H+1 SP), we recorded hemodynamic parameters (heart rate and mean arterial pressure), arterial blood gas (pH, PaO_2, $PaCO_2$, saturation of arterial oxygen (SaO_2), PaO_2:FiO_2 ratio), ventilator parameters (V_t, RR, PEEP, P_{peak}, P_{plat}, V_M, FiO_2, and C_{RS}), and vv-ECMO parameters (vv-ECMO blood flow, sweep gas, and FmO_2).

2.9. Assessment of Safety of Prone Position

In the COVID-19 cohort, we recorded and compared pre-specified adverse events potentially associated with PP maneuvers, including severe hypoxemia (SpO_2 < 80% for at least 5 min), decrease in vv-ECMO blood flow > 20% of baseline; mean arterial pressure < 55 mmHg for at least 5 min; pneumothorax; tracheal tube obstruction; and vv-ECMO cannula, intravenous catheter, or endotracheal tube dislodgment.

2.10. Statistical Analysis

No sample size was calculated. However, we planned to include 25 patients in the COVID-19 ambispective cohort. For the non-COVID-19 retrospective cohort, we extracted available data of interest from a previous study [12].

Qualitative variables were expressed as numbers and percentages. Comparisons between groups were performed with the chi^2 test or Fisher test as appropriate.

Quantitative variables were expressed as median (interquartile range) or mean ± standard deviation. Comparisons between groups were performed with the U Mann–Whitney test or the Student t test as appropriate.

Comparisons between times were performed with the Kruskal–Wallis test or with ANOVA as appropriate. Post hoc tests were performed with the Tukey and Bonferroni tests.

A p value < 0.05 was considered as significant.

All statistics were calculated and figures were created with SPSS 20.0 (IBM, Armonk, NY, USA).

3. Results

Eighty-five patients were included, 60 in the non-COVID-19 ARDS cohort and 25 in the COVID-19 ARDS cohort.

3.1. Baseline Characteristics and Outcomes

The baseline characteristics of the two cohorts are displayed in Table 1.

Table 1. Baseline characteristics of the two cohorts.

	COVID-19 ARDS N = 25	Non-COVID-19 ARDS N = 60	p Value
Age, median (IQR)	55 (45–61)	51 (38–64)	0.79
Male sex, n (%)	18 (72)	44 (74)	0.80
Body mass index (kg/m^2), median (IQR)	30 (27.6–35.2)	28.7 (25.5–35.4)	0.38
SAPS 2 at admission, median (IQR)	41 (31–49)	47 (42–55)	0.006
SOFA score at inclusion, median (IQR)	7 (4–9)	10 (8–12)	0.001
Cause of ARDS			
COVID-19	25 (100)	0 (0)	
Viral non-COVID-19	0 (0)	13 (22)	
Bacterial	0 (0)	35 (58)	<0.001
Aspiration	0 (0)	2 (3.5)	
Pulmonary—others	0 (0)	8 (13)	
Extrapulmonary sepsis	0 (0)	2 (3.5)	
Comorbidity, n (%)			
Immunocompromised	3 (12)	0 (0)	0.07
Hypertension	11 (44)	14 (24)	0.06
Diabetes mellitus	4 (16)	8 (14)	0.77
Chronic renal failure	1 (4)	2 (3.5)	0.89
Chronic obstructive pulmonary disease	7 (28)	11 (19)	0.34

Table 1. Cont.

	COVID-19 ARDS N = 25	Non-COVID-19 ARDS N = 60	p Value
Before vv-ECMO			
Duration of mechanical ventilation, median (IQR)	5 (1–7)	3 (1–7)	0.47
Prone position, n (%)	25 (100)	44 (74)	0.005
Inhaled nitric oxide, n (%)	20 (80)	26 (44)	0.002
PaO$_2$:FiO$_2$ ratio, mmHg, median (IQR)	68 (50–74)	66 (50–81)	0.93
Renal replacement therapy, n (%)	1 (4)	2 (3.5)	0.89
Referred from other ICUs, n (%)	24 (96)	56 (95)	0.83
Retrieved by vv-ECMO mobile team, n (%)	21 (84)	48 (81)	0.77
vv-ECMO configuration, n (%)			
Femoro-jugular	25 (100)	55 (92)	
Femoro-femoral	0 (0)	4 (7)	0.32
Jugulo-jugular	0 (0)	1 (1)	
Outcomes			
ECMO days before PP, median (IQR)	2 (1–3)	5 (3–7)	<0.001
Number of PP sessions on vv-ECMO, median (IQR)	4 (3–6)	2 (1–4)	<0.001
vv-ECMO duration, days, median (IQR)	23 (15–34)	20 (13–36)	0.75
vv-ECMO weaning rate, n (%)	18 (72)	38 (64)	0.50
ICU mortality rate, n (%)	12 (48)	32 (54)	0.60
Hospital mortality rate, n (%)	12 (48)	36 (61)	0.27

Definition of abbreviations: IQR = interquartile range; SAPS 2 = simplified acute physiology score; SOFA = sequential organ failure assessment score; ARDS = acute respiratory distress syndrome; COVID-19 = coronavirus disease 2019; vv-ECMO = venovenous extracorporeal membrane oxygenation; PP = prone position; PaO$_2$:FiO$_2$ ratio = ratio of the partial pressure of arterial oxygen to the fraction of inspired oxygen; ICU = intensive care unit.

Besides obvious differences in ARDS etiology, the non-COVID-19 ARDS cohort had higher severity scores and less frequently received adjunctive therapy (PP or iNO) before vv-ECMO implantation as compared with the COVID-19 ARDS group.

In the COVID-19 ARDS cohort, 12 patients (48%) had thoracic CT scans realized at ECMO initiation. The percentage of lung consolidation was 75 (55–90)%.

Concerning the pre-specified outcomes, there was no difference in the vv-ECMO duration, vv-ECMO weaning rate, ICU mortality, and hospital mortality between the two groups.

First PP was considered after a median of 4 days of vv-ECMO. This delay was shorter in the COVID-19 ARDS cohort as compared with the non-COVID-19 ARDS cohort.

3.2. Effects of the First PP under vv-ECMO in the COVID-19 ARDS Group

No significant effect was observed among the respiratory mechanics variables, the vv-ECMO settings, and gas exchanges during the first PP under vv-ECMO (Table 2, Figures 1 and 2). Concerning hemodynamics, we found a significant variation in mean arterial pressure with an increase during PP.

Definition of abbreviations and formula: Pplat = plateau airway pressure; RS compliance = respiratory system compliance calculated by tidal volume divided by driving pressure; mechanical power calculated by the simplified equation of Gattinoni (0.098 × tidal volume (L) × respiratory rate (cycles/min) × peak inspiratory pressure less driving pressure divided by 2); PP = prone position.

Definition of abbreviations: FmO$_2$ = oxygen fraction delivered by the membrane oxygenator of the vv-ECMO; FiO$_2$: oxygen fraction inspired delivered by the ventilator; PaO$_2$ = partial pressure of arterial oxygen; PaCO$_2$ = partial pressure of arterial carbon dioxide; PP = prone position.

Table 2. Evolution of respiratory mechanics, vv-ECMO settings, arterial blood gas, and hemodynamics during the first prone position in the COVID-19 ARDS cohort.

	Baseline Supine H-1 PP	Start of Prone H+1 PP	End of Prone H-1 SP	Return to Supine H+1 SP	*p* Value
Ventilatory parameters					
Tidal volume, mL, median (IQR)	150 (106–215)	145 (100–220)	150 (115–200)	160 (100–230)	0.97
Plateau airway pressure, cm H_2O, median (IQR)	25 (21–26)	25 (22–26)	23 (23–24)	25 (22–26)	0.48
Peak inspiratory pressure, cm H_2O, median (IQR)	27 (23–29)	29 (26–32)	26 (25–30)	29 (25–31)	0.36
PEEP, cm H_2O, median (IQR)	12 (9–14)	12 (10–14)	12 (10–14)	12 (10–14)	0.93
Driving pressure, cm H_2O, median (IQR)	12 (10–15)	13 (9–15)	12 (8–14)	13 (11–14)	0.68
Respiratory rate, cycles/min, median (IQR)	15 (13–17)	15 (13–16)	15 (12–16)	15 (13–19)	0.89
Minute ventilation, L/min, median (IQR)	2.2 (1.5–3.7)	2 (1.5–3.6)	2.1 (1.5–3.4)	2.4 (1.5–3.8)	0.94
Respiratory system compliance, mL/cm H_2O, median (IQR)	11 (10–17)	13 (10–21)	13 (10–21)	11 (9–17)	0.83
Mechanical power, J/min, median (IQR)	4.1 (2.8–7.2)	4.7 (3.4–9)	4.2 (3.1–8.2)	4.3 (3.4–9)	0.94
Inspired fraction of oxygen, %, median (IQR)	50 (40–75)	60 (45–80)	50 (40–70)	55 (35–75)	0.76
vv-ECMO parameters					
vv-ECMO blood flow, L/min, median (IQR)	3.8 (3.3–4.7)	4 (3.3–4.4)	3.8 (3.2–4.8)	3.9 (3.2–4.6)	0.99
Sweep gas flow, L/min, median (IQR)	5 (3.5–6)	5 (4–6)	5 (3.5–7)	5 (3.7–6.5)	0.93
Membrane lung fraction of oxygen, %, median (IQR)	100 (100–100)	100 (100–100)	100 (100–100)	100 (100–100)	-
Arterial blood gas					
PaO_2, mmHg, median (IQR)	75 (69–81)	78 (69–85)	77 (70–83)	77 (67–89)	0.33
$PaCO_2$, mmHg, median (IQR)	54 (43–58)	51 (43–55)	53 (45–56)	48 (44–54)	0.57
$PaO_2:FiO_2$ ratio, mmHg, median (IQR)	140 (95–185)	142 (98–186)	144 (127–207)	147 (95–221)	0.74
pH, median (IQR)	7.40 (7.36–7.42)	7.42 (7.37–7.43)	7.40 (7.35–7.44)	7.42 (7.39–7.45)	0.11
Hemodynamic parameters					
Heart rate, bpm, median (IQR)	89 (71–116)	92 (73–111)	96 (76–105)	81 (70–105)	0.70
Mean arterial pressure, mmHg, median (IQR)	80 (73–90)	87 (80–100) *	87 (77–100) *	73 (67–86)	0.002

Definition of abbreviations and formula: IQR = interquartile range; PEEP = positive end-expiratory pressure; mechanical power calculated by the simplified equation of Gattinoni (0.098 × tidal volume (L) × respiratory rate (cycles/min) × peak inspiratory pressure less driving pressure divided by 2); vv-ECMO: venovenous extracorporeal membrane oxygenation; PaO_2 = partial pressure of arterial oxygen; $PaCO_2$ = partial pressure of arterial carbon dioxide; $PaO_2:FiO_2$ ratio = ratio of the partial pressure of arterial oxygen to the fraction of inspired oxygen; PP = prone position; SP = supine position. * $p < 0.05$ compared with return to supine with post hoc Tukey and Bonferroni tests.

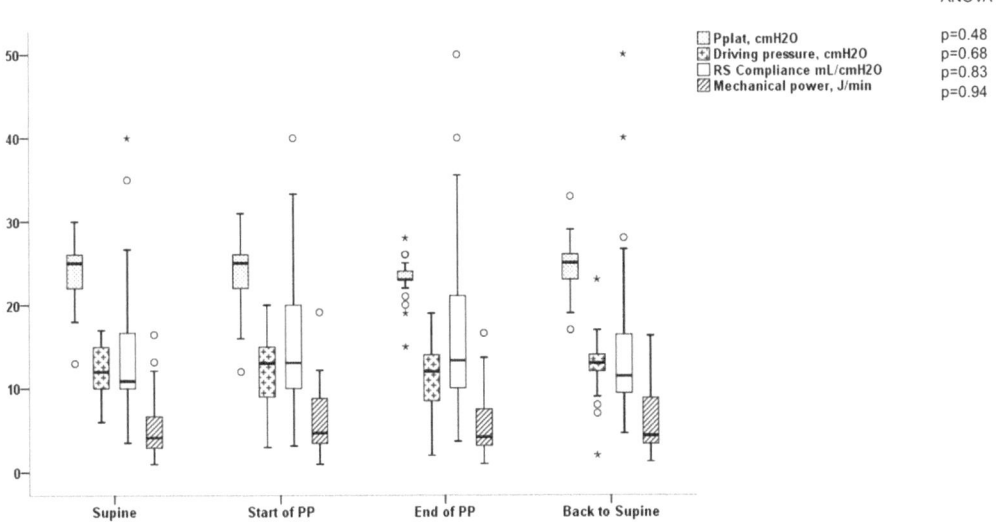

Figure 1. Variation in respiratory mechanics parameters during the first PP under vv-ECMO in patients with COVID-19 ARDS. The empty circles represent the outliers and the black stars represent the extreme values.

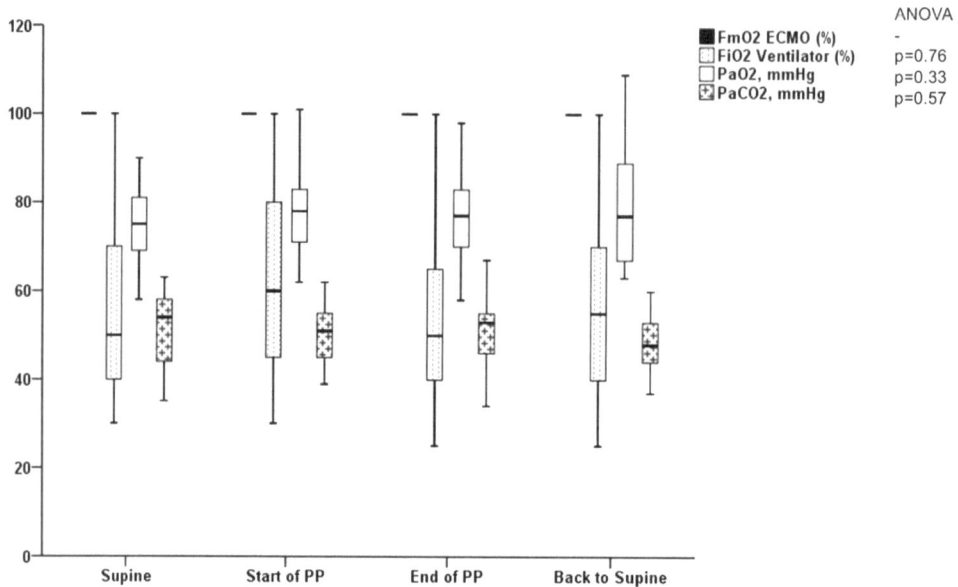

Figure 2. Variation in gas exchange during the first prone positioning under vv-ECMO for COVID-19 ARDS.

3.3. Effects of the First PP under vv-ECMO in the Non-COVID-19 ARDS Group

Respiratory mechanics, vv-ECMO settings, and arterial blood gas before and after the first PP under vv-ECMO in the non-COVID-19 ARDS cohort are displayed in Table 3.

Table 3. Evolution of respiratory mechanics, vv-ECMO settings, and arterial blood gas before and after the first prone position in the non-COVID-19 ARDS cohort (N = 60).

	Supine before Proning	Supine after Proning	*p* Value
Ventilatory parameters			
Tidal volume, mL, mean ± sd	206 ± 110	201 ± 99	0.79
Plateau airway pressure, cm H_2O, mean ± sd	25 ± 4	25 ± 4	0.21
PEEP, cm H_2O, mean ± sd	15 ± 3	15 ± 3	0.85
Driving pressure, cm H_2O, mean ± sd	11 ± 4	10 ± 4	0.28
Respiratory rate, cycles/min, mean ± sd	14 ± 6	13 ± 5	0.79
Minute ventilation, L/min, mean ± sd	2.9 ± 2.1	2.8 ± 2.2	0.84
Respiratory system compliance, mL/cm H_2O, mean ± sd	22.4 ± 12.3	22.5 ± 12.3	0.95
Inspired fraction of oxygen, %, mean ± sd	63 ± 22	54 ± 18	0.022
vv-ECMO parameters			
vv-ECMO blood flow, L/min, mean ± sd	4 ± 0.8	3.8 ± 0.8	0.35
Sweep gas flow, L/min, mean ± sd	6 ± 2	6 ± 2	0.90
Membrane lung fraction of oxygen, %, mean ± sd	100 ± 0	100 ± 0	-
Arterial blood gas			
PaO_2, mmHg, mean ± sd	75 ± 14	84 ± 22	0.002
$PaCO_2$, mmHg, mean ± sd	45 ± 10	43 ± 9	0.32
PaO_2:FiO_2 ratio, mmHg, mean ± sd	135 ± 57	176 ± 72	0.001

Definition of abbreviations: sd = standard deviation; PEEP = positive end-expiratory pressure; vv-ECMO: venovenous extracorporeal membrane oxygenation; PaO_2 = partial pressure of arterial oxygen; $PaCO_2$ = partial pressure of arterial carbon dioxide; PaO_2:FiO_2 ratio = ratio of the partial pressure of arterial oxygen to the fraction of inspired oxygen.

No significant change in respiratory mechanics was observed, whereas PaO_2 and the PaO_2:FiO_2 ratio increased significantly from 75 ± 14 mmHg to 84 ± 22 mmHg (p = 0.02) and from 135 ± 57 mmHg to 176 ± 72 mmHg (p = 0.001), respectively. We performed a sensitivity analysis restricted to the non-COVID-19 cohort who received PP before ECMO (N = 44) and found no difference except for a slight decrease in ECMO blood flow after the first PP (4 ± 0.9 L/min and 3.7 ± 1 L/min, p = 0.03).

3.4. Comparison between COVID-19 ARDS Group and Non-COVID-19 ARDS Group before and after the First PP under vv-ECMO

Comparisons of respiratory mechanics, vv-ECMO settings, and arterial blood gas before and after the first PP under vv-ECMO between COVID-19 ARDS and non-COVID-19 ARDS are displayed in Table 4.

Table 4. Comparisons of respiratory mechanics, vv-ECMO settings, and arterial blood gas before and after the first prone position between COVID-19 ARDS and non-COVID-19 ARDS.

	Supine before Proning		p Value	Supine after Proning		p Value
	COVID-19 ARDS N = 25	Non-COVID-19 ARDS N = 60		COVID-19 ARDS N = 25	Non-COVID-19 ARDS N = 60	
Ventilatory parameters						
Tidal volume, mL, median (IQR)	150 (106–215)	170 (150–243)	0.08	160 (115–240)	170 (130–250)	0.31
Plateau airway pressure, cm H_2O, median (IQR)	25 (21–26)	26 (23–28)	0.06	25 (22–26)	25 (22–26)	0.90
PEEP, cm H_2O, median (IQR)	12 (9–14)	15 (12–18)	<0.001	12 (10–14)	15 (12–18)	0.002
Driving pressure, cm H_2O, median (IQR)	12 (10–15)	10 (7–13)	0.06	13 (11–14)	9 (7–12)	0.001
Respiratory rate, cycles/min, median (IQR)	15 (13–17)	12 (10–15)	0.01	15 (13–19)	12 (10–15)	0.006
Minute ventilation, L/min, median (IQR)	2.2 (1.5–3.7)	2.1 (1.5–3.3)	0.84	2.4 (1.5–3.8)	2.0 (1.5–3.0)	0.44
Respiratory system compliance, mL cm H_2O, median (IQR)	11 (10–17)	20 (12–31)	0.009	11 (9–17)	21 (13–30)	0.005
Inspired fraction of oxygen, %, median (IQR)	50 (40–75)	60 (40–80)	0.19	55 (35–75)	50 (40–60)	0.35
ECMO parameters						
vv-ECMO blood flow, L/min, median (IQR)	3.8 (3.3–4.7)	3.8 (3.2–4.6)	0.76	3.9 (3.2–4.5)	3.7 (3.2–4.5)	0.53
Sweep gas flow, L/min, median (IQR)	5 (3.5–6)	6 (5–7)	0.04	5 (4–6)	6 (5–7)	0.24
Membrane lung fraction of oxygen, %, median (IQR)	100 (100–100)	100 (100–100)	1	100 (100–100)	100 (100–100)	1
Arterial blood gas						
PaO_2, mmHg, median (IQR)	75 (69–81)	71 (64–82)	0.42	77 (67–89)	77 (68–92)	0.66
$PaCO_2$, mmHg, median (IQR)	54 (43–58)	43 (39–49)	0.006	48 (44–54)	42 (38–50)	0.008
$PaO_2:FiO_2$ ratio, mmHg, median (IQR)	140 (95–185)	127 (92–162)	0.27	147 (95–221)	160 (125–214)	0.31

Definition of abbreviations: IQR = interquartile range; PEEP = positive end-expiratory pressure; vv-ECMO: venovenous extracorporeal membrane oxygenation; PaO_2 = partial pressure of arterial oxygen; $PaCO_2$ = partial pressure of arterial carbon dioxide; $PaO_2:FiO_2$ ratio = ratio of the partial pressure of arterial oxygen to the fraction of inspired oxygen; ARDS = acute respiratory distress syndrome; COVID-19 = coronavirus disease 2019.

Before the first PP under vv-ECMO, PEEP and C_{RS} were higher in patients with non-COVID-19 ARDS as compared with patients with COVID-19 ARDS. Conversely, ΔP was lower in the non-COVID-19 ARDS cohort. These differences were consistent after the first PP.

In addition, no difference was observed for P_{plat} and Vt. A slightly higher respiratory rate was used in the COVID-19 ARDS cohort with no difference in minute ventilation. Before the first PP, higher sweep gas flow and RR resulting in lower $PaCO_2$ were found in the non-COVID-19 ARDS cohort. These differences were also consistent after the first PP. A limited increase in C_{RS} in the non-COVID-19 ARDS group and a limited decrease in C_{RS} resulted in a significant difference in ΔP between groups after the first PP.

3.5. Assessment of Safety in the COVID-19 Cohort

Among pre-specified safety concerns, no patient presented a serious adverse event during the first PP under vv-ECMO.

4. Discussion

In our retrospective and ambispective single-center cohort study, we observed distinct responses to the first PP in severe ARDS supported by vv-ECMO depending on COVID-19 etiology.

Whereas no significant difference among C_{RS} and other respiratory mechanics variables was observed, a significant increase in oxygenation parameters was ensured by PP only in the non-COVID-19 ARDS cohort.

vv-ECMO is a valuable therapeutic option for patients with very severe ARDS and refractory hypoxemia when a strategy associating lung-protective ventilation with low tidal volume and low plateau pressure associated with prolonged and repeated prone position fails [5].

While PP and vv-ECMO have been proven to individually decrease mortality, the combination of both has not been investigated in a randomized clinical study.

In our cohort of patients with non-COVID-19 ARDS, we found an improvement in oxygenation-related parameters after the first PP under vv-ECMO. The increase in PaO_2 and PaO_2:FiO_2 ratio may be the result of an improvement of the ventilation/perfusion ratio by homogenization of transpulmonary pressures and decreasing lung strain rather than an increase in alveolar recruitment since we did not observe an increase in C_{RS}.

An increase in oxygenation during PP during vv-ECMO has been reported in a previous meta-analysis both in COVID and non-COVID-19 patients and seems consistent [14]. Despite a significant decrease in driving pressure, the global effect on C_{RS} was not significant.

This could be due to the delay in proning the patient during ECMO. Indeed, Giani et al. found that non-COVID-19 ARDS patients who were proned after 5 days of vv-ECMO start did not improve in C_{RS} despite improvement in oxygenation [15].

Despite a shorter delay in proning the patients in the COVID-19 cohort, it was not associated with improvement in oxygenation or C_{RS}. Our COVID-19 ARDS cohort had notably a lower C_{RS} but similar oxygenation severity compared to the non-COVID-19 ARDS cohort. We cannot exclude that those patients had a higher degree of secondary lung fibrosis limiting the beneficial effects of the prone position [16].

In addition, the assessment of the first PP under vv-ECMO may be insufficient to demonstrate an effect on oxygenation and/or on C_{RS}.

A positive effect of PP has been demonstrated after the repetition of sessions regardless of the effect on oxygenation [17]. Therefore, we can hypothesize the potential protective effects of PP on ventilator-induced lung injuries at a non-clinically measurable level.

Contrary to the hypothesis raised at the beginning of the pandemic, large studies and a systematic review have demonstrated that C_{RS} measured close to the time of the initiation of invasive mechanical ventilation was normally distributed [18,19] and was comparable to that in non-COVID-19 ARDS patients [20]. This does not support the concept of distinct phenotypes in COVID-19-related ARDS. Finally, in the late stage of the disease (from the third week), the likelihood of oxygenation improving with prone positioning becomes extremely low [20–22].

No major complication related to PP during vv-ECMO was reported in our study. In the cohort of COVID-19 patients, a significant increase in mean arterial pressure in the PP position was observed. This effect may be related to an increase in venous return and mean systemic pressure [23].

One hundred percent of the COVID-19 cohort but only 74% of the non-COVID-19 cohort had a first PP attempt before ECMO implementation. This could be also taken into account regarding the lack of response for the COVID-19 cohort.

Several limitations in our study should be noted. First, due to the design of the study, a significant proportion (36%) of the non-COVID-19 cohort with missing respiratory mechanics variables or gas exchange data was not included. In addition, we included a relatively small sample size in the COVID-19 cohort to minimize the missing data. Therefore, the risk of type II error should be mentioned. Second, the decision to perform or not perform PP was at the discretion of the medical team in charge. No threshold for the PaO$_2$:FiO$_2$ ratio (which is difficult to interpret during vv-ECMO) was determined in the design of the protocol. It cannot be ruled out that a number of PP sessions were performed as a rescue therapy and not routinely when the PaO$_2$:FiO$_2$ ratio was below 150 mmHg, which may, at least partly, explain the non-significance of the study. Third, the COVID-19 variants during successive surges may have played a role in response to PP. Finally, the possible beneficial effect of pursuing PP during vv-ECMO on vv-ECMO duration or mortality reported in a very recently terminated randomized clinical trial [24] needs urgent confirmation.

5. Conclusions

We did not observe changes in C_{RS} during the first PP performed in two distinct cohorts of ARDS patients supported by vv-ECMO. In non-COVID-19 patients, PP was associated with improvement in oxygenation. We cannot exclude beneficial effects at a non-clinical level (e.g., on biotrauma), and these effects need further investigation.

Author Contributions: L.T., I.G.-C., F.D., S.V., C.S. and C.G. collected and analyzed the data. L.T., L.P., J.-M.F., S.H., A.R. and C.G. analyzed and interpreted the data more precisely. C.G. performed the statistical analysis. L.T. and C.G. wrote the manuscript. All authors have read and agreed to the published version of the manuscript.

Funding: This research received no external funding.

Institutional Review Board Statement: The study was approved by the French Intensive Care Society (SRLF) Ethics Committee (Commission d'Ethique de la SRLF, reference CE SRLF 21-47, Approved date: 4 October 2021) which waived the need for written consent according to French legislation. The study was also declared and approved by the "Portail d'Accès aux Données de Santé, Assistance Publique-Hôpitaux de Marseille" (Registration number PADS21-89).

Informed Consent Statement: Patients and their relatives were informed of the possibility of the use of their medical data, and their opposition was researched.

Data Availability Statement: The datasets used and/or analyzed during the current study are available from the corresponding author on reasonable request.

Conflicts of Interest: Christophe Guervilly reports personal consulting fees from Xenios FMC outside the submitted work. The other authors declare no conflict of interest.

Abbreviations

APRV	airway pressure release ventilation
ARDS	acute respiratory distress syndrome
BMI	body mass index
COVID-19	coronavirus disease 2019
C_{RS}	compliance of respiratory system
ΔP	driving pressure
FiO$_2$	fraction of inspired oxygen
FmO$_2$	oxygen fraction delivered by the membrane oxygenator
ICU	intensive care unit
iNO	inhaled nitric oxide
MP	mechanical power
PaCO$_2$	partial pressure of arterial carbon dioxide
PaO$_2$	partial pressure of arterial oxygen
PaO$_2$:FiO$_2$ ratio	ratio of partial pressure of arterial oxygen to fraction of inspired oxygen
PEEP	positive end-expiratory pressure
PP	prone position
P$_{peak}$	peak inspiratory pressure
P$_{plat}$	plateau pressure
RR	respiratory rate
SARS-CoV-2	severe acute respiratory syndrome coronavirus 2

SP	supine position
SaO$_2$	saturation of arterial oxygen
VILI	ventilator-induced lung injury
V$_M$	minute ventilation
V$_T$	tidal volume
vv-ECMO	venovenous extracorporeal membrane oxygenation

References

1. ARDS Definition Task Force; Ranieri, V.M.; Rubenfeld, G.D.; Thompson, B.; Ferguson, N.; Caldwell, E.; Fan, E.; Camporota, L.; Slutsky, A.S. Acute respiratory distress syndrome: The Berlin Definition. *JAMA* **2012**, *307*, 2526–2533.
2. Fan, E.; Del Sorbo, L.; Goligher, E.C.; Hodgson, C.L.; Munshi, L.; Walkey, A.J.; Adhikari, N.K.; Amato, M.B.; Branson, R.; Brower, R.G.; et al. An Official American Thoracic Society/European Society of Intensive Care Medicine/Society of Critical Care Medicine Clinical Practice Guideline: Mechanical Ventilation in Adult Patients with Acute Respiratory Distress Syndrome. *Am. J. Respir. Crit. Care Med.* **2017**, *195*, 1253–1263. [CrossRef] [PubMed]
3. Slutsky, A.S.; Ranieri, V.M. Ventilator-induced lung injury. *N. Engl. J. Med.* **2013**, *369*, 2126–2136. [CrossRef] [PubMed]
4. Schmidt, M.; Pham, T.; Arcadipane, A.; Agerstrand, C.; Ohshimo, S.; Pellegrino, V.; Vuylsteke, A.; Guervilly, C.; McGuinness, S.; Pierard, S.; et al. Mechanical Ventilation Management during Extracorporeal Membrane Oxygenation for Acute Respiratory Distress Syndrome. An International Multicenter Prospective Cohort. *Am. J. Respir. Crit. Care Med.* **2019**, *200*, 1002–1012. [CrossRef] [PubMed]
5. Combes, A.; Hajage, D.; Capellier, G.; Demoule, A.; Lavoué, S.; Guervilly, C.; Da Silva, D.; Zafrani, L.; Tirot, P.; Veber, B.; et al. Extracorporeal Membrane Oxygenation for Severe Acute Respiratory Distress Syndrome. *N. Engl. J. Med.* **2018**, *378*, 1965–1975. [CrossRef] [PubMed]
6. Available online: https://covid19.who.int/ (accessed on 20 May 2023).
7. Lorusso, R.; Combes, A.; Coco, V.L.; De Piero, M.E.; Belohlavek, J.; on behalf of the EuroECMO COVID-19 WorkingGroup; Euro-ELSO Steering Committee. ECMO for COVID-19 patients in Europe and Israel. *Intensive Care Med.* **2021**, *47*, 344–348. [CrossRef]
8. Nesseler, N.; Fadel, G.; Mansour, A.; Para, M.; Falcoz, P.E.; Mongardon, N.; Porto, A.; Bertier, A.; Levy, B.; Cadoz, C.; et al. Extracorporeal Membrane Oxygenation for Respiratory Failure Related to COVID-19: A Nationwide Cohort Study. *Anesthesiology* **2022**, *136*, 732–748. [CrossRef]
9. Schmidt, M.; Hajage, D.; Lebreton, G.; Monsel, A.; Voiriot, G.; Levy, D.; Baron, E.; Beurton, A.; Chommeloux, J.; Meng, P.; et al. Extracorporeal membrane oxygenation for severe acute respiratory distress syndrome associated with COVID-19: A retrospective cohort study. *Lancet Respir. Med.* **2020**, *8*, 1121–1131. [CrossRef]
10. Lorusso, R.; De Piero, M.E.; Mariani, S.; Di Mauro, M. Determinants of long-term outcomes in patients with COVID-19 supported with ECMO—Authors' reply. *Lancet Respir. Med.* **2023**. epub ahead of print. [CrossRef] [PubMed]
11. Roch, A.; Hraiech, S.; Masson, E.; Grisoli, D.; Forel, J.M.; Boucekine, M.; Morera, P.; Guervilly, C.; Adda, M.; Dizier, S.; et al. Outcome of acute respiratory distress syndrome patients treated with extracorporeal membrane oxygenation and brought to a referral center. *Intensive Care Med.* **2014**, *40*, 74–83. [CrossRef]
12. Guervilly, C.; Prud'homme, E.; Pauly, V.; Bourenne, J.; Hraiech, S.; Daviet, F.; Adda, M.; Coiffard, B.; Forel, J.M.; Roch, A.; et al. Prone positioning and extracorporeal membrane oxygenation for severe acute respiratory distress syndrome: Time for a randomized trial? *Intensive Care Med.* **2019**, *45*, 1040–1042. [CrossRef]
13. Gattinoni, L.; Tonetti, T.; Cressoni, M.; Cadringher, P.; Herrmann, P.; Moerer, O.; Protti, A.; Gotti, M.; Chiurazzi, C.; Carlesso, E.; et al. Ventilator-related causes of lung injury: The mechanical power. *Intensive Care Med.* **2016**, *42*, 1567–1575. [CrossRef] [PubMed]
14. Poon, W.H.; Ramanathan, K.; Ling, R.R.; Yang, I.X.; Tan, C.S.; Schmidt, M.; Shekar, K. Prone positioning during venovenous extracorporeal membrane oxygenation for acute respiratory distress syndrome: A systematic review and meta-analysis. *Crit. Care* **2021**, *25*, 292. [CrossRef]
15. Giani, M.; Rezoagli, E.; Guervilly, C.; Rilinger, J.; Duburcq, T.; Petit, M.; Textoris, L.; Garcia, B.; Wengenmayer, T.; Bellani, G.; et al. Timing of Prone Positioning during Venovenous Extracorporeal Membrane Oxygenation for Acute Respiratory Distress Syndrome. *Crit. Care Med.* **2023**, *51*, 25–35. [CrossRef] [PubMed]
16. Compagnone, N.; Palumbo, D.; Cremona, G.; Vitali, G.; De Lorenzo, R.; Calvi, M.R.; Del Prete, A.; Baiardo Redaelli, M.; Calamarà, S.; Belletti, A.; et al. Residual lung damage following ARDS in COVID-19 ICU survivors. *Acta Anaesthesiol. Scand.* **2022**, *66*, 223–231. [CrossRef]
17. Albert, R.K.; Keniston, A.; Baboi, L.; Ayzac, L.; Guérin, C.; Proseva Investigators. Prone position-induced improvement in gas exchange does not predict improved survival in the acute respiratory distress syndrome. *Am. J. Respir. Crit. Care Med.* **2014**, *189*, 494–496. [CrossRef] [PubMed]
18. Vandenbunder, B.; Ehrmann, S.; Piagnerelli, M.; Sauneuf, B.; Serck, N.; Soumagne, T.; Textoris, J.; Vinsonneau, C.; Aissaoui, N.; Blonz, G.; et al. Static compliance of the respiratory system in COVID-19 related ARDS: An international multicenter study. *Crit. Care* **2021**, *25*, 52. [CrossRef] [PubMed]

19. Reddy, M.P.; Subramaniam, A.; Chua, C.; Ling, R.R.; Anstey, C.; Ramanathan, K.; Slutsky, A.S.; Shekar, K. Respiratory system mechanics, gas exchange, and outcomes in mechanically ventilated patients with COVID-19-related acute respiratory distress syndrome: A systematic review and meta-analysis. *Lancet Respir. Med.* **2022**, *10*, 1178–1188. [CrossRef]
20. Fusina, F.; Albani, F.; Crisci, S.; Morandi, A.; Tansini, F.; Beschi, R.; Rosano, A.; Natalini, G. Respiratory system compliance at the same PEEP level is similar in COVID and non-COVID ARDS. *Respir. Res.* **2022**, *23*, 7. [CrossRef] [PubMed]
21. Gattinoni, L.; Camporota, L.; Marini, J.J. Prone Position and COVID-19: Mechanisms and Effects. *Crit Care Med.* **2022**, *50*, 873–875. [CrossRef]
22. Rossi, S.; Palumbo, M.M.; Sverzellati, N.; Busana, M.; Malchiodi, L.; Bresciani, P.; Ceccarelli, P.; Sani, E.; Romitti, F.; Bonifazi, M.; et al. Mechanisms of oxygenation responses to proning and recruitment in COVID-19 pneumonia. *Intensive Care Med.* **2022**, *48*, 56–66. [CrossRef] [PubMed]
23. Lai, C.; Adda, I.; Teboul, J.L.; Persichini, R.; Gavelli, F.; Guérin, L.; Monnet, X. Effects of Prone Positioning on Venous Return in Patients with Acute Respiratory Distress Syndrome. *Crit. Care Med.* **2021**, *49*, 781–789. [CrossRef] [PubMed]
24. Available online: https://clinicaltrials.gov/ct2/show/NCT04607551 (accessed on 20 May 2023).

Disclaimer/Publisher's Note: The statements, opinions and data contained in all publications are solely those of the individual author(s) and contributor(s) and not of MDPI and/or the editor(s). MDPI and/or the editor(s) disclaim responsibility for any injury to people or property resulting from any ideas, methods, instructions or products referred to in the content.

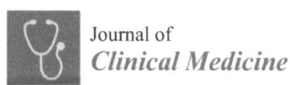

Article

Increased Alveolar Epithelial Damage Markers and Inflammasome-Regulated Cytokines Are Associated with Pulmonary Superinfection in ARDS

Konrad Peukert [1,†], Andrea Sauer [1,†], Benjamin Seeliger [2], Caroline Feuerborn [1], Mario Fox [1], Susanne Schulz [1], Lennart Wild [1], Valeri Borger [3], Patrick Schuss [3,4], Matthias Schneider [3], Erdem Güresir [3,5], Mark Coburn [1], Christian Putensen [1], Christoph Wilhelm [6] and Christian Bode [1,*]

[1] Department of Anesthesiology and Intensive Care Medicine, University Hospital Bonn, Venusberg-Campus 1, 53127 Bonn, Germany
[2] Department of Respiratory Medicine and German Centre of Lung Research (DZL), Hannover Medical School, Carl-Neuberg-Str. 1, 30635 Hannover, Germany
[3] Department of Neurosurgery, University Hospital Bonn, Venusberg-Campus 1, 53127 Bonn, Germany
[4] Department of Neurosurgery, BG Klinikum Unfallkrankenhaus Berlin gGmbH, Warener Str. 7, 12683 Berlin, Germany
[5] Department of Neurosurgery, University Hospital Leipzig, Liebig Str. 20, Haus 4, 04103 Leipzig, Germany
[6] Institute of Clinical Chemistry and Clinical Pharmacology, University Hospital Bonn, Venusberg-Campus 1, 53127 Bonn, Germany
* Correspondence: christian.bode@ukbonn.de; Tel.: +49-228-287-14114; Fax: +49-228-287-11332
† These authors contributed equally to this work.

Abstract: Acute respiratory distress syndrome (ARDS) is a life-threatening form of respiratory failure defined by dysregulated immune homeostasis and alveolar epithelial and endothelial damage. Up to 40% of ARDS patients develop pulmonary superinfections, contributing to poor prognosis and increasing mortality. Understanding what renders ARDS patients highly susceptible to pulmonary superinfections is therefore essential. We hypothesized that ARDS patients who develop pulmonary superinfections display a distinct pulmonary injury and pro-inflammatory response pattern. Serum and BALF samples from 52 patients were collected simultaneously within 24 h of ARDS onset. The incidence of pulmonary superinfections was determined retrospectively, and the patients were classified accordingly. Serum concentrations of the epithelial markers soluble receptor for advanced glycation end-products (sRAGE) and surfactant protein D (SP-D) and the endothelial markers vascular endothelial growth factor (VEGF) and angiopoetin-2 (Ang-2) as well as bronchoalveolar lavage fluid concentrations of the pro-inflammatory cytokines interleukin 1ß (IL-1ß), interleukin 18 (IL-18), interleukin 6 (IL-6), and tumor necrosis factor-alpha (TNF-a) were analyzed via multiplex immunoassay. Inflammasome-regulated cytokine IL-18 and the epithelial damage markers SP-D and sRAGE were significantly increased in ARDS patients who developed pulmonary superinfections. In contrast, endothelial markers and inflammasome-independent cytokines did not differ between the groups. The current findings reveal a distinct biomarker pattern that indicates inflammasome activation and alveolar epithelial injury. This pattern may potentially be used in future studies to identify high-risk patients, enabling targeted preventive strategies and personalized treatment approaches.

Keywords: pulmonary superinfection; inflammasome; molecular phenotyping; acute respiratory distress syndrome; precision medicine; pneumonia; influenza

Citation: Peukert, K.; Sauer, A.; Seeliger, B.; Feuerborn, C.; Fox, M.; Schulz, S.; Wild, L.; Borger, V.; Schuss, P.; Schneider, M.; et al. Increased Alveolar Epithelial Damage Markers and Inflammasome-Regulated Cytokines Are Associated with Pulmonary Superinfection in ARDS. *J. Clin. Med.* **2023**, *12*, 3649. https://doi.org/10.3390/jcm12113649

Academic Editors: David Barnes, Paolo Pelosi and Denise Battaglini

Received: 14 March 2023
Revised: 9 April 2023
Accepted: 18 May 2023
Published: 24 May 2023

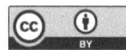

Copyright: © 2023 by the authors. Licensee MDPI, Basel, Switzerland. This article is an open access article distributed under the terms and conditions of the Creative Commons Attribution (CC BY) license (https://creativecommons.org/licenses/by/4.0/).

1. Introduction

Acute respiratory distress syndrome (ARDS) is a heterogeneous syndrome characterized by a dysregulated inflammatory host response leading to severe alveolar epithelial and endothelial injury. A subsequent loss of alveolar–capillary barrier integrity results in the accumulation of protein-rich edema fluid in the lung interstitium and critical arterial hypoxemia in ARDS patients [1]. One of the main complications of ARDS is the development of pulmonary superinfections contributing to negative outcomes and excess mortality. Up to 40% of patients suffering from ARDS develop pulmonary superinfections over the course of treatment [2,3]. Major risk factors include a loss of epithelial barrier function, prolonged mechanical ventilation, and prone positioning which might facilitate microbial dissemination and increase the risk for abundant microaspiration of gastric contents. Pulmonary dysbiosis in combination with defects in innate and adaptive immunity may further explain the high incidence of pulmonary superinfection [4–6]. Hence, it is imperative to understand what predisposes ARDS patients to pulmonary superinfections to tailor future clinical trials and to be able to adjust treatment accordingly.

Several biomarkers indicating lung endothelial and epithelial damage as well as pulmonary inflammation in ARDS patients have been identified so far and are promising tools to refine molecular phenotyping, assess prognosis, and evaluate treatment response [7,8]. Although biomarkers have been validated for ARDS, little is known about their predictive value for pulmonary superinfections in ARDS.

Serum surfactant protein D (SP-D) and soluble receptor for advanced glycation endproducts (sRAGE) are both promising markers of alveolar epithelial injury which have both been linked to poor prognosis in ARDS [9–11]. Furthermore, external validation of biomarkers and a clinical prediction model for hospital mortality in ARDS patients included SP-D in a variety of clinical settings and may be useful in risk assessments for clinical trial enrolment [12]. In contrast, vascular endothelial growth factor (VEGF) and Angiopoetin-2 (Ang-2) reflect endothelial injury in ARDS [13,14] and predict ARDS onset as well as increased mortality [15,16].

Lung injury including epithelial and endothelial damage is mediated by inflammatory cytokines [1]. In particular, inflammasome activation and its downstream cytokines IL-1ß and IL-18 are major contributors to lung injury in ARDS and correlate with an unfavorable outcome [17–20]. Inflammasomes are pivotal components of the innate immune system that consist of a sensor NOD-, LRR-, and pyrin-domain-containing protein 3 (NLRP3), an adaptor-apoptosis-associated speck-like protein containing a CARD (ASC), and an effector (caspase-1) [8,21]. Its activation is tightly controlled by a two-step mechanism. Step one or the priming signal is initiated by pattern recognition receptors (PRRs) such as TLRs (toll-like receptors) that sense a diverse set of microbial molecules, termed pathogen-associated molecular patterns (PAMPs), such as bacterial lipopolysaccharides (LPS) or endogenous damage-associated molecular patterns (DAMPs) including ATP, mitochondrial DNA, and fibrinogen. As a result of, e.g., TLR-4 sensing LPS, transcription factor nuclear factor kappa B (NF-κb) becomes activated leading to the subsequent upregulation of the sensor NLRP3 and pro-interleukin-1ß (pro-IL-1ß). A plethora of stimuli including extracellular ATP, pathogen-associated RNA, and bacterial pore-forming toxins can activate NLRP3, triggering inflammasome assembly via the recruitment of adaptor protein ASC (step two). The assembled inflammasome includes activated caspase 1 which cleaves pro-IL-1ß and pro-IL-18 into their biologically active forms IL-1ß and IL-18, inducing pyroptosis, a form of alternative inflammatory cell death [8,22,23]. Excess inflammation and deleterious pyroptosis are major drivers of pulmonary injury and may predispose ARDS patients to pulmonary superinfections [1,5,24].

We hypothesize that ARDS patients who develop pulmonary superinfections exhibit a distinct pulmonary injury and inflammatory response pattern. To test this hypothesis, we analyzed epithelial and endothelial damage markers as well as pro-inflammatory markers in ARDS patients with and without pulmonary superinfections.

2. Materials and Methods

2.1. Study Design and Population

We performed a single-center, retrospective analysis of ARDS patients hospitalized at the University Hospital Bonn, Bonn, Germany. ARDS was diagnosed according to the Berlin definition of the 2012 announcement which defines ARDS as the acute onset of hypoxemia with bilateral infiltrates and no evidence of left atrial hypertension [25]. Bronchoalveolar lavage fluid (BALF) and serum samples were collected within 24 h of disease onset. The incidence of pulmonary superinfection was then determined in a retrospective analysis via electronic health records.

If ARDS was already present at the time of hospital admission, we defined ARDS onset as the time of symptom onset. Pulmonary superinfection was defined as any secondary pulmonary infection caused by bacterial, viral, or fungal pathogens that occurred within 28 days after ARDS onset. Diagnosis of pulmonary superinfection was confirmed by pathogen detection in microbial cultures or via RT-PCR accompanied by increased secondary white cell count and procalcitonin (PCT) as well as the presence of new or progressive pulmonary infiltrates on chest radiographs or chest computed tomography (CT) scans.

BALF and serum samples were obtained from ARDS patients of the University Hospital Bonn, Bonn, Germany, with approval of the Institutional Review Board of the University Hospital Bonn, Bonn, Germany (No.088/16). The study was conducted according to the guidelines of the Declaration of Helsinki. Written informed consent was obtained from all participants prior to inclusion in this study.

2.2. Sample Collection and Processing

BALF and serum samples were collected simultaneously within 24 h of ARDS onset. Blood samples were collected from ARDS patients using serum gel monovettes (S-Monovette, Sarstedt AG & Co. KG, Nuembrecht, Germany). After centrifugation at $2500 \times g$ and room temperature for 10 min, the serum samples were aliquoted into cryotubes and stored at $-80\,°C$ until further processing.

A standard bronchoscopy protocol was used to obtain BALF for bacterial and virological testing as described before [8]. In brief, bronchoalveolar lavage (BAL) was performed with a flexible bronchoscope wedged in a segment of the right middle lobe. A total quantity of 200 mL of normal saline was instilled in 4 aliquots with a 50 mL syringe and added tubing, and BALF was recovered by manual aspiration. The BALF samples were immediately placed on ice after collection and centrifuged at $400 \times g$ and $4\,°C$ for 5 min. The supernatant was stored at $-80\,°C$ until further processing. Levels of SP-D, RAGE, Ang-2, VEGF, IL-18, IL-1ß, TNF-α, and IL-6 were analyzed by multiplex immunoassay (Luminex Assay, Bio-Techne, Minneapolis, MN, USA).

2.3. Data Collection

The data collected from electronic health records included patient demographics (age, gender), epidemiology, comorbidities, physiological and laboratory parameters (white cell count, procalcitonin, and blood gas analysis), including those used to calculate the Sequential Organ Failure Assessment (SOFA) score, microbiology and virology results (respiratory tract cultures and viral RT-PCRs), ventilatory parameters, immunosuppressive medication administration, and short- and long-term outcomes. The electronic health records of all ARDS patients included in this study were reviewed by several researchers to ensure clinical significance.

2.4. Statistical Analysis

The statistical analysis and calculations were performed with GraphPad Prism Software (Version 9.0, La Jolla, CA, USA); a p-value < 0.05 was considered statistically significant. The patient characteristics were compared by the Kruskal–Wallis test or Fisher's exact test and expressed as median, 25% percentile, and 75% percentile. For better comparability and to achieve normal distribution, the biomarker data were log-transformed and presented as an individual value with mean $\pm$ SD. Comparisons between groups were analyzed by an unpaired t-test.

3. Results

3.1. Patient Characteristics

Fifty-two ARDS patients who were treated at the University Hospital Bonn, Bonn, Germany, from October 2018 until October 2020 were included in this retrospective study. A total quantity of 25 ARDS patients developed pulmonary superinfections over the course of treatment. The main characteristics of the ARDS patients with and without superinfections are shown in Table 1 and Table S1. No significant differences in demographics, comorbidities, immunocompromised conditions, ventilatory settings, inflammatory parameters, disease severity, and mortality were observed between the ARDS patients that developed or did not show pulmonary superinfections.

Table 1. Characteristics of ARDS patients with and without pulmonary superinfections.

Characteristics	ARDS (Superinfection) (n = 25)	ARDS (No Superinfection) (n = 27)	p
Age (y)	60 (45–69)	53 (44–58)	0.158
Male (%)	68	85	0.1933
BMI (kg/m^2)	31.1 (27–37.6)	29.39 (27.2–34.1)	0.4315
Diabetes (%)	12	18.5	0.705
Immunosuppression (%)	8	7.4	>0.9999
Steroids (%)	20	37	0.2274
PaO$_2$/FiO$_2$ ratio (mmHg)	80 (68.5–116.5)	92 (64.9–161.5)	0.4642
PEEP (cmH$_2$O)	19 (15–20)	18 (15–20)	0.7482
Driving pressure (cmH$_2$O)	10 (7.5–13.5)	9 (6–12)	0.33
Tidal volume (ml/kg predicted body weight)	2.5 1.7–4.1	3.3 (1.9–6.4)	0.3555
Procalcitonin (µg/L)	17.1 (1.4–43,6)	5.57 (1.2–45.8)	0.7714
Lactate (mmol/L)	1.9 (1.6–4.6)	1.68 (1.2–3.1)	0.5276
SOFA score (best assumed)	8 (7–10.5)	8 (6–11)	0.6636
ICU mortality (%)	36	33.3	>0.9999

The data are presented as median, 25% percentile, and 75% percentile using the Kruskall–Wallis test or Fisher's exact test. Abbreviations: BMI, body mass index; PEEP, positive end-expiratory pressure; SOFA score, sepsis-related organ failure assessment score (best assumed for CNS).

3.2. Epithelial Damage Markers Differ in ARDS Patients with and without Secondary Pulmonary Infection

Epithelial barrier function plays an important role in preventing superinfections. Both sRAGE and SP-D have previously been described as promising biomarkers to assess epithelial damage in ARDS patients and are associated with an unfavorable prognosis in ARDS patients [9–11]. To investigate whether these lung epithelial damage markers are also associated with pulmonary superinfections in ARDS patients, we determined the levels of sRAGE and SP-D in serum samples drawn within 24 h of ARDS onset. As shown in Figure 1A, the serum concentrations of SP-D and sRAGE were both significantly increased in ARDS patients with pulmonary superinfections compared to ARDS patients who did not develop pulmonary superinfections ($p = 0.0397$ and $p = 0.0495$, respectively). We next tested whether endothelial damage might also be associated with pulmonary superinfections. Ang-2 and VEGF both play a central role in activating endothelial cells and increasing microvascular permeability. We therefore monitored the endothelial injury molecules Ang-2 and VEGF and did not observe any differences in serum levels between ARDS patients with and without pulmonary superinfections. Altogether, we found that epithelial rather than endothelial damage markers were increased in patients with secondary infections.

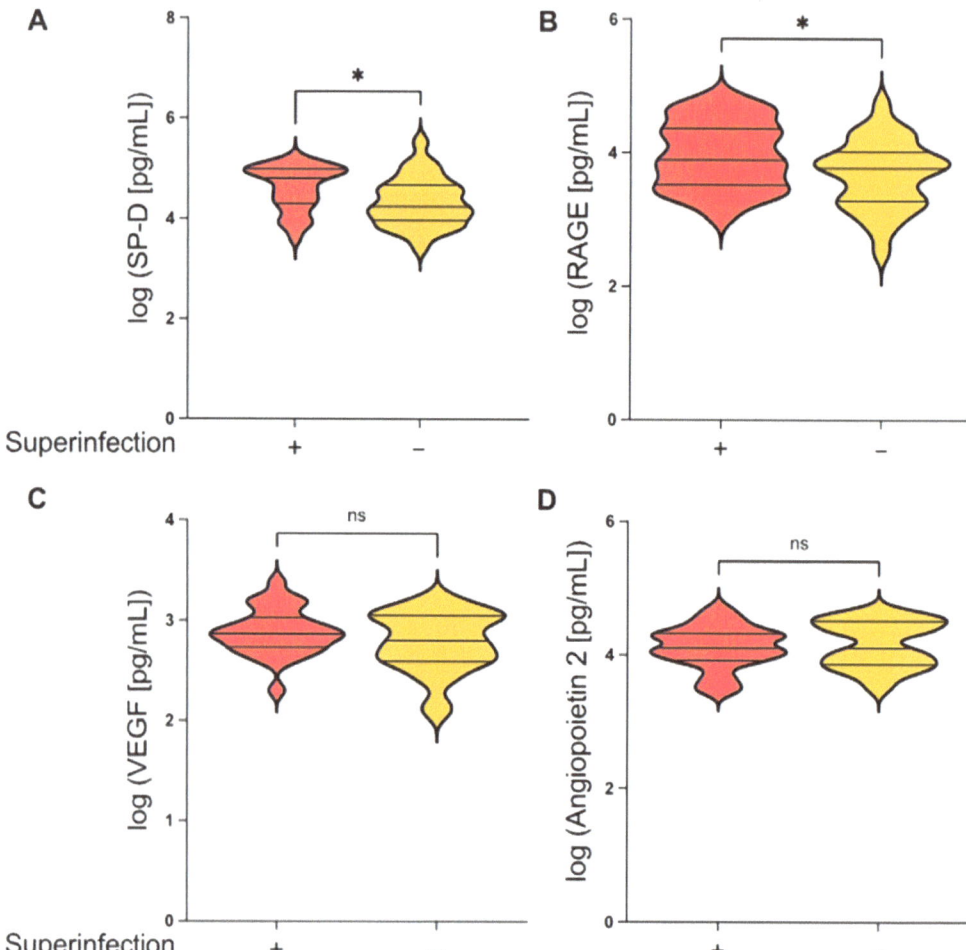

Figure 1. Epithelial damage markers are differentially expressed in ARDS patients with and without pulmonary superinfections. Violin plots of (**A**) SP-D, (**B**) sRage, (**C**) VEGF, and (**D**) Angiopoetin-2 serum levels in ARDS patients with and without pulmonary superinfections. Blood samples were collected from ARDS patients within 24 h of disease onset and analyzed via multiplex immunoassay. A total of 25 ARDS patients with pulmonary superinfections and 27 ARDS patients without pulmonary superinfections were included in this study. Mean ± SD of log-transformed data; unpaired t-test; * $p \leq 0.05$; ns = not significant; red violin plot = ARDS with superinfection; yellow violin plot = ARDS without superinfection.

3.3. Inflammasome-Regulated Cytokines Differ in ARDS Patients with and without Secondary Pulmonary Infection

As inflammation is a modulator of host susceptibility to pulmonary superinfections [5], we investigated the local pro-inflammatory cytokine milieu in the lungs. In particular, the inflammasome-regulated cytokines IL-1ß and IL-18 are crucial mediators of pulmonary hyperinflammation in ARDS [8,17]. We therefore determined the BALF levels of IL-1ß and IL-18 as well as TNF-α and IL-6 which are known to be elevated in ARDS patients with fatal outcomes [11,20]. Interestingly, the inflammasome-regulated cytokine IL-18 (but not IL-1ß) was significantly increased in ARDS patients who developed pulmonary superinfections compared to patients without a secondary infection (p = 0.0271). In contrast, no significant differences between the groups were detected for the inflammasome-independent mediators TNF-α and IL-6 (Figure 2).

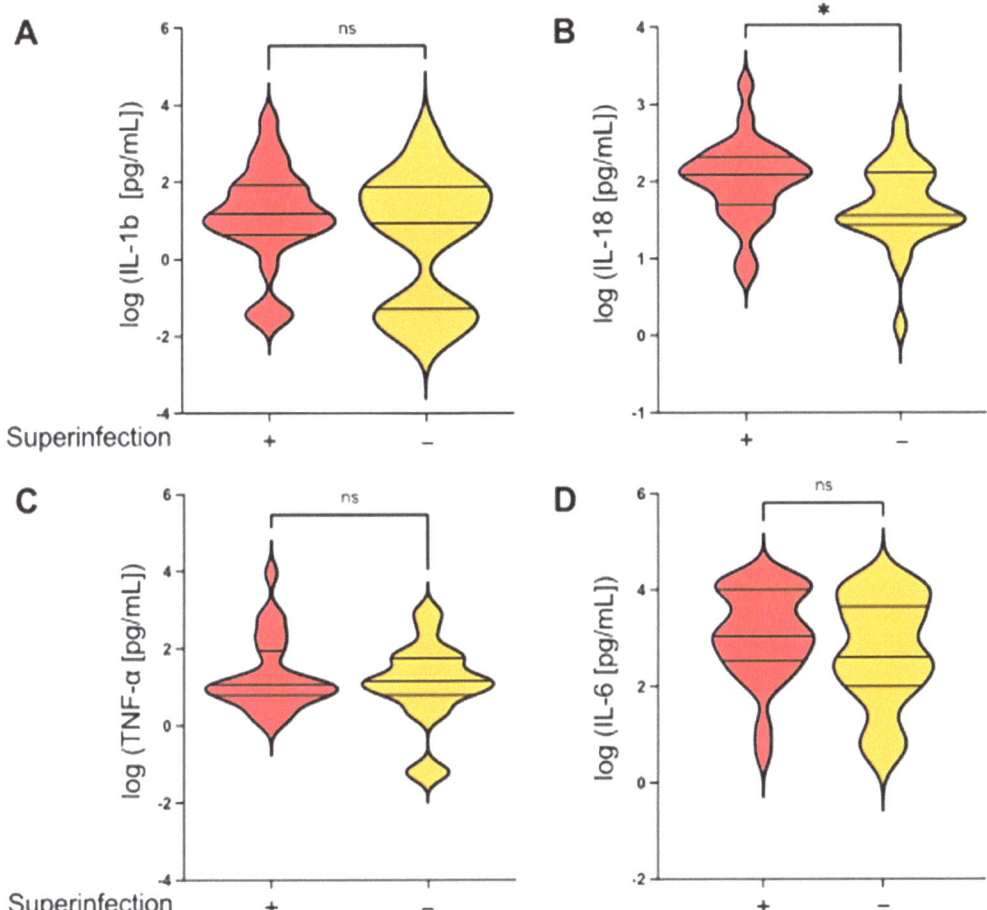

Figure 2. Pulmonary superinfections in patients with ARDS are associated with the increased production of inflammasome-dependent cytokines. Flexible fiberoptic bronchoscopy was performed within 24 h of disease onset. Bronchoalveolar lavage fluid (BALF) samples were collected in the right middle lobe and analyzed afterward via multiplex immunoassay. BALF concentrations of (**A**) IL-1ß, (**B**) IL-18, (**C**) TNF-α, and (**D**) IL-6 compared between ARDS patients with and without pulmonary superinfections. Mean ± SD of log-transformed data; unpaired t-test; * $p \leq 0.05$; ns = not significant; red violin plot = ARDS with superinfection; yellow violin plot = ARDS without superinfection.

4. Discussion

Pulmonary superinfection significantly influences patients' outcomes. Although the pathogenesis of ARDS development is well studied, the underlying mechanisms of the development of pulmonary superinfection remain not well understood. Besides the loss of epithelial barrier function, prolonged mechanical ventilation, and prone positioning, pulmonary dysbiosis in combination with altered immune defenses are major risk factors [4–6].

In this study, we showed that the alveolar epithelial damage markers sRAGE and SP-D were significantly increased in ARDS patients who developed pulmonary superinfections while the levels of the endothelial injury markers VEGF and Ang-2 did not differ between the groups (Figure 1). Furthermore, ARDS patients with pulmonary superinfections demonstrated increased levels of inflammasome-regulated IL-18 but not Il-1ß (Figure 2B).

To the best of our knowledge, the current study is the first report that links alveolar epithelial damage markers in ARDS to pulmonary superinfection. Yet, whether sRAGE and SP-D are direct injurious mediators or just markers of tissue damage that lead to pulmonary superinfection is unknown. sRAGE and SP-D are both elevated in ARDS patients and correlate with increased mortality and the severity of disease [9,26–28]. Patients with pneumonia or ARDS caused by influenza A virus infection are highly susceptible to co-infections and are characterized by increased SP-D and sRAGE levels [4,11,29–32]. This might be explained by multifactorial pathogenesis. Elevated levels of SP-D and sRAGE may indicate a loss of barrier function rendering patients more susceptible to pulmonary superinfections by forming new bacterial attachment sites and allowing bacterial translocation [6]. Furthermore, SP-D strongly potentiates the neutrophil respiratory burst in the presence of the influenza A virus by increasing the neutrophil uptake of the influenza A virus [33]. Similar to SP-D, sRAGE has been shown to promote a pro-inflammatory response by activating Nf-Kb. A side effect of RAGE signaling is the induction of reactive oxygen species (ROS), which can also activate Nf-Kb and boost other pro-inflammatory pathways such as cellular apoptosis [34]. Nf-Kb and ROS serve as key inflammasome activators triggering inflammasome assembly which mediates caspase-1 activation and subsequently the release of pro-inflammatory IL-1ß and IL-18 [21].

Inflammasome activation and consecutive IL-1ß and IL-18 production play a major role in the development of ARDS by driving tissue inflammation and a rapid, pro-inflammatory form of cell death called pyroptosis [8,17,35,36]. The subsequent loss of pulmonary epithelial cells might lead to immune barrier dysfunction, thereby increasing the susceptibility to pulmonary superinfections [37]. Accordingly, we observed significantly increased IL-18 concentrations and lung epithelial damage in ARDS patients who developed pulmonary superinfections in comparison to patients without pulmonary superinfections. Consistent with this, murine studies suggest that the production of inflammasome-regulated cytokines including IL-18 may contribute to the increased susceptibility to pulmonary superinfections [24,38,39]. Furthermore, inflammasome adaptor $ASC^{-/-}$ mice possessing a dysfunctional inflammasome function were protected from bacterial superinfection and associated lethality [40]. Yet, the current study found no differences in IL-1ß concentrations between ARDS patients with and without pulmonary superinfections. This might be explained by the extremely short half-life of IL-1ß, which is therefore often undetectable even in human pathologies that are clearly mediated by IL-1ß [40–43]. In addition, the immunopathological activity of IL-1β in ARDS patients might also be confined to local secretion and paracrine signaling that cannot be captured by a universal detection method such as BAL [43–45]. Therefore, previous studies that investigated the role of inflammasome activation in ARDS also focused on IL-18 production as a readout [17,46].

This study has several limitations, primarily its small sample size and single-center status which do not allow us to draw far-reaching conclusions from the results. The data from this study should be regarded as hypothesis-generating and used to design future confirmatory trials with larger cohorts which may allow us to define cut-off values for pulmonary superinfection biomarkers. Due to the retrospective nature of this study, routine systematic testing for pulmonary superinfection was not performed. Moreover, the decision to obtain microbiological and virological testing depended heavily on the treating physician and disease severity of the patient which might have indirectly created selection bias. The sensitivity of quantitative BAL cultures is as high as 90% for the diagnosis of bacterial infection and up to 80% in mycobacterial, fungal, and most viral infections [47]. However, false negative rates vary among studies possibly due to the lack of a uniform threshold for positive BAL cultures. The use of RT-PCR was also mostly limited to virological testing while multiplex PCR, which has shown superior sensitivity for the detection of respiratory lower tract infections compared to quantitative bacterial cultures [48], has rarely been performed. Hence, the number of pulmonary superinfections may be underestimated in our study. Another limitation is the lack of a universal, valid definition of pulmonary superinfection making it a challenging diagnosis. Timing, chest imaging, laboratory values, and microbiology and/or virology results in conjunction with clinical parameters should be incorporated into the definition. Lastly, the complexity and host susceptibility for pulmonary superinfection cannot be fully mirrored by biomarkers measured in serum and BALF at one specific time point. Although the identification of a unique time point can be easily implemented into clinical trials and routine practice, it may not fully reflect the intricate release kinetics of each individual biomarker, thus suggesting the superiority of serial measurements vs. single measurements. Serial measurements at the time of ICU admission and over the course of treatment may provide better prognostic information and ensure reliability. In addition, SP-D, sRAGE, and Ang-2, for example, are biomarkers that display high sensitivity and specificity for the diagnosis or outcome prediction of ARDS but have not been evaluated for pulmonary superinfections in ARDS patients [7].

5. Conclusions

In summary, the current study demonstrates that ARDS patients who develop pulmonary superinfections may exhibit a distinct biomarker pattern that indicates epithelial injury and inflammasome activation upon ICU admission. Our findings raise the question of whether this biomarker pattern could potentially be utilized to identify high-risk patients, possibly implementing targeted prevention and facilitating personalized treatment approaches.

Supplementary Materials: The following supporting information can be downloaded at: https://www.mdpi.com/article/10.3390/jcm12113649/s1. Table S1: Origin of ARDS in patients with and without pulmonary superinfection.

Author Contributions: Conceptualization, K.P., A.S. and C.B.; data curation, A.S., K.P., S.S., M.F., C.F. and C.B.; formal analysis, K.P., B.S. and C.B.; funding acquisition, K.P., M.C. and C.B.; investigation, K.P., A.S. and C.B.; methodology, K.P. and C.B.; project administration, K.P.; resources, P.S., M.S., E.G., B.S., V.B. and C.P.; supervision, C.B.; writing—original draft, K.P., A.S. and C.B.; writing—review and editing, A.S., K.P., L.W., C.F., M.C., C.P. and C.W. All authors have read and agreed to the published version of the manuscript.

Funding: This research was funded by grants and fellowships from the University of Bonn (BONFOR) and the B. Braun Foundation.

Institutional Review Board Statement: The study was conducted in accordance with the Declaration of Helsinki and approved by the Ethics Review Board of the University Hospital Bonn (protocol code 088/16, date of approval: 29 April 2016).

Informed Consent Statement: Written informed consent for participation was obtained to publish this paper.

Data Availability Statement: The study materials and datasets are available from the corresponding author upon reasonable request.

Conflicts of Interest: The authors declare no conflict of interest.

References

1. Matthay, M.A.; Zemans, R.L.; Zimmerman, G.A.; Arabi, Y.M.; Beitler, J.R.; Mercat, A.; Herridge, M.; Randolph, A.G.; Calfee, C.S. Acute respiratory distress syndrome. Nat Rev Dis Primer. *Nat. Publ. Group* **2019**, *5*, 18.
2. Ayzac, L.; Girard, R.; Baboi, L.; Beuret, P.; Rabilloud, M.; Richard, J.C.; Guérin, C. Ventilator-associated pneumonia in ARDS patients: The impact of prone positioning. A secondary analysis of the PROSEVA trial. *Intensive Care Med.* **2016**, *42*, 871–878. [CrossRef] [PubMed]
3. Forel, J.-M.; Voillet, F.; Pulina, D.; Gacouin, A.; Perrin, G.; Barrau, K.; Jaber, S.; Arnal, J.-M.; Fathallah, M.; Auquier, P.; et al. Ventilator-associated pneumonia and ICU mortality in severe ARDS patients ventilated according to a lung-protective strategy. *Crit. Care* **2012**, *16*, R65. [CrossRef]
4. Luyt, C.-E.; Bouadma, L.; Morris, A.C.; Dhanani, J.A.; Kollef, M.; Lipman, J.; Martin-Loeches, I.; Nseir, S.; Ranzani, O.T.; Roquilly, A.; et al. Pulmonary infections complicating ARDS. *Intensive Care Med.* **2020**, *46*, 2168–2183. [CrossRef]

5. Aguilera, E.R.; Lenz, L.L. Inflammation as a Modulator of Host Susceptibility to Pulmonary Influenza, Pneumococcal, and Co-Infections. *Front. Immunol.* **2020**, *11*, 105. [CrossRef] [PubMed]
6. Paget, C.; Trottein, F. Mechanisms of Bacterial Superinfection Post-influenza: A Role for Unconventional T Cells. *Front. Immunol.* **2019**, *10*, 336. [CrossRef] [PubMed]
7. Spadaro, S.; Park, M.; Turrini, C.; Tunstall, T.; Thwaites, R.; Mauri, T.; Ragazzi, R.; Ruggeri, P.; Hansel, T.T.; Caramori, G.; et al. Biomarkers for Acute Respiratory Distress syndrome and prospects for personalised medicine. *J. Inflamm.* **2019**, *16*, 1. [CrossRef]
8. Peukert, K.; Fox, M.; Schulz, S.; Feuerborn, C.; Frede, S.; Putensen, C.; Wrigge, H.; Kümmerer, B.M.; David, S.; Seeliger, B.; et al. Inhibition of Caspase-1 with Tetracycline Ameliorates Acute Lung Injury. *Am. J. Respir. Crit. Care Med.* **2021**, *204*, 53–63. [CrossRef]
9. Jabaudon, M.; Blondonnet, R.; Pereira, B.; Cartin-Ceba, R.; Lichtenstern, C.; Mauri, T.; Determann, R.M.; Drabek, T.; Hubmayr, R.D.; Gajic, O.; et al. Plasma sRAGE is independently associated with increased mortality in ARDS: A meta-analysis of individual patient data. *Intensive Care Med.* **2018**, *44*, 1388–1399. [CrossRef] [PubMed]
10. Eisner, M.; Parsons, P.; Matthay, M.; Ware, L.; Greene, K. Plasma surfactant protein levels and clinical outcomes in patients with acute lung injury. *Thorax* **2003**, *58*, 983–988. [CrossRef]
11. Peukert, K.; Seeliger, B.; Fox, M.; Feuerborn, C.; Sauer, A.; Schuss, P.; Schneider, M.; David, S.; Welte, T.; Putensen, C.; et al. SP-D Serum Levels Reveal Distinct Epithelial Damage in Direct Human ARDS. *J. Clin. Med.* **2021**, *10*, 737. [CrossRef]
12. Zhao, Z.; Wickersham, N.; Kangelaris, K.N.; May, A.K.; Bernard, G.R.; Matthay, M.A.; Calfee, C.S.; Koyama, T.; Ware, L.B. External validation of a biomarker and clinical prediction model for hospital mortality in acute respiratory distress syndrome. *Intensiv. Care Med.* **2017**, *43*, 1123–1131. [CrossRef]
13. Fremont, R.D.; Koyama, T.; Calfee, C.S.; Wu, W.; Dossett, L.A.; Bossert, F.R.; Mitchell, D.; Wickersham, N.; Bernard, G.R.; Matthay, M.A.; et al. Acute Lung Injury in Patients with Traumatic Injuries: Utility of a Panel of Biomarkers for Diagnosis and Pathogenesis. *J. Trauma* **2010**, *68*, 1121–1127. [CrossRef] [PubMed]
14. Terpstra, M.L.; Aman, J.; van Nieuw Amerongen, G.P.; Groeneveld, A.B.J. Plasma biomarkers for acute respiratory distress syndrome: A systematic review and meta-analysis. *Crit Care Med.* **2014**, *42*, 691–700. [CrossRef] [PubMed]
15. Agrawal, A.; Matthay, M.A.; Kangelaris, K.N.; Stein, J.; Chu, J.C.; Imp, B.M.; Cortez, A.; Abbott, J.; Liu, K.D.; Calfee, C.S. Plasma angiopoietin-2 predicts the onset of acute lung injury in critically ill patients. *Am. J. Respir. Crit. Care Med.* **2013**, *187*, 736–742. [CrossRef] [PubMed]
16. Wada, T.; Jesmin, S.; Gando, S.; Yanagida, Y.; Mizugaki, A.; Sultana, S.N.; Zaedi, S.; Yokota, H. The role of angiogenic factors and their soluble receptors in acute lung injury (ALI)/acute respiratory distress syndrome (ARDS) associated with critical illness. *J. Inflamm.* **2013**, *10*, 6. [CrossRef]
17. Dolinay, T.; Kim, Y.S.; Howrylak, J.; Hunninghake, G.M.; An, C.H.; Fredenburgh, L.; Massaro, A.F.; Rogers, A.; Gazourian, L.; Nakahira, K.; et al. Inflammasome-regulated cytokines are critical mediators of acute lung injury. *Am. J. Respir. Crit. Care Med.* **2012**, *185*, 1225–1234. [CrossRef]
18. RRogers, A.J.; Guan, J.; Trtchounian, A.; Hunninghake, G.M.; Kaimal, R.; Desai, M.; Kozikowski, L.-A.; DeSouza, L.; Mogan, S.; Liu, K.D.; et al. Association of Elevated Plasma Interleukin-18 Level With Increased Mortality in a Clinical Trial of Statin Treatment for Acute Respiratory Distress Syndrome. *Crit. Care Med.* **2019**, *47*, 1089–1096. [CrossRef]
19. Grailer, J.J.; Canning, B.A.; Kalbitz, M.; Haggadone, M.D.; Dhond, R.M.; Andjelkovic, A.V.; Zetoune, F.S.; Ward, P.A. Critical role for the NLRP3 inflammasome during acute lung injury. *J. Immunol.* **2014**, *192*, 5974–5983. [CrossRef]
20. Meduri, G.U.; Kohler, G.; Headley, S.; Tolley, E.; Stentz, F.; Postlethwaite, A. Inflammatory cytokines in the BAL of patients with ARDS. Persistent elevation over time predicts poor outcome. *Chest* **1995**, *108*, 1303–1314. [CrossRef]
21. McVey, M.J.; Steinberg, B.E.; Goldenberg, N.M. Inflammasome activation in acute lung injury. *Am. J. Physiol. Lung Cell Mol. Physiol. Am. Physiol. Soc.* **2021**, *320*, L165–L178. [CrossRef] [PubMed]
22. Guo, H.; Callaway, J.B.; Ting, J.P.-Y. Inflammasomes: Mechanism of action, role in disease, and therapeutics. *Nat. Med.* **2015**, *21*, 677–687. [CrossRef] [PubMed]
23. Hornung, V.; Latz, E. Critical functions of priming and lysosomal damage for NLRP3 activation. *Eur. J. Immunol.* **2010**, *40*, 620–623. [CrossRef]
24. Robinson, K.M.; Ramanan, K.; Clay, M.; McHugh, K.J.; Pilewski, M.J.; Nickolich, K.L.; Corey, C.; Shiva, S.; Wang, J.; Alcorn, J.F. The inflammasome potentiates influenza/Staphylococcus aureus superinfection in mice. *J. Clin. Investig.* **2018**, *3*, 97470. [CrossRef]
25. Force, A.D.T.; Ranieri, V.M.; Rubenfeld, G.D.; Thompson, B.; Ferguson, N.; Caldwell, E.; Fan, E.; Camporota, L.; Slutsky, A.S. The ARDS Definition Task Force. Acute Respiratory Distress Syndrome: The Berlin Definition. *JAMA* **2012**, *307*, 2526–2533.
26. Agustama, A.; Surgean Veterini, A.; Utariani, A. Correlation of Surfactant Protein-D (SP-D) Serum Levels with ARDS Severity and Mortality in Covid-19 Patients in Indonesia. *Acta Medica Acad.* **2022**, *51*, 21–28. [CrossRef] [PubMed]
27. Dahmer, M.K.; Flori, H.; Sapru, A.; Kohne, J.; Weeks, H.M.; Curley, M.A.; Matthay, M.A.; Quasney, M.W.; Bateman, S.T.; Berg, M.; et al. Surfactant Protein D Is Associated with Severe Pediatric ARDS, Prolonged Ventilation, and Death in Children with Acute Respiratory Failure. *Chest* **2020**, *158*, 1027–1035. [CrossRef]
28. Lim, A.; Radujkovic, A.; Weigand, M.A.; Merle, U. Soluble receptor for advanced glycation end products (sRAGE) as a biomarker of COVID-19 disease severity and indicator of the need for mechanical ventilation, ARDS and mortality. *Ann. Intensiv. Care* **2021**, *11*, 50. [CrossRef]

29. Delgado, C.; Krötzsch, E.; Jiménez-Alvarez, L.A.; Ramírez-Martínez, G.; Márquez-García, J.E.; Cruz-Lagunas, A.; Morán, J.; Hernández, C.; Sierra-Vargas, P.; Avila-Moreno, F.; et al. Serum surfactant protein D (SP-D) is a prognostic marker of poor outcome in patients with A/H1N1 virus infection. *Lung* **2014**, *193*, 25–30. [CrossRef]
30. Klein, E.Y.; Monteforte, B.; Gupta, A.; Jiang, W.; May, L.; Hsieh, Y.; Dugas, A. The frequency of influenza and bacterial coinfection: A systematic review and meta-analysis. *Influenza Other Respir. Viruses* **2016**, *10*, 394–403. [CrossRef]
31. Park, J.; Pabon, M.; Choi, A.M.K.; Siempos, I.I.; Fredenburgh, L.E.; Baron, R.M.; Jeon, K.; Chung, C.R.; Yang, J.H.; Park, C.-M.; et al. Plasma surfactant protein-D as a diagnostic biomarker for acute respiratory distress syndrome: Validation in US and Korean cohorts. *BMC Pulm. Med.* **2017**, *17*, 204. [CrossRef] [PubMed]
32. van Zoelen, M.A.; van der Sluijs, K.F.; Achouiti, A.; Florquin, S.; Braun-Pater, J.M.; Yang, H.; Nawroth, P.P.; Tracey, K.J.; Bierhaus, A.; van der Poll, T. Receptor for advanced glycation end products is detrimental during influenza A virus pneumonia. *Virology* **2009**, *391*, 265–273. [CrossRef] [PubMed]
33. White, M.R.; Crouch, E.; Vesona, J.; Tacken, P.J.; Batenburg, J.J.; Leth-Larsen, R.; Holmskov, U.; Hartshorn, K.L. Respiratory innate immune proteins differentially modulate the neutrophil respiratory burst response to influenza A virus. *Am. J. Physiol. Cell. Mol. Physiol.* **2005**, *289*, L606–L616. [CrossRef] [PubMed]
34. Oczypok, E.A.; Perkins, T.N.; Oury, T.D. All the "RAGE" in lung disease: The receptor for advanced glycation endproducts (RAGE) is a major mediator of pulmonary inflammatory responses. *Paediatr. Respir. Rev.* **2017**, *23*, 40–49. [CrossRef] [PubMed]
35. Tsai, Y.; Chiang, K.; Hung, J.; Chang, W.; Lin, H.; Shieh, J.; Chong, I.; Hsu, Y. Der f1 induces pyroptosis in human bronchial epithelia via the NLRP3 inflammasome. *Int. J. Mol. Med.* **2018**, *41*, 757–764. [CrossRef]
36. Latz, E.; Xiao, T.S.; Stutz, A. Activation and regulation of the inflammasomes. *Nat. Rev. Immunol.* **2013**, *13*, 397–411. [CrossRef]
37. Major, J.; Crotta, S.; Llorian, M.; McCabe, T.M.; Gad, H.H.; Priestnall, S.L.; Hartmann, R.; Wack, A. Type I and III interferons disrupt lung epithelial repair during recovery from viral infection. *Science* **2020**, *369*, 712–717. [CrossRef]
38. Robinson, K.M.; Choi, S.M.; McHugh, K.J.; Mandalapu, S.; Enelow, R.I.; Kolls, J.K.; Alcorn, J.F. Influenza A Exacerbates Staphylococcus aureus Pneumonia by Attenuating IL-1β Production in Mice. *J. Immunol.* **2013**, *191*, 5153–5159. [CrossRef]
39. Ataide, M.A.; Andrade, W.A.; Zamboni, D.S.; Wang, D.; Souza, M.D.C.; Franklin, B.S.; Elian, S.; Martins, F.S.; Pereira, D.; Reed, G.; et al. Malaria-Induced NLRP12/NLRP3-Dependent Caspase-1 Activation Mediates Inflammation and Hypersensitivity to Bacterial Superinfection. *PLoS Pathog.* **2014**, *10*, e1003885. [CrossRef]
40. Buszko, M.; Park, J.-H.; Verthelyi, D.; Sen, R.; Young, H.A.; Rosenberg, A.S. The dynamic changes in cytokine responses in COVID-19: A snapshot of the current state of knowledge. *Nat. Immunol.* **2020**, *21*, 1146–1151. [CrossRef]
41. Kudo, S.; Mizuno, K.; Hirai, Y.; Shimizu, T. Clearance and tissue distribution of recombinant human interleukin 1 beta in rats. *Cancer Res.* **1990**, *50*, 5751–5755. [PubMed]
42. Dinarello, C.A. Interleukin-1 in the pathogenesis and treatment of inflammatory diseases. *Blood* **2011**, *117*, 3720–3732. [CrossRef] [PubMed]
43. Pascual, V.; Allantaz, F.; Arce, E.; Punaro, M.; Banchereau, J. Role of interleukin-1 (IL-1) in the pathogenesis of systemic onset juvenile idiopathic arthritis and clinical response to IL-1 blockade. *J. Exp. Med.* **2005**, *201*, 1479–1486. [CrossRef]
44. Merad, M.; Martin, J.C. Pathological inflammation in patients with COVID-19: A key role for monocytes and macrophages. *Nat. Rev. Immunol.* **2020**, *20*, 355–362. [CrossRef]
45. Vora, S.M.; Lieberman, J.; Wu, H. Inflammasome activation at the crux of severe COVID-19. *Nat. Rev. Immunol.* **2021**, *21*, 694–703. [CrossRef] [PubMed]
46. Sefik, E.; Qu, R.; Junqueira, C.; Kaffe, E.; Mirza, H.; Zhao, J.; Brewer, J.R.; Han, A.; Steach, H.R.; Israelow, B.; et al. Inflammasome activation in infected macrophages drives COVID-19 pathology. *Nature* **2022**, *606*, 585–593. [CrossRef]
47. Stanzel, F. Bronchoalveolar Lavage. In *Principles and Practice of Interventional Pulmonology*; Springer: New York, NY, USA, 2012; pp. 165–176. [CrossRef]
48. Salina, A.; Schumann, D.M.; Franchetti, L.; Jahn, K.; Purkabiri, K.; Müller, R.; Strobel, W.; Khanna, N.; Tamm, M.; Stolz, D. Multiplex bacterial PCR in the bronchoalveolar lavage fluid of non-intubated patients with suspected pulmonary infection: A quasi-experimental study. *ERJ Open Res.* **2022**, *8*, 00595–2021. [CrossRef]

Disclaimer/Publisher's Note: The statements, opinions and data contained in all publications are solely those of the individual author(s) and contributor(s) and not of MDPI and/or the editor(s). MDPI and/or the editor(s) disclaim responsibility for any injury to people or property resulting from any ideas, methods, instructions or products referred to in the content.

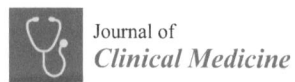

Article

Application of Neuromuscular Blockers in Patients with ARDS in ICU: A Retrospective Study Based on the MIMIC-III Database

Xiaojun Pan [†], Jiao Liu [†], Sheng Zhang, Sisi Huang, Limin Chen, Xuan Shen and Dechang Chen *

Department of Critical Care Medicine, Ruijin Hospital, Shanghai Jiao Tong University School of Medicine, No. 197, Ruijin 2nd Road, Shanghai 200025, China
* Correspondence: cdc12064@rjh.com.cn
† These authors contributed equally to this work.

Abstract: Background: Although neuromuscular blocker agents (NMBAs) are recommended by guidelines as a treatment for ARDS patients, the efficacy of NMBAs is still controversial. Our study aimed to investigate the association between cisatracurium infusion and the medium- and long-term outcomes of critically ill patients with moderate and severe ARDS. Methods: We performed a single-center, retrospective study of 485 critically ill adult patients with ARDS based on the Medical Information Mart for Intensive Care III (MIMIC-III) database. Propensity score matching (PSM) was used to match patients receiving NMBA administration with those not receiving NMBAs. The Cox proportional hazards model, Kaplan–Meier method, and subgroup analysis were used to evaluate the relationship between NMBA therapy and 28-day mortality. Results: A total of 485 moderate and severe patients with ARDS were reviewed and 86 pairs of patients were matched after PSM. NMBAs were not associated with reduced 28-day mortality (hazard ratio (HR) 1.44; 95% CI: 0.85~2.46; $p = 0.20$), 90-day mortality (HR = 1.49; 95% CI: 0.92~2.41; $p = 0.10$), 1-year mortality (HR = 1.34; 95% CI: 0.86~2.09; $p = 0.20$), or hospital mortality (HR = 1.34; 95% CI: 0.81~2.24; $p = 0.30$). However, NMBAs were associated with a prolonged duration of ventilation and the length of ICU stay. Conclusions: NMBAs were not associated with improved medium- and long-term survival and may result in some adverse clinical outcomes.

Keywords: intensive care unit; ARDS; NMBAs; mortality

1. Introduction

Acute respiratory distress syndrome (ARDS) affects approximately 3 million patients globally every year [1] and accounts for approximately 10% of intensive care unit (ICU) inpatients [2,3]. Although we have made progress in our understanding of the disease, the treatment options for ARDS are still limited. The mortality of ARDS patients ranges from 40% to 60% depending on the severity of the disease, which is usually high [1,4–7].

ARDS is defined as an acute inflammatory lung injury caused by a variety of diseases, resulting in refractory hypoxemia and ultimately leading to pulmonary dysfunction, which threatens the patient's life [2,3]. Mechanical ventilation is a key element of the treatment process for ARDS and can reduce mortality among ARDS patients [8]. Although the low-tidal-volume ventilation strategy may protect the lungs from a ventilation-related lung injury, both high pressure and a large tidal volume may occur through the spontaneous breathing effort of the patients [9].

Neuromuscular blocking agents (NMBAs) are a class of therapeutic drugs that act on the skeletal neuromuscular junction (NMJ) by inducing muscle paralysis, which can reduce the consumption of oxygen and patient–ventilator asynchrony [10]. NMBAs can improve oxygenation and decrease ventilator-induced lung injury and the work required for breathing, prevent ventilator asynchrony, and reduce airway pressure and lung stress [11].

However, NMBA therapy may not affect oxygen consumption in patients under appropriate sedation [12]. Moreover, it may result in a variety of adverse outcomes such as ICU-acquired weakness, polyneuropathy, atelectasis, muscle paralysis, etc. [10,13]. A randomized control trial (RCT) showed that continuous cisatracurium infusion can improve oxygenation in patients with ARDS [14]. Another RCT demonstrated that cisatracurium can significantly reduce the inflammatory response in ARDS patients [15]. In 2010, the ACURASYS trial recruited 339 patients and found that the early administration of cisatracurium to patients with moderate and severe ARDS improved the hospital mortality rate [11]. The PETAL trial reported that there was no significant difference in all-cause mortality on day 90 between ARDS patients who received early or continuous cisatracurium administration and those who received usual care [16].

Therefore, NMBA infusion in patients with ARDS remains controversial. The aim of this study was to evaluate the efficacy and middle- and long-term outcomes of early cisatracurium infusion in moderate and severe ARDS patients.

2. Materials and Methods

2.1. Sources of Data

Data for the study were derived from the MIMIC-III database (Medical Information Mart for Intensive Care, version 1.4). The database was approved by the Institutional Review Board (IRB) of the Massachusetts Institute of Technology (MIT). After full completion of the National Institutes of Health web-based training course and the Protecting Human Research Participants examination (NO. 35209874), permission to extract data from MIMIC-III was provided. The database is funded by the National Institutes of Health (NIH), Beth Israel Deaconess Medical Center, the Massachusetts Institute of Technology (MIT), Oxford University, and Massachusetts General Hospital (MGH), having been created by emergency doctors, intensive physicians, computer science experts, etc. The database records the data of patients admitted to the Beth Israel Deaconess Medical Center from June 2001 to October 2012. It contains more than 58,000 inpatient data points representing 38,645 adult individuals and 7875 newborns. These data are organized into tables in CSV format for research inquiries and include almost all the data of the patients during ICU treatment, such as demographic characteristics, vital signs recorded every hour, operation records, the administration time and dose of the drug used, the amount of fluid passing in and out, the results of microbiological examinations, care records, the outcomes of the patients (inpatient deaths, out-of-hospital deaths, and discharges), etc.

2.2. Study Cohort

We conducted a single-center, retrospective study of ARDS patients according to the Berlin definition. All the data were extracted based on the method established by Johnson et al. [13,14]. The inclusion criteria were as follows: (1) moderate and severe ARDS patients; (2) patients first admitted to ICU; (3) age $\geq$ 16 years old; (4) patients receiving mechanical ventilation for more than 48 h; and (5) patients receiving cisatracurium therapy. The exclusion criteria were as follows: (1) patients who died within the first 48 h; (2) removal of the endotracheal tube within 48 h; and (3) missing key data. Data were extracted from the MIMIC-III database using Structured Query Language (SQL). The following data were collected on the first day of ICU admission: weight, gender, age, admission type, ethnicity (White, Hispanic, Black, or Other), mechanical ventilation, use of NMBAs and vasopressors, renal replacement therapy (RRT), ARDS severity, simplified acute physiology score II (SAPS II) and sequential organ failure assessment (SOFA) score, heart rate, saturation of pulse oxygen (SPO2), respiratory rate, positive end-expiratory pressure (PEEP), and comorbidities. The definitions of moderate and severe ARDS were in accordance with the Berlin definition.

2.3. Endpoints

The primary endpoint was the 28-day mortality. The secondary endpoints were the 90-day mortality, 1-year mortality, hospital mortality, length of stay in the ICU and hospital, and ventilation duration. Moreover, we extracted the vital signs (including the heart rate, blood pressure, body temperature, and SpO2), respiratory mechanic indicators (including the tidal volume, plateau pressure, peak inspiratory pressure, PEEP, respiratory rate, and PaO2/FiO2 (P/F) ratio), Ramsay sedation scores (RASS), and total amount of fluid input and urine output of the patients from the first day of hospital admission to the seventh day.

2.4. Statistical Analysis

Continuous variables are summarized as the mean and standard deviation or median and interquartile range according to the data distribution, and categorical variables are presented as numbers and percentages. The Shapiro–Wilk test was used to test for a normal distribution. A Wilcoxon rank-sum test, Student's t-test, or Chi-square test was performed to compare the differences between groups where appropriate. The Cox hazards model was conducted to evaluate the difference in mortality outcomes between the two groups and the confounding variables were defined according to a p-value < 0.05 based on univariate analysis and clinical expert judgment. Kaplan–Meier curves were created for the pre-matched and matched cohorts to assess the survival of the NMBA and non-NMBA groups.

To control the confounding factors between the two groups, propensity-score matching (PSM) was used. The propensity score of an individual was determined based on the given covariates of age, gender, ethnicity, admission type, SOFA and SAPS II scores, ARDS severity, heart rate, respiratory rate, RASS score, first-day use of vasopressors, ventilation and RRT, chronic disease of the liver, chronic obstructive pulmonary disease (COPD), chronic heart failure (CHF), and malignancy using a generalized linear model. We used random forest imputation to process the missing data before PSM. When the missing data amounted to less than 5%, random forest was performed using the "randomForest" package in R. Patients were matched in a 1:1 ratio using the nearest neighbor algorithm with a caliper of 0.2. After matching, the standardized mean differences (SMDs) between the two groups were calculated. Statistical significance was considered to be indicated by a two-sided $p < 0.05$. All the statistical analyses mentioned above were performed using RStudio (version 4.0.5).

3. Results

3.1. Baseline Characteristics

After reviewing 61,532 subjects from the MIMIC-III database, we identified ARDS in 1349 subjects according to the Berlin definition, and 485 patients were enrolled after the application of the exclusion criteria (Figure 1). A total of 115 patients (23.71%) received NMBA therapy and 370 (76.29%) did not, as shown in Table 1. There were no significant differences in weight, gender, admission type, ethnicity, first-day use of ventilation and RRT, the SAPS II score, CHF, AFIB, CAD, malignancy, stroke, and chronic disease of the liver or renal between the two groups. The most common comorbidities were chronic heart failure and COPD, which were observed at lower frequencies in the NMBA group than in the non-NMBA group. After PSM, 86 patients who received NMBAs were matched with 86 patients who did not. The baseline was well balanced between the two groups (shown in Table 2 and Figure S1).

3.2. Relationship between NMBAs and Outcomes

In our study, the 28-day mortality, 90-day mortality, and 1-year mortality were 29.48%, 35.05%, and 43.09%, respectively. The results of the pre-matched cohort showed that the 28-day mortality (HR = 1.62; 95% CI: 1.14–2.30; $p < 0.01$), 90-day mortality (HR = 1.58; 95% CI: 1.14–2.19; $p < 0.01$), 1-year mortality (HR = 1.40; 95% CI: 1.04–1.90; $p = 0.03$), and hospital mortality (HR = 1.41; 95% CI: 0.99–2.00; $p = 0.06$) were associated with NMBA therapy in the original cohort. After being adjusted for the confounders (including gender, age, SOFA, SAPS II, ethnicity, ARDS severity, chronic disease of the liver, malignancy, and respiratory rate) with two COX models, NMBAs were still associated with the 28-day, 90-day, or 1-year mortality (Table 3). The median lengths of hospital stay and ICU stay were 17.09 and 10.98 days, respectively, and the median duration of ventilation was 7.59 days (Table 4). The duration of ICU stay and ventilation were longer among patients who received NMBA therapy.

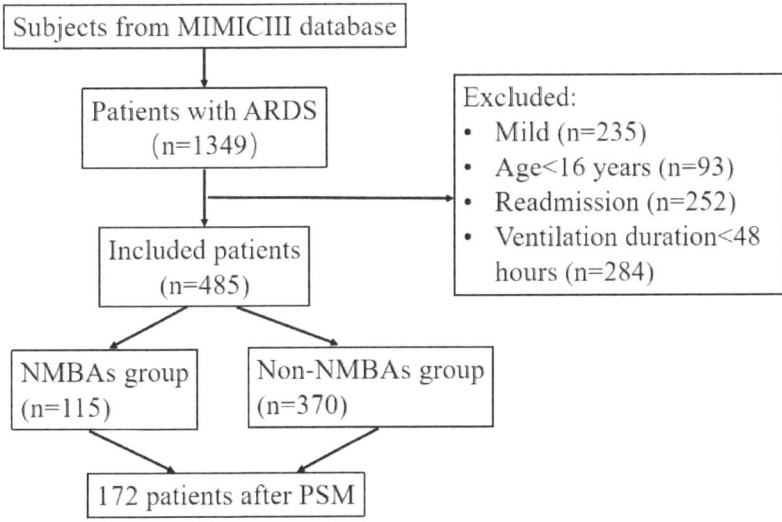

Figure 1. Flowchart of included patients. MIMIC-III: Multiparameter Intelligent Monitoring in Intensive Care Database III; ICU: intensive care unit; PSM: propensity-score matching.

Table 1. Baseline characteristics of the original cohort.

	All (n = 485)	Non-NMBAs (n = 370)	NMBAs (n = 115)	p-Value
Weight	80.00 [68.45, 95.00]	80.20 [68.00, 95.00]	80.00 [69.15, 94.95]	0.90
Gender (%)				0.05
Male	284 (58.56)	207 (55.95)	77 (66.96)	
Female	201 (41.44)	163 (44.05)	38 (33.04)	
Age (years)	58.52 [46.04, 72.22]	59.85 [47.02, 75.20]	56.47 [40.64, 66.45]	0.01
Admission type (%)				0.42
Elective	31 (6.39)	22 (5.95)	9 (7.83)	
Emergency	432 (89.07)	329 (88.92)	103 (89.57)	
Urgent	22 (4.54)	19 (5.14)	3 (2.61)	
Ethnicity (%)				0.96
White	307 (63.30)	236 (63.78)	71 (61.74)	
Hispanic	17 (3.51)	13 (3.51)	4 (3.48)	
Black	31 (6.39)	24 (6.49)	7 (6.09)	
Other	130 (26.80)	97 (26.22)	33 (28.70)	
Mechanical ventilation (%)	426 (87.84)	323 (87.30)	103 (89.57)	0.63
Vasopressors (%)	249 (51.34)	173 (46.76)	76 (66.09)	<0.01
RRT (%)	30 (6.19)	20 (5.41)	10 (8.70)	0.29
ARDS severity (%)				<0.01
Moderate	250 (51.55)	214 (57.84)	36 (31.30)	
Severe	235 (48.45)	156 (42.16)	79 (68.70)	
SAPS II	43.00 [33.00, 54.00]	43.00 [33.00, 53.00]	44.00 [34.50, 59.00]	0.28
SOFA	7.00 [5.00, 10.00]	7.00 [5.00, 9.00]	9.00 [6.00, 12.00]	<0.01
Heart rate (bpm)	93.27 (17.94)	92.12 (16.99)	96.99 (20.35)	0.01

Table 1. Cont.

	All (n = 485)	Non-NMBAs (n = 370)	NMBAs (n = 115)	p-Value
SpO2	96.73 [95.43, 97.89]	97.03 [95.70, 98.08]	96.08 [94.67, 97.40]	<0.01
Respiratory rate (bpm)	22.35 (4.93)	21.64 (4.85)	24.61 (4.52)	<0.01
PEEP	8.78 [5.84, 11.22]	8.33 [5.00, 10.24]	11.70 [8.57, 14.94]	<0.01
RASS score	−1.20 [−1.44, −0.83]	−1.07 [−1.20, −0.75]	−1.72 [−2.30, −1.20]	<0.01
Co-morbidities (%)				
CHF	171 (35.26)	142 (37.40)	29 (25.22)	0.08
AFIB	115 (23.71)	92 (24.86)	23 (20.00)	0.34
CAD	44 (9.07)	35 (9.46)	9 (7.83)	0.73
Malignancy	85 (17.53)	71 (19.19)	14 (12.17)	0.11
Kidney	36 (7.42)	28 (7.57)	8 (6.96)	>0.99
Liver	31 (6.39)	24 (6.49)	7 (6.09)	>0.99
COPD	66 (13.60)	60 (16.22)	6 (5.22)	0.01
Stroke	44 (9.07)	34 (9.19)	10 (8.70)	>0.99

Abbreviations: NMBAs, neuromuscular blocking agents. ARDS, acute respiratory distress syndrome. RRT, renal replacement therapy. SAPS II, simplified acute physiology score II. SOFA, sequential organ failure assessment. PEEP, positive end-expiratory pressure. RASS sore, Richmond agitation–sedation scale score. CHF, chronic heart failure. AFIB, atrial fibrillation. CAD, coronary artery disease. COPD, chronic obstructive pulmonary disease. bpm, beats per minute. All covariates were reported as the mean (standard deviation) and median (IQR). Mechanical ventilation, vasopressors, and RRT were received on the first day of therapy. All data were extracted in the first 24 h of ICU admission.

Table 2. Baseline characteristics of the matched cohort.

	Matched Cohort		
	Non-NMBAs	NMBAs	SMD
n	86	86	
Gender (%)			0.12
Male	58 (67.44)	53 (61.63)	
Female	28 (32.56)	33 (38.37)	
Age (years)	52.69 (19.88)	54.45 (16.28)	0.10
Admission type (%)			0.14
Elective	5 (5.81)	7 (8.14)	
Emergency	76 (88.37)	76 (88.37)	
Urgent	5 (5.81)	3 (3.49)	
Ethnicity (%)			0.08
White	52 (60.47)	54 (62.79)	
Hispanic	5 (5.81)	4 (4.65)	
Black	5 (5.81)	4 (4.65)	
Other	24 (27.91)	24 (27.91)	
Ventilation (%)	77 (89.53)	77 (89.53)	<0.01
RRT (%)	6 (6.98)	7 (8.14)	0.04
Vasopressors (%)	57 (66.28)	51 (59.30)	0.15
ARDS severity (%)			<0.01
Moderate	29 (33.72)	29 (33.72)	
Severe	57 (66.28)	57 (66.28)	
SAPS II	45.00 (14.68)	45.62 (16.83)	0.04
SOFA	8.65 (3.60)	8.63 (3.85)	<0.01
Heart rate (bpm)	94.52 (18.08)	95.94 (19.27)	0.08
Respiratory rate (bpm)	24.49 (4.77)	24.21 (4.24)	0.06
RASS	2.69 (0.62)	2.65 (0.48)	0.07
Co-morbidities (%)			
CHF	24 (27.91)	21 (24.42)	0.08
Renal			
Liver	7 (8.14)	6 (6.98)	0.04
COPD	3 (3.49)	5 (5.81)	0.11
Stroke	9 (10.47)	9 (10.47)	<0.01

Abbreviation: SMD, standardized mean difference. All covariates are reported as the mean and standard deviation.

Table 3. Outcomes of NMBAs and non-NMBA patients and sensitivity analysis.

	HR	Low 95% CI	High 95% CI	p-Value
Pre-matched cohort				
28-day mortality	1.62	1.14	2.30	<0.01
Adjusted model I	1.78	1.23	2.56	<0.01
Adjusted model II	1.39	0.94	2.04	<0.01
90-day mortality	1.58	1.14	2.19	<0.01
Adjusted model I	1.75	1.25	2.45	<0.01
Adjusted model II	1.49	1.03	2.14	<0.01
One-year mortality	1.40	1.04	1.90	0.03
Adjusted model I	1.41	1.03	1.92	<0.01
Adjusted model II	1.39	1.00	1.95	<0.01
Hospital mortality	1.41	0.99	2.00	0.06
Adjusted model I	1.60	1.11	2.30	<0.01
Adjusted model II	1.32	0.90	1.95	<0.01
Matched cohort				
28-day mortality	1.44	0.85	2.46	0.20
Adjusted model I	1.39	0.81	2.39	0.23
Adjusted model II	1.47	0.84	2.56	0.17
90-day mortality	1.49	0.92	2.41	0.10
Adjusted model I	1.54	0.94	2.54	0.09
Adjusted model II	1.61	0.97	2.67	0.06
One-year mortality	1.34	0.86	2.09	0.20
Adjusted model I	1.34	0.85	2.10	0.20
Adjusted model II	1.41	0.89	2.22	0.15
Hospital mortality	1.34	0.81	2.24	0.30
Adjusted model I	1.39	0.83	2.32	0.21
Adjusted model II	1.48	0.87	2.52	0.15

Abbreviations: CI, confidence interval. HR, hazard ratio; All models were obtained by Cox proportional hazards model analysis of the relationship between NMBA therapy and all-cause mortality. Model I was adjusted for gender, age, admission type, and ethnicity. Model II was adjusted for gender, age, SOFA, SAPS II, ethnicity, ARDS severity, chronic disease of the liver, malignancy, and respiratory rate.

Table 4. Other outcomes.

	Overall	Non-NMBAs	NMBAs	p-Value
Pre-matched cohort	N = 485	N = 370	N = 115	
Length of hospital stay (days)	17.09 [10.11, 24.90]	16.80 [10.12, 23.76]	18.09 [9.48, 29.80]	0.21
Length of ICU stay (days)	10.98 [6.14, 18.76]	10.20 [5.96, 16.18]	14.92 [7.29, 26.79]	<0.01
Duration of ventilation (days)	7.59 [4.42, 14.00]	7.12 [4.17, 11.97]	12.29 [5.53, 20.33]	<0.01
Matched cohort	N = 172	N = 86	N = 86	
Length of hospital stay (days)	17.15 [9.62, 26.70]	14.92 [9.43, 22.02]	18.05 [11.56, 28.95]	0.06
Length of ICU stay (days)	11.22 [6.02, 19.94]	9.37 [5.47, 12.86]	14.67 [7.96, 26.22]	<0.01
Duration of ventilation (days)	8.72 [4.42, 15.59]	6.40 [3.40, 10.48]	12.38 [5.55, 19.77]	<0.01

Data are represented by median (IQR).

After PSM, NMBA therapy use was not associated with a reduced 28-day, 90-day, 1-year, or hospital mortality in the matched cohort (Table 3). Moreover, NMBA therapy was not associated with the 28-day, 90-day, 1-year, or hospital mortality after adjusting for the possible confounding factors in the matched cohort (Table 3). However, the ventilation duration and ICU stay were 8.72 and 11.22 days, which were prolonged by NMBA administration (Table 4). Kaplan–Meier survival curves were plotted to evaluate the effect of NMBA treatment using the log-rank test, and the results are shown in Figure 2. The 28-day, 90-day, and 1-year mortality were higher in the NMBA group in the original cohort ($p < 0.01$, $p < 0.01$, $p = 0.03$). However, there was no difference in the 28-day, 90-day, or 1-year mortality between the groups in the matched cohort ($p = 0.84$, $p = 0.95$, $p = 0.78$).

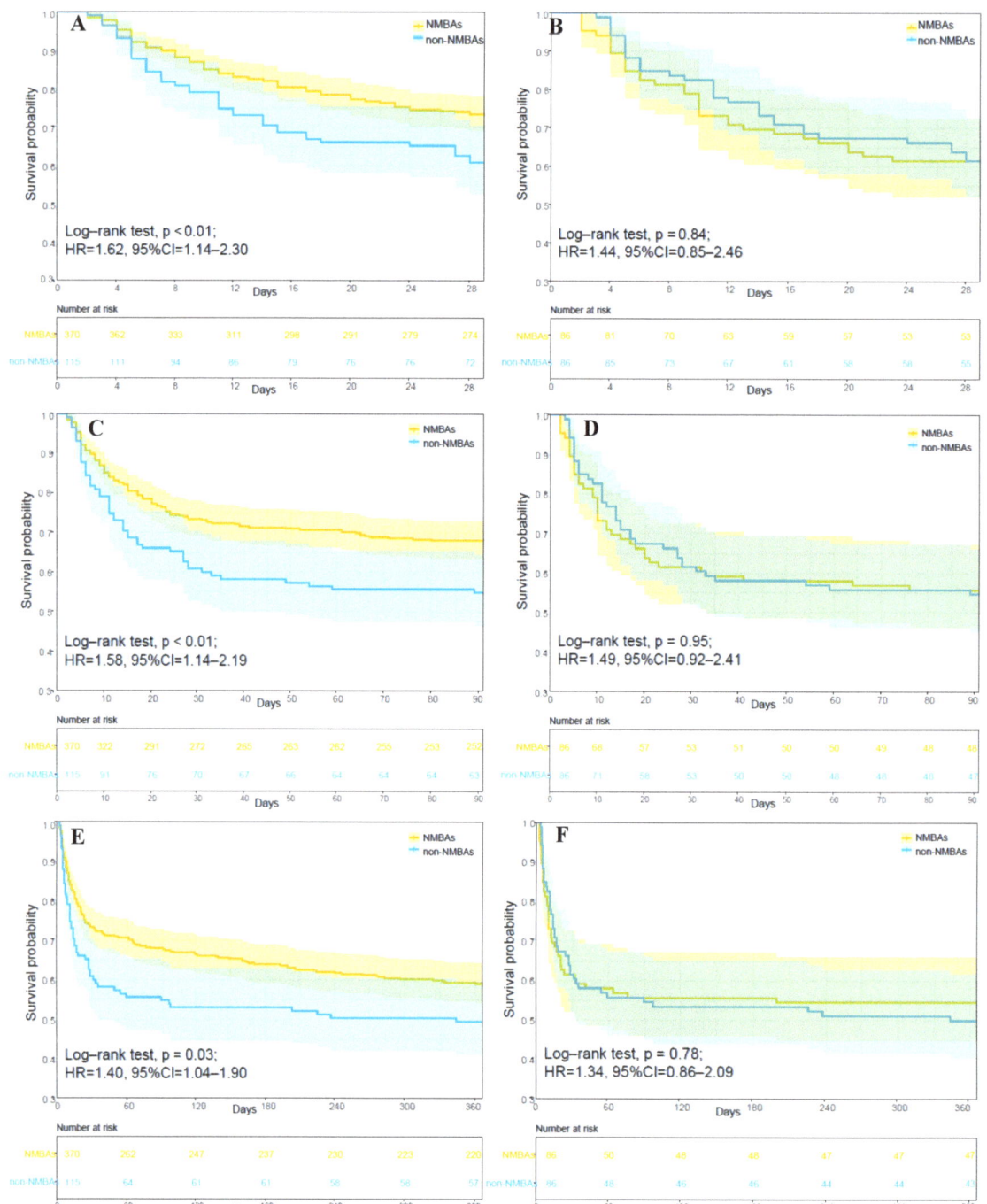

Figure 2. Survival analysis of NMBA and non-NMBA groups. Kaplan–Meier survival curves for the 28-day (**A**,**B**), 90-day (**C**,**D**), and 1-year (**E**,**F**) mortality among all patients are shown. Kaplan–Meier survival curves for pre-matched cohort (**A**,**C**,**E**) and matched cohort (**B**,**D**,**F**).

The univariate COX analysis results of the 28-day mortality are shown in Table S1. Age, the SAPSII and SOFA scores, ARDS severity, comorbidities associated with the liver and malignancy, body temperature, and respiratory rate were the risk factors for 28-day mortality. The vital signs, respiratory mechanic indicators, RASS scores, and total amount of fluid input and urine output of the patients from the first day of admission to the ICU to the seventh day are shown in Figures S2–S4.

3.3. Subgroup Analysis

The results of the subgroup analysis of the 28-day mortality are shown in Figure 3. There were no differences in NMBA treatment between the subgroups.

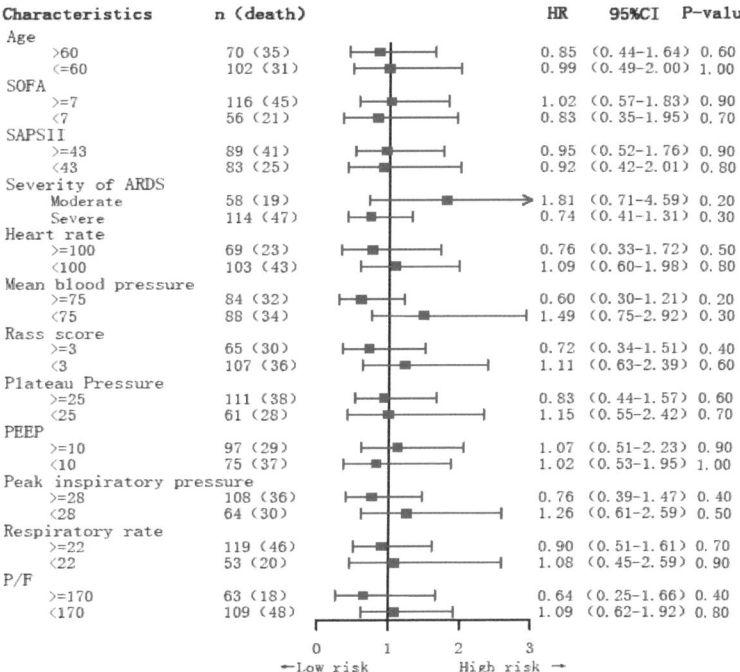

Figure 3. The association between NMBA administration and 28-day mortality in the subgroups.

4. Discussion

NMBAs are used in 25–45% of ARDS patients through either intermittent or continuous infusion [17]. Cisatracurium is a competitive antagonist of the nicotinic acetylcholine receptors that prevents acetylcholine from binding to the receptors in order to induce reversible muscular paresis. It undergoes Hofmann elimination, which means that its metabolism does not depend on renal or hepatic function; hence, it is preferred for critically ill patients [18]. However, the data used to evaluate the efficacy of NMBAs in ARDS patients are inconsistent. The ACURASYS study showed that the early administration of neuromuscular blocking agents improved the 90-day survival rate and decreased the duration of mechanical ventilation [11]. Nevertheless, the recent PETAL trial found that early therapy with NMBAs was not significantly associated with 90-day mortality [16]. A meta-analysis showed that NMBA therapy may be beneficial for short-term mortality among patients with ARDS but not for mid- or long-term mortality [19]. Herein, we retrospectively reviewed a cohort of 485 ARDS patients from the MIMIC-III database and demonstrated that NMBAs were not associated with an increased risk of 28-day, 90-day, 1-year, or hospital mortality but may prolong the ventilation duration and length of ICU stay.

Our study showed different results from the ACURASYS trial, mainly because we used the Berlin definition, which is in contrast to the definition of the American–European Consensus Conference used in the ACURASYS trial but is the same as the definition used in the PETAL trial. Thus, there is slight heterogeneity between the population of our study and that of the ACURASYS trial. The pathophysiological process of ARDS is divided into three stages, the exudative, repaired, and proliferative phases [20]. NMBAs may also inhibit the release of inflammatory factors (IL-1β, IL-6, and IL-8, etc.) and improve the outcomes of patients in the early stage of ARDS [15,21,22]. NMBAs improved the mechanical compliance of the chest wall and induced a change in the ventilation/perfusion ratio, which could be responsible for improvements in gas exchange and oxygenation [19]. Gainnier et al. showed a significant benefit of NMBA therapy in influencing the PaO2/FiO2 ratio [14], whereas the ACURASYS study showed that the PaO2/FiO2 ratio was higher on day 7 in patients receiving NMBAs [11]. Furthermore, an increase in thoracic–pulmonary compliance in ARDS patients can increase their functional residual capacity (FRC) and decrease the degree of intrapulmonary shunt [23]. Moreover, NMBA administration improved asynchrony, which contributed to patient comfort, rendered ventilation more effective, decreased the airway pressure and work required for breathing, and prevented muscle fatigue [11,24]. Tidal volumes can be closely regulated with NMBA therapy, thus decreasing the barotrauma and volutrauma caused by the overinflation of the alveoli, which may minimize the manifestations of ventilator-induced lung injury (VILI) [11]. There are inherent risks of NMBA therapy for ICU patients following the discontinuation of neuromuscular blocking agents such as ICU-acquired weakness (ICUAW), prolonged paralysis, the development of critical illness myopathy, polyneuropathy, etc. [25]. Patients who were paralyzed and subjected to NMBA administration underwent more serious adverse events such as hypoxia and hypercarbia, causing cardiopulmonary collapse [26]. More seriously, NMBAs led to the inhibition of the cough reflex, which hindered secretion clearance, and thus may prolong the ventilation duration and length of ICU stay. Moreover, NMBAs have very complex interactions with other drugs, such as corticosteroids, beta-blockers, calcium channel blockers, vancomycin, clindamycin, and so on, causing even more alterations in the pH and electrolyte levels [27]. Therefore, NMBAs may not result in clinical benefits due to their side effects after the exudative stage [28]. The present study did not exclude patients who used NMBAS for more than 48 h. Long-term NMBA infusion is associated with muscle paralysis [29] and ICU-acquired weakness, which may increase mortality among critically ill patients [30,31]. A prolonged length of ICU stay and mechanical ventilation duration were associated with higher mortality [32,33]. Thus, the inclusion of patients who received long-term NMBA therapy may have resulted in negative results in this study.

Another important factor may be differences in the sedation strategy. In patients who have received NMBA therapy, deep sedation may result in higher mortality and a prolonged duration of extubation [34]. The early deep sedation level is associated with higher mortality in critically ill patients who have received mechanical ventilation [34–37], whereas a light sedation strategy may improve the clinical outcomes of mechanically ventilated patients in the early stage [35,36]. Although the RASS scores on the first day of admission to the ICU were carefully propensity-score matched between the two groups, it is possible that the patients who underwent NMBA infusion were more deeply sedated than the patients who did receive NMBAs on the second day (following the first day of admission). The sedation level is associated with the prognosis of patients with ARDS [28].

5. Limitations

Most notably, the MIMIC-III database used in our study only contains the data of critically ill patients admitted between 2001 and 2012. Secondly, the different treatment strategies for critically ill patients, including ventilation strategies, nutritional support, and fluid management, may have influenced the outcomes of the ARDS patients. Thirdly, our study had a single-center, retrospective design; thus, the results of the present study still require further validation using external datasets. Despite our careful propensity-score matching, residual confounding factors cannot be fully excluded. Therefore, the risk of confounding factors should be taken into account when interpreting the results.

6. Conclusions

The use of NMBAs was not associated with reduced 28-day or 90-day mortality and may prolong the duration of ventilation and length of ICU stay. Due to their many side effects, we should use NMBAs with caution.

Supplementary Materials: The following supporting information can be downloaded at: https://www.mdpi.com/article/10.3390/jcm12051878/s1, Table S1: Univariate COX analysis of 28-day mortality; Figure S1: Standardized mean difference (SMD) of variables before and after propensity score matching; Figure S2: The vital signs of patients from the first day to seventh day. (A). Heart rate. (B). Blood pressure. (C). Body temperature. (D). SpO2. E. RASS score; Figure S3: The respiratory mechanics indicators of patients from the first day to seventh day. (A). Tidal volume. (B). Plateau pressure. (C). Peak inspiratory pressure. (D). PEEP. (E). Respiratory rate. (F). P/F ratio; Figure S4: The total amount of fluid input and urine output of patients from the first day admitted to ICU to seventh day. (A). Fluid input. (B). Urine output.

Author Contributions: X.P. and J.L. designed the study, collected and analyzed the data, and contributed to the writing of this manuscript. S.Z. and S.H. collected and analyzed the data. L.C. and X.S. helped with the data analysis. D.C. designed and supervised the study and drafted the manuscript. All authors have read and agreed to the published version of the manuscript.

Funding: This work was supported by the National Natural Science Foundation of China (grant No. 82172152, No. 81873944).

Institutional Review Board Statement: The MIMIC-III database used in the present study was approved by the Institutional Review Board (IRB) of the Massachusetts Institute of Technology and does not contain protected health information (NO. 35209874).

Informed Consent Statement: Not applicable.

Data Availability Statement: The datasets used in the present study are available from the authors upon reasonable request.

Conflicts of Interest: The authors declare that they have no competing interests.

References

1. Rubenfeld, G.D.; Caldwell, E.; Peabody, E.; Weaver, J.; Martin, D.P.; Neff, M.; Stern, E.J.; Hudson, L.D. Incidence and outcomes of acute lung injury. *N. Engl. J. Med.* **2005**, *353*, 1685–1693. [CrossRef]
2. Bellani, G.; Laffey, J.G.; Pham, T.; Fan, E.; Brochard, L.; Esteban, A.; Gattinoni, L.; van Haren, F.; Larsson, A.; McAuley, D.F.; et al. Epidemiology, Patterns of Care, and Mortality for Patients With Acute Respiratory Distress Syndrome in Intensive Care Units in 50 Countries. *JAMA* **2016**, *315*, 788–800. [CrossRef]
3. Fan, E.; Brodie, D.; Slutsky, A.S. Acute Respiratory Distress Syndrome: Advances in Diagnosis and Treatment. *JAMA* **2018**, *319*, 698–710. [CrossRef] [PubMed]
4. Bernard, G.R. Acute respiratory distress syndrome: A historical perspective. *Am. J. Respir. Crit. Care. Med.* **2005**, *172*, 798–806. [CrossRef]
5. Brun-Buisson, C.; Minelli, C.; Bertolini, G.; Brazzi, L.; Pimentel, J.; Lewandowski, K.; Bion, J.; Romand, J.A.; Villar, J.; Thorsteinsson, A.; et al. Epidemiology and outcome of acute lung injury in European intensive care units. Results from the ALIVE study. *Intensive Care Med.* **2004**, *30*, 51–61. [CrossRef] [PubMed]
6. Esteban, A.; Ferguson, N.D.; Meade, M.O.; Frutos-Vivar, F.; Apezteguia, C.; Brochard, L.; Raymondos, K.; Nin, N.; Hurtado, J.; Tomicic, V.; et al. Evolution of mechanical ventilation in response to clinical research. *Am. J. Respir. Crit. Care Med.* **2008**, *177*, 170–177. [CrossRef]
7. Esteban, A.; Anzueto, A.; Frutos, F.; Alia, I.; Brochard, L.; Stewart, T.E.; Benito, S.; Epstein, S.K.; Apezteguia, C.; Nightingale, P.; et al. Characteristics and outcomes in adult patients receiving mechanical ventilation: A 28-day international study. *JAMA* **2002**, *287*, 345–355. [CrossRef]
8. Sahetya, S.K.; Mallow, C.; Sevransky, J.E.; Martin, G.S.; Girard, T.D.; Brower, R.G.; Checkley, W.; Society of Critical Care Medicine Discovery Network Critical Illness Outcomes Study Investigators. Association between hospital mortality and inspiratory airway pressures in mechanically ventilated patients without acute respiratory distress syndrome: A prospective cohort study. *Crit. Care* **2019**, *23*, 367. [CrossRef]

9. Brower, R.G.; Matthay, M.A.; Morris, A.; Schoenfeld, D.; Thompson, B.T.; Wheeler, A. Ventilation with lower tidal volumes as compared with traditional tidal volumes for acute lung injury and the acute respiratory distress syndrome. *N. Engl. J. Med.* **2000**, *342*, 1301–1308. [CrossRef]
10. Bennett, S.; Hurford, W.E. When should sedation or neuromuscular blockade be used during mechanical ventilation? *Respir. Care* **2011**, *56*, 168–176; discussion 176–180. [CrossRef] [PubMed]
11. Papazian, L.; Forel, J.M.; Gacouin, A.; Penot-Ragon, C.; Perrin, G.; Loundou, A.; Jaber, S.; Arnal, J.M.; Perez, D.; Seghboyan, J.M.; et al. Neuromuscular blockers in early acute respiratory distress syndrome. *N. Engl. J. Med.* **2010**, *363*, 1107–1116. [CrossRef] [PubMed]
12. Terao, Y.; Miura, K.; Saito, M.; Sekino, M.; Fukusaki, M.; Sumikawa, K. Quantitative analysis of the relationship between sedation and resting energy expenditure in postoperative patients. *Crit. Care Med.* **2003**, *31*, 830–833. [CrossRef] [PubMed]
13. Renew, J.R.; Ratzlaff, R.; Hernandez-Torres, V.; Brull, S.J.; Prielipp, R.C. Neuromuscular blockade management in the critically Ill patient. *J. Intensive Care* **2020**, *8*, 37. [CrossRef] [PubMed]
14. Gainnier, M.; Roch, A.; Forel, J.M.; Thirion, X.; Arnal, J.M.; Donati, S.; Papazian, L. Effect of neuromuscular blocking agents on gas exchange in patients presenting with acute respiratory distress syndrome. *Crit. Care Med.* **2004**, *32*, 113–119. [CrossRef] [PubMed]
15. Forel, J.M.; Roch, A.; Marin, V.; Michelet, P.; Demory, D.; Blache, J.L.; Perrin, G.; Gainnier, M.; Bongrand, P.; Papazian, L. Neuromuscular blocking agents decrease inflammatory response in patients presenting with acute respiratory distress syndrome. *Crit. Care Med.* **2006**, *34*, 2749–2757. [CrossRef]
16. Moss, M.; Huang, D.T.; Brower, R.G.; Ferguson, N.D.; Ginde, A.A.; Gong, M.N.; Grissom, C.K.; Gundel, S.; Hayden, D.; Hite, R.D.; et al. Early Neuromuscular Blockade in the Acute Respiratory Distress Syndrome. *N. Engl. J. Med.* **2019**, *380*, 1997–2008. [CrossRef]
17. Bourenne, J.; Hraiech, S.; Roch, A.; Gainnier, M.; Papazian, L.; Forel, J.M. Sedation and neuromuscular blocking agents in acute respiratory distress syndrome. *Ann. Transl. Med.* **2017**, *5*, 291. [CrossRef]
18. Fodale, V.; Santamaria, L.B. Laudanosine, an atracurium and cisatracurium metabolite. *Eur. J. Anaesthesiol.* **2002**, *19*, 466–473. [CrossRef]
19. Alhazzani, W.; Alshahrani, M.; Jaeschke, R.; Forel, J.M.; Papazian, L.; Sevransky, J.; Meade, M.O. Neuromuscular blocking agents in acute respiratory distress syndrome: A systematic review and meta-analysis of randomized controlled trials. *Crit. Care* **2013**, *17*, R43. [CrossRef]
20. Meyer, N.J.; Gattinoni, L.; Calfee, C.S. Acute respiratory distress syndrome. *Lancet* **2021**, *398*, 622–637. [CrossRef]
21. Brochard, L. Ventilation-induced lung injury exists in spontaneously breathing patients with acute respiratory failure: Yes. *Intensive Care Med.* **2017**, *43*, 250–252. [CrossRef] [PubMed]
22. Fanelli, V.; Morita, Y.; Cappello, P.; Ghazarian, M.; Sugumar, B.; Delsedime, L.; Batt, J.; Ranieri, V.M.; Zhang, H.; Slutsky, A.S. Neuromuscular Blocking Agent Cisatracurium Attenuates Lung Injury by Inhibition of Nicotinic Acetylcholine Receptor-α1. *Anesthesiology* **2016**, *124*, 132–140. [CrossRef]
23. Hurford, W.E. Neuromuscular Blockade Applicability in Early Acute Respiratory Distress Syndrome. *Anesthesiology* **2020**, *132*, 1577–1584. [CrossRef]
24. Trapani, G.; Altomare, C.; Liso, G.; Sanna, E.; Biggio, G. Propofol in anesthesia. Mechanism of action, structure-activity relationships, and drug delivery. *Curr. Med. Chem.* **2000**, *7*, 249–271. [CrossRef] [PubMed]
25. Latronico, N.; Bolton, C.F. Critical illness polyneuropathy and myopathy: A major cause of muscle weakness and paralysis. *The Lancet. Neurology* **2011**, *10*, 931–941. [CrossRef]
26. Grawe, E.S.; Bennett, S.; Hurford, W.E. Early Paralysis for the Management of ARDS. *Respir. Care* **2016**, *61*, 830–838. [CrossRef] [PubMed]
27. Greenberg, S.B.; Vender, J. The use of neuromuscular blocking agents in the ICU: Where are we now? *Crit. Care Med.* **2013**, *41*, 1332–1344. [CrossRef]
28. Shao, S.; Kang, H.; Tong, Z. Early neuromuscular blocking agents for adults with acute respiratory distress syndrome: A systematic review, meta-analysis and meta-regression. *BMJ Open* **2020**, *10*, e037737. [CrossRef]
29. Dodson, B.A.; Kelly, B.J.; Braswell, L.M.; Cohen, N.H. Changes in acetylcholine receptor number in muscle from critically ill patients receiving muscle relaxants: An investigation of the molecular mechanism of prolonged paralysis. *Crit. Care Med.* **1995**, *23*, 815–821. [CrossRef]
30. Saccheri, C.; Morawiec, E.; Delemazure, J.; Mayaux, J.; Dubé, B.P.; Similowski, T.; Demoule, A.; Dres, M. ICU-acquired weakness, diaphragm dysfunction and long-term outcomes of critically ill patients. *Ann. Intensive Care* **2020**, *10*, 1. [CrossRef]
31. Baek, M.S.; Kim, J.H.; Lim, Y.; Kwon, Y.S. Neuromuscular blockade in mechanically ventilated pneumonia patients with moderate to severe hypoxemia: A multicenter retrospective study. *PloS ONE* **2022**, *17*, e0277503. [CrossRef] [PubMed]
32. Dong, Z.H.; Yu, B.X.; Sun, Y.B.; Fang, W.; Li, L. Effects of early rehabilitation therapy on patients with mechanical ventilation. *World J. Emerg. Med.* **2014**, *5*, 48–52. [CrossRef] [PubMed]
33. Yosef-Brauner, O.; Adi, N.; Ben Shahar, T.; Yehezkel, E.; Carmeli, E. Effect of physical therapy on muscle strength, respiratory muscles and functional parameters in patients with intensive care unit-acquired weakness. *Clin. Respir. J.* **2015**, *9*, 1–6. [CrossRef]
34. Shehabi, Y.; Bellomo, R.; Reade, M.C.; Bailey, M.; Bass, F.; Howe, B.; McArthur, C.; Seppelt, I.M.; Webb, S.; Weisbrodt, L. Early intensive care sedation predicts long-term mortality in ventilated critically ill patients. *Am. J. Respir. Crit. Care Med.* **2012**, *186*, 724–731. [CrossRef] [PubMed]

35. Shehabi, Y.; Chan, L.; Kadiman, S.; Alias, A.; Ismail, W.N.; Tan, M.A.; Khoo, T.M.; Ali, S.B.; Saman, M.A.; Shaltut, A.; et al. Sedation depth and long-term mortality in mechanically ventilated critically ill adults: A prospective longitudinal multicentre cohort study. *Intensive Care Med.* **2013**, *39*, 910–918. [CrossRef] [PubMed]
36. Shehabi, Y.; Bellomo, R.; Kadiman, S.; Ti, L.K.; Howe, B.; Reade, M.C.; Khoo, T.M.; Alias, A.; Wong, Y.L.; Mukhopadhyay, A.; et al. Sedation Intensity in the First 48 Hours of Mechanical Ventilation and 180-Day Mortality: A Multinational Prospective Longitudinal Cohort Study. *Crit. Care Med.* **2018**, *46*, 850–859. [CrossRef]
37. Balzer, F.; Weiß, B.; Kumpf, O.; Treskatsch, S.; Spies, C.; Wernecke, K.D.; Krannich, A.; Kastrup, M. Early deep sedation is associated with decreased in-hospital and two-year follow-up survival. *Crit. Care* **2015**, *19*, 197. [CrossRef]

Disclaimer/Publisher's Note: The statements, opinions and data contained in all publications are solely those of the individual author(s) and contributor(s) and not of MDPI and/or the editor(s). MDPI and/or the editor(s) disclaim responsibility for any injury to people or property resulting from any ideas, methods, instructions or products referred to in the content.

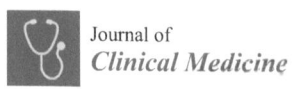

Article

Biological Markers to Predict Outcome in Mechanically Ventilated Patients with Severe COVID-19 Living at High Altitude

Jorge Luis Vélez-Páez [1,2,3,†], Paolo Pelosi [4,5], Denise Battaglini [5,*] and Ivan Best [6,†]

1. Facultad de Ciencias Médicas, Universidad Central de Ecuador, Quito 170129, Ecuador
2. Laboratorio de Inmunología, Facultad de Ciencias y Filosofía, Departamento de Ciencias Celulares y Moleculares, Universidad Peruana Cayetano Heredia, Lima 15074, Peru
3. Unidad de Terapia Intensiva, Hospital Pablo Arturo Suárez, Centro de Investigación Clínica, Quito 170129, Ecuador
4. Department of Surgical Sciences and Integrated Diagnostics, University of Genoa, 16132 Genoa, Italy
5. Anesthesiology and Critical Care, San Martino Policlinico Hospital, 16132 Genoa, Italy
6. Carrera de Medicina Humana, Facultad de Ciencias de la Salud, Universidad San Ignacio de Loyola, Lima 15024, Peru
* Correspondence: battaglini.denise@gmail.com
† These authors contributed equally to this work.

Abstract: Background: There is not much evidence on the prognostic utility of different biological markers in patients with severe COVID-19 living at high altitude. The objective of this study was to determine the predictive value of inflammatory and hematological markers for the risk of mortality at 28 days in patients with severe COVID-19 under invasive mechanical ventilation, living at high altitude and in a low-resource setting. Methods: We performed a retrospective observational study including patients with severe COVID-19, under mechanical ventilation and admitted to the intensive care unit (ICU) located at 2850 m above sea level, between 1 April 2020 and 1 August 2021. Inflammatory (interleukin-6 (IL-6), ferritin, D-dimer, lactate dehydrogenase (LDH)) and hematologic (mean platelet volume (MPV), neutrophil/lymphocyte ratio (NLR), MPV/platelet ratio) markers were evaluated at 24 h and in subsequent controls, and when available at 48 h and 72 h after admission to the ICU. The primary outcome was the association of inflammatory and hematological markers with the risk of mortality at 28 days. Results: We analyzed 223 patients (median age (1st quartile [Q1]–3rd quartile [Q3]) 51 (26–75) years and 70.4% male). Patients with severe COVID-19 and with IL-6 values at 24 h $\geq$ 11, NLR values at 24 h $\geq$ 22, and NLR values at 72 h $\geq$ 14 were 8.3, 3.8, and 3.8 times more likely to die at 28 days, respectively. The SOFA and APACHE-II scores were not able to independently predict mortality. Conclusions: In mechanically ventilated patients with severe COVID-19 and living at high altitude, low-cost and immediately available blood markers such as IL-6 and NLR may predict the severity of the disease in low-resource settings.

Keywords: SARS-CoV-2; coronavirus infection; mortality; biomarkers; COVID-19

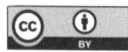

1. Introduction

Biomarkers can be helpful for prognostic enrichment and for testing the efficacy of therapies according to biological sub-phenotypes in acute respiratory distress syndrome (ARDS) [1–3]. In patients with severe coronavirus disease 2019 (COVID-19), the search for biomarkers associated with clinical progression and prognosis could be considered as a possible option to clarify the evaluation, severity, and therapeutic management processes. Ferritin [4,5] and interleukin-6 (IL-6) [6–9] have shown their clinical utility; however, their high cost and the use of specialized equipment for the analysis may limit their use and clinical applicability in low-resource settings. Both inflammatory and hematological markers have been evaluated in series of patients with COVID-19 and various conditions of severity [4,7,10–16], although there is less evidence in critically ill patients undergoing invasive mechanical ventilation, as well as those patients that live at high altitudes. Some studies suggest lower mortality and severity rates of SARS-CoV-2 infection at higher geographical altitudes, probably due to acclimatization to hypobaric hypoxia and other determinants that have not yet been clarified [17,18]. Previous studies in critically ill patients with COVID-19 living at high altitude showed that interleukin-6 (IL-6) together with the neutrophil/lymphocyte ratio (NLR) and lactate dehydrogenase (LDH) were independent predictors of mortality [8]. The objective of this study was to determine the predictive value of inflammatory and hematologic markers on the risk of mortality at 28 days in patients with severe COVID-19 under mechanical ventilation and admitted to the intensive care unit (ICU), at high altitude and in a low-resource setting.

2. Materials and Methods

2.1. Study Design and Criteria of Inclusion

This was a retrospective observational study including patients with severe COVID-19 admitted to the ICU from 1 April 2020, to 1 August 2021. The study was approved by the ethics committee of the Universidad Peruana Cayetano Heredia, Lima, Peru (Code N° 301-30-21), and performed in the Pablo Arturo Suárez General Provincial Hospital located in Quito, Ecuador, at 2850 m above sea level (m.a.s.l.), which is an exclusive care center for symptomatic respiratory patients with COVID-19 who require hospitalization. A confirmed case of COVID-19 was defined in the presence of a nasal swab with a positive real-time reverse transcription polymerase chain reaction (RT-PCR) test. The inclusion criteria were the following: (1) age older than 18 years; (2) admission to the ICU requiring invasive mechanical ventilation. The study participants were retrospectively classified as survivors and non-survivors at the time of discharge from the ICU. Informed consent was waived due to the retrospective nature of this study in accordance with local regulations.

2.2. Data Collection

Information was collected from the electronic clinical records on clinical–epidemiological variables, including age, gender, comorbidities (diabetes mellitus (DM), arterial hypertension, obesity), clinical scales of organ failure and severity such as the sequential organ failure assessment (SOFA) and acute physiology and chronic health evaluation (APACHE) II, as well as inflammatory (D-dimer, ferritin, LDH, and IL-6) and hematological markers (mean platelet volume (MPV), NLR, MPV/platelet ratio). These variables were obtained at 24 h from admission to the ICU and in subsequent controls, and when available at 48 and 72 h. Routine blood counts and MPV values were measured using an automated hematology analyzer (Advia 2120i, Tarrytown, NY, USA), while ferritin and IL-6 were evaluated via chemiluminescence testing (Inmulite 2000 XPi, Malvern, PA, USA). LDH was measured via photometry (Advia 1800, Malvern, PA, USA) and D-dimer via enzyme-linked immunosorbent assay (ELISA).

2.3. Statistical Analysis

No formal sample size calculation was performed due to the exploratory, descriptive, and retrospective nature of the study. The variables are reported as medians (1st and 3rd quartiles) or absolute or relative frequencies (percentages) as appropriate. The Shapiro–Wilk test was used to assess the normal distribution of the data. For the quantitative variables, the Student's t-test for independent samples or the Mann–Whitney test for a comparison between survivor and non-survivor groups was used as appropriate. The estimation of any association between the laboratory variables and survivors versus non-survivors was assessed with a preliminary univariate analysis (Chi-square test with Yates correction or Fisher's exact test), followed by a multivariate logistic regression model adjusted for all baseline variables. Significant variables to the binary logistic regression model were entered in the multivariate model with the odds ratio (OR) and the 95% confidence interval (CI) as

3. Results

3.1. Demographic and Clinical Characteristics of Patients with Severe COVID-19

Overall, 240 patients were assessed for eligibility. Of these, 17 patients did not meet the inclusion criteria due to having an unconfirmed diagnosis and variables not being entered. Therefore, 223 patients were included in this study. At the time of ICU discharge, 145 (65.1%) patients survived, and 78 patients had died (34.9%) (Figure 1).

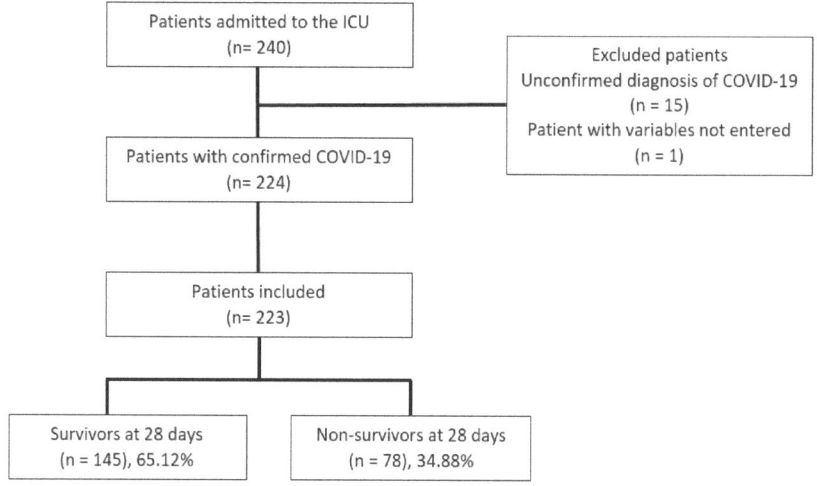

Figure 1. Flowchart of study inclusion and exclusion criteria. ICU: intensive care unit.

The median (1st quartile (Q1)–3rd quartile (Q3)) age of all patients was 51 (26–75) years. The non-survivors were significantly older (median age (Q1-Q3) years, 56 (31–79) years) than the survivors (48 (25–72) years) ($p = 0.000$). The most frequent comorbidity was obesity, followed by hypertension and diabetes mellitus, without differences between survivors and non-survivors. At ICU admission, a significantly higher APACHE II score was found in non-survivors compared to survivors ($p = 0.010$). SOFA, at 24, 48, and 72 h after ICU admission, was significantly higher in non-survivors compared to survivors ($p < 0.001$). In both survivors and non-survivors, the trend of SOFA scores showed higher values at 24 h, with decreasing values at 48 and 72 h. On average, corticosteroids were used in 90.1% of the patients, and 77.5% required low molecular weight heparin (LMWH) as an anticoagulant. The median (Q1–Q3) hospital stay was 10 (6–15) days, with no significant differences between survivors (10 (6–14)) and non-survivors (12.5 (6.8–12.3)) ($p = 0.129$). Table 1 shows the demographic and clinical characteristics of the overall population, survivors, and non-survivors in the ICU.

3.2. Inflammatory and Hematological Markers in Patients with Severe COVID-19

At 24 and 48 h after admission to the ICU, the D-dimer and ferritin concentrations were not significantly different, while LDH was significantly higher ($p < 0.05$) in non-survivors compared to survivors. At 24 h, IL-6 was significantly higher in non-survivors compared to survivors ($p < 0.01$). The median (Q1–Q3) IL-6 concentrations were 21.6 (9.7–55.4) and 35.1 (15.0–107.0) pg/mL for survivors and non-survivors, respectively. Table 2 presents the inflammatory markers in the overall population as well as in survivors and non-survivors from the ICU.

Table 1. Demographic and clinical characteristics in the overall population as well as in survivors and non-survivors in the intensive care unit. Data are expressed as medians (1st quartile (Q1)–3rd quartile (Q3)) or numbers (percentages). * Significant differences between survivors and non-survivors based on Student's t-test [1], Chi-square test, or Fisher's exact statistic [2] and Mann–Whitney U test [3]. DM: diabetes mellitus; SOFA: sequential organ failure assessment; APACHE II: acute physiology and chronic health II.

Clinical Features	All Patients	Survivors	Non-Survivors	p-Value
	(n = 223)	(n = 145)	(n = 78)	
Median age (Q1–Q3), years [1]	51 (26–75)	48 (25–72)	56 (31–79)	0.000 *
Sex, n (%) [2]				
Male	157 (70.4)	99 (68.3)	58 (74.4)	0.343
Female	66 (29.6)	46 (31.7)	20 (25.6)	
DM, n (%) [2]	28 (12.6)	16 (11.0)	12 (15.4)	0.350
Hypertension, n (%) [2]	32 (14.4)	16 (11.0)	16 (20.5)	0.054
Obesity, n (%) [2]	74 (33.2)	50 (34.5)	24 (30.8)	0.574
APACHE II, 24 h [3]	16 (12–20)	16 (12–19.5)	18 (14–22)	0.010 *
SOFA [3]				
24 h	7 (5–9)	7 (5–8)	8 (6–11)	0.001 *
48 h	5 (3–7)	5 (3–7)	7 (5–8)	0.000 *
72 h	4 (3–7)	4 (2–6)	6 (4–8)	0.000 *
Corticosteroid use, n (%) [2]	201 (90.1)	131 (90.3)	70 (89.7)	0.886
Heparin use, n (%) [2]	172 (77.5)	109 (75.2)	63 (81.8)	0.259
Hospitalization, days [3]	10 (6–15)	10 (6–14)	12.5 (6.8–16.3)	0.129

Table 2. Inflammatory markers in the overall population, as well as in survivors and non-survivors in the intensive care unit. Data are expressed as medians (1st quartile (Q1)–3rd quartile (Q3)). * Significant differences between survivors and non-survivors based on Mann–Whitney U test; LDH: lactate dehydrogenase; IL-6: interleukin-6.

Inflammatory Markers	All Patients	Survivors	Non-Survivors	p-Value
	(n = 223)	(n = 145)	(n = 78)	
D-dimer 24 h, ng/mL	1161 (751.6–2684.5)	1055 (733.8–1910.8)	1318 (821.5–3257)	0.085
D-dimer 48 h, ng/mL	1227 (718–2704)	1221.5 (691.8–2099.2)	1311 (813–4290)	0.108
Ferritin 24 h, ng/mL	1137 (668.5–1650)	1040.5 (614.5–1650)	1348.5 (874.6–1650)	0.088
Ferritin 48 h, ng/mL	1140 (802–1500)	1075.8 (690.4–1500)	1187.1 (916.8–1500)	0.136
LDH 24 h, U/L	820 (671.5–1001.5)	773 (633–948)	887 (745.3–1103.3)	0.001 *
LDH 48 h, U/L	686.5 (579–859.5)	661 (559.8–820.8)	770 (624.5–910.5)	0.010 *
IL-6 24 h, pg/mL	25.2 (12.2–65.1)	21.6 (9.7–55.4)	35.1 (15.0–107.0)	0.001 *

The hematological markers in the overall population as well as in survivors and non-survivors from ICU are shown in Table 3. At 24, 48, and 72 h after admission to the ICU, the MPV values were not significantly different between survivors and non-survivors. Significant decreases in lymphocyte counts were observed at 24, 48, and 72 h after ICU admission in non-survivors compared to survivors ($p = 0.000$), while the non-survivors showed significant increases in NLR values at 24, 48, and 72 compared to survivors ($p = 0.000$). The MPV/platelet ratios were higher in non-survivors compared to survivors at 48 and 72 h after ICU admission ($p < 0.001$).

Table 3. Hematological markers in the overall population, as well as survivors and non-survivors in the intensive care unit. Data are expressed as medians (1st quartile (Q1)–3rd quartile (Q3)). * Significant differences between survivors and non-survivors based on Mann–Whitney U test. MPV: mean platelet volume; NLR: neutrophil/lymphocyte ratio.

Hematology Markers	All Patients	Survivors	Non-Survivors	p-Value
	(n = 223)	(n = 145)	(n = 78)	
MPV, 24 h	8.9 (8.5–9.6)	8.9 (8.5–9.5)	8.9 (8.4–9.6)	0.650
MPV, 48 h	8.9 (8.5–9.4)	8.9 (8.5–9.4)	9 (8.5–9.6)	0.419
MPV, 72 h	9 (8.5–9.6)	8.9 (8.6–9.5)	9 (8.5–9.7)	0.502
Lymphocytes, 24 h (cells/mL)	620 (410–900)	660 (465–930)	465 (340–712.5)	0.000 *
Lymphocytes, 48 h (cells/mL)	520 (400–820)	620 (455–840)	455 (290–607.5)	0.000 *
Lymphocytes, 72 h (cells/mL)	555 (350–882)	630 (395–970)	430 (300–600)	0.000 *
NLR, 24 h	15.6 (9.6–23.4)	13.7 (8.4–20.1)	21.7 (12.7–33.1)	0.000 *
NLR, 48 h	15.6 (9.8–22.7)	13.1 (8.7–18.4)	22.0 (14.3–29.5)	0.000 *
NLR, 72 h	15.4 (9.1–25.9)	13.2 (7.8–21.3)	20.6 (14.1–31.7)	0.000 *
MPV/platelet, 24 h	2.8 (2.2–3.6)	2.7 (2.1–3.5)	2.9 (2.4–4.1)	0.052
MPV/platelet, 48 h	2.7 (2.1–3.6)	2.6 (2–3.3)	3.0 (2.3–4.3)	0.004 *
MPV/platelet, 72 h	2.7 (2.1–3.5)	2.5 (2.0–3.3)	3.1 (2.3–3.9)	0.003 *

3.3. Predictors of 28-Day Mortality

I the multivariate analysis, IL-6 values at 24 h $\geq$ 11, NLR values at 24 h $\geq$ 22, and NLR values at 72 h $\geq$ 14, were associated with 28-day mortality in patients with severe COVID-19 living at high altitude ($p < 0.05$). Consequently, we found that patients with severe COVID-19 with IL-6 values at 24 h $\geq$ 11, NLR values at 24 h $\geq$ 22, and NLR values at 72 h $\geq$ 14 were 8.3, 3.8, and 3.8 times more likely to die at 28 days, respectively (Table 4).

Table 4. Multivariate regression model to predict mortality at 28 days in patients with severe COVID-19 admitted to the intensive care unit. * Mortality predictor variable, $p < 0.05$; ** significant risk CI does not include the value 1. MPV = mean platelet volume; NLR = neutrophil/lymphocyte ratio; CI = confidence interval; OR = odds ratio.

Variables	OR	95% CI	p-Value
SOFA 24 h $\geq$ 8	1.0	0.4–2.8	0.990
SOFA 48 h $\geq$ 6	1.1	0.3–3.8	0.825
SOFA 72 h $\geq$ 4	1.7	0.5–5.7	0.395
IL-6 24 h $\geq$ 11 **	8.3	1.5–44.6	0.014 *
LDH 24 h $\geq$ 781	1.7	0.6–4.4	0.301
LDH 48 h $\geq$ 709	2.0	0.7–5.6	0.180
NLR 24 h $\geq$ 22 **	3.8	1.3–10.9	0.015 *
NLR 48 h $\geq$ 18	0.8	0.3–2.5	0.746
NLR 72 h $\geq$ 14 **	3.8	1.3–11.0	0.013 *
MPV/Platelets 48 h $\geq$ 4	1.6	0.4–6.1	0.470
MPV/Platelets 72 h $\geq$ 3	1.4	0.5–4.0	0.480

4. Discussion

The main finding of our study is that in mechanically ventilated patients admitted to the ICU with severe COVID-19 in low-resource settings and living at high altitude, low-cost and immediately available blood biomarkers such as IL-6 and NLR can predict mortality in the ICU.

A homogeneous population of severe mechanically ventilated COVID-19 patients admitted to the ICU was included in the analysis. Several inflammatory and hematological biomarkers were systematically analyzed at different timings from the ICU admission as potential predictors of the outcome. COVID-19 is a heterogeneous disease with high potential for multiple organ failure and impaired outcomes in patients admitted to an ICU. It has been hypothesized that the multisystem involvement in COVID-19 can be caused by an unbalanced immune response that facilitates the progression of the disease to multiple organs. This hypothesis has been confirmed by the presence of altered biomarkers and cytokines as the manifestation of inflammatory and thromboembolic disorders at high risk of progression to multiorgan failure [3]. Some biomarkers showed an optimal ability to predict the outcome in critically ill patients without COVID-19, but little is known about the specific biomarkers that can be used to predict survival in severe COVID-19. To the best of our knowledge, this is one of the first studies confirming the existence of low-cost and easily available prognostic biomarkers as predictors of mortality in this patient population.

In the present study, the patients with severe COVID-19 who died were older, more clinically severe, and with higher risk of organ failure (as measured by the APACHE-II and SOFA scores) than those who survived. Although there was a predominance of males over females as non-survivors as compared to survivors, the mortality rates did not differ by gender. This is in agreement with previous studies where age and severity were associated with worse clinical outcomes, with a predominance of male gender in the hospital admissions [19,20].

We found that pro-inflammatory markers such as IL-6 (at 24 h) and hematological markers such as NLR (at 24 and 72 h, respectively) were independent predictors of 28-day mortality in patients with severe COVID-19 living at high altitude in a low-resource setting. IL-6 is a pro-inflammatory cytokine that is produced by stromal cells and released by the activation of pro-inflammatory cytokines, especially IL-1β and tumor necrosis factor-α (TNF-α), and by lung macrophages after stimulation of toll-like receptors (TLR) [21]. In patients with non-COVID-19 ARDS, the persistent elevation of IL-6 levels was a consistent and efficient predictor of the outcome over time [22]. In COVID-19, an increase in IL-6 levels has been associated with the development of lung injury and hypoxemia, representing an important prognostic biomarker of severity [7,8,23]. However, the value of IL-6 as a predictor of the outcome in critically ill patients with COVID-19 is still controversial. Therefore, IL-6 has been proposed as a possible biological target for clinical and therapeutic decision-making, such as the use of IL-6 receptor blocker drugs [24]. Our results are in line with the available literature on the prognostic utility of this cytokine in patients with severe COVID-19 [7,8,23].

The severe inflammation observed in severe COVID-19 stimulates the production of neutrophils and induces apoptosis of the lymphocytes. This phenomenon is commonly observed in coronaviruses and Middle East respiratory syndrome coronavirus disease (MERS-CoV) infections, and the hematological change in leukocyte populations adequately predicted mortality [25]. In hospitalized patients with COVID-19, high neutrophil and low lymphocyte counts were independent predictors of mortality [26,27]. Some studies agree that by merging these two parameters into a unique biomarker (NLR), a more robust predictor of severity [14,28–31] and mortality at the time of ICU admission can be obtained [32]. The NLR has been recently investigated as a potential prognostic biomarker in COVID-19, influenza, and respiratory syncytial virus infections, showing significant associations with poor clinical outcomes only in patients with COVID-19 [33]. This suggests that the prognostic value of the NLR is specific to certain sub-populations of critically ill patients such as in COVID-19. A study from South America showed the better prognostic performance of NLRs > 5.5 over other inflammatory markers such as CRP, LDH, ferritin, and lymphocyte counts [34]. Furthermore, a retrospective study that analyzed more than 4000 patients living at high altitudes demonstrated a significant association of this marker with the severity and need for ICU admission [19]. Our results are consistent with the previous evidence [8,14,30–34], confirming the biological value of this biomarker, similarly to IL-6, which is a strong predictor of severity and mortality in COVID-19. Corticosteroids represent now a standard of care for critically ill patients with COVID-19 [35]. The effects include changes in blood cell counts, such as neutrophilia and lymphopenia, possibly explaining the increase in the NLR. In our series, the use of corticosteroids did not differ between non-survivors and survivors. Therefore, NLR changes can be attributed to the severity of COVID-19 and not to other confounding variables.

Platelets participate in the endothelial and thrombotic alterations of SARS-CoV-2 [36,37]. When dysregulated, platelets interact with neutrophils, forming neutrophil extracellular traps (NETs) to trigger immune–thrombosis and microcirculation disturbances. In COVID-19, the platelets are activated and aggregate chaotically, being consumed with possible increases in mean volume and decreases in the absolute count [26,38,39]. In our study, unlike other reports [10], the MPV was not associated with mortality. However, the MPV/platelet ratio was associated with mortality at 48 and 72 h, despite not being an independent predictor in the multivariate analysis. High altitudes seem to decrease the severity and mortality of SARS-CoV-2 infection [18,40]; however, the biological responses of biomarkers, especially those derived from blood counts, are different compared to at sea level. A preliminary study performed in a high-altitude city could not demonstrate the predictive performance of platelet counts, although they did not assess other platelet indices, in determining associations with mortality in critical patients with COVID-19 [8]. High altitudes are associated with a prothrombotic subphenotype [14]. At high altitudes, hypoxia generates hyperreactivity and increased platelet aggregation in response to adenosine diphosphate (ADP) and tends to increase other platelet indices [14]. This could explain the low predictive capacity of the MPV and the MPV/platelet ratio, which would allow us to hypothesize a lower performance rate for the platelet indices compared to that observed at sea level. However, the NLR, which is also derived from the blood count, has high prognostic potential for the prediction of mortality in critical patients with COVID-19. This is supposedly because unlike the platelets, lymphocytes, and neutrophils, the NLR does not participate in the coagulation but reflects inflammation only. In COVID-19, some validated scoring systems, such as the SCOPE score, which is based on biomarkers such as C-reactive protein (CRP), ferritin, D-dimer, and IL-6, demonstrated good prediction of the progression of COVID-19 pneumonia to severe respiratory failure or death within 14 days. This allowed therapeutic choices to be made, such as the administration of anakinra when the score was ≥ 6 [41]. In the present study, neither ferritin and D-dimer values nor scores of severity (APACHE-II and SOFA) could predict mortality in patients with severe COVID-19 living at high altitudes, so low-cost alternative markers such as NLR and IL-6 values could contribute to obtaining a score to predict mortality in this group of patients under these geographic conditions. The APACHE-II and SOFA scores are usually adopted to assess the severity of illness in critically ill patients. In our study, within this specific sub-population of COVID-19 patients, we sought to determine whether these scores have the same value for the prediction of the outcome as in critically ill subjects without COVID-19. We found that patients who had lower APACHE-II and SOFA scores died at similar rates to those with higher scores. Investigating this association in the multivariate analysis, we found that these scores seem to not be very effective for predicting mortality in critically ill patients with COVID-19. Therefore, we can assume that the APACHE-II and SOFA scores have differing prognostic value, depending on the population under study. Accordingly, some important features of COVID-19 that may be responsible for patients' critical illnesses are not investigated by the APACHE-II and SOFA scores, including thromboembolic disorders.

Finally, the strengths of this research lie in the fact that it was determined that the IL-6 and NLR values, which are immediately available, low-cost, affordable laboratory markers in basic instrumentation laboratories, represent prognostic alternatives for critically ill patients with severe COVID-19 at high altitude in low-resource settings.

Limitations

The present study has several limitations that need to be addressed. First, the retrospective design of the study limited the causative association with the outcome, and the study also lacked a validation sample. Second, only a few specific inflammatory and hematological markers are usually measured in high-, middle-, and low-income countries. We cannot exclude that other markers may be differently associated with the outcome. Third, the study population included patients with specific clinical characteristics admitted to the ICU and undergoing invasive mechanical ventilation, which would limit the extension of the present findings to different groups of COVID-19 patients with different disease severity levels. Fourth, we did not investigate COVID-19 variants that may have affected our findings, although our cohort was studied in a relative short period of time corresponding to the first peaks of the pandemic, when the beta and alpha variants were preponderant. Fifth, our findings are limited to a specific cohort of patients living at high altitude. Therefore, similar conclusions may not be obtained at sea level.

5. Conclusions

In the present retrospective study, low-cost markers such as IL-6 and the NLR could be used as potential predictors of the outcome in mechanically ventilated patients with severe COVID-19 admitted to the ICU living at high altitude. Further investigations are warranted to corroborate these findings.

Author Contributions: Conceptualization, J.L.V.-P.; methodology, J.L.V.-P. and I.B.; software, J.L.V.-P. and I.B.; validation, J.L.V.-P. and I.B.; formal analysis, J.L.V.-P. and I.B.; investigation, J.L.V.-P. and I.B.; resources, J.L.V.-P. and I.B.; data curation, J.L.V.-P. and I.B.; writing—original draft preparation, J.L.V.-P. and I.B.; writing—review and editing, J.L.V.-P., I.B., D.B. and P.P.; visualization, J.L.V.-P., I.B., D.B. and P.P.; supervision, J.L.V.-P., I.B., D.B. and P.P.; project administration, J.L.V.-P. and I.B. All authors have read and agreed to the published version of the manuscript.

Funding: This research received no external funding.

Institutional Review Board Statement: The study was conducted in accordance with the Declaration of Helsinki and approved by the Institutional Review Board of the Universidad Peruana Cayetano Heredia, Lima, Peru (Code N° 301-30-21).

Informed Consent Statement: Informed consent was waived due to the retrospective nature of this study in accordance with the local regulations.

Data Availability Statement: The data are available from the corresponding author under reasonable request.

Acknowledgments: We thank the staff of the Pablo Arturo Suárez General Provincial Hospital, Quito, Ecuador.

Conflicts of Interest: The authors declare no conflict of interest.

References

1. Bos, L.D.J.; Laffey, J.G.; Ware, L.B.; Heijnen, N.F.L.; Sinha, P.; Patel, B.; Jabaudon, M.; Bastarache, J.A.; McAuley, D.F.; Summers, C.; et al. Towards a Biological Definition of ARDS: Are Treatable Traits the Solution? *Intensive Care Med. Exp.* **2022**, *10*, 8. [CrossRef] [PubMed]
2. Battaglini, D.; Al-Husinat, L.; Normando, A.G.; Leme, A.P.; Franchini, K.; Morales, M.; Pelosi, P.; Rocco, P.R. Personalized Medicine Using Omics Approaches in Acute Respiratory Distress Syndrome to Identify Biological Phenotypes. *Respir. Res.* **2022**, *23*, 318. [CrossRef] [PubMed]
3. Battaglini, D.; Lopes-Pacheco, M.; Castro-Faria-Neto, H.C.; Pelosi, P.; Rocco, P.R.M. Laboratory Biomarkers for Diagnosis and Prognosis in COVID-19. *Front. Immunol.* **2022**, *13*, 857573. [CrossRef] [PubMed]
4. Mehta, P.; McAuley, D.F.; Brown, M.; Sanchez, E.; Tattersall, R.S.; Manson, J.J. COVID-19: Consider Cytokine Storm Syndromes and Immunosuppression. *Lancet* **2020**, *395*, 1033–1034. [CrossRef]

5. Fox, S.E.; Akmatbekov, A.; Harbert, J.L.; Li, G.; Quincy Brown, J.; Vander Heide, R.S. Pulmonary and Cardiac Pathology in African American Patients with COVID-19: An Autopsy Series from New Orleans. *Lancet Respir. Med.* **2020**, *8*, 681–686. [CrossRef] [PubMed]
6. Liu, T.; Zhang, J.; Yang, Y.; Ma, H.; Li, Z.; Zhang, J.; Cheng, J.; Zhang, X.; Zhao, Y.; Xia, Z.; et al. The Role of Interleukin-6 in Monitoring Severe Case of Coronavirus Disease 2019. *EMBO Mol. Med.* **2020**, *12*, e12421. [CrossRef]
7. Herold, T.; Jurinovic, V.; Arnreich, C.; Lipworth, B.J.; Hellmuth, J.C.; von Bergwelt-Baildon, M.; Klein, M.; Weinberger, T. Elevated Levels of IL-6 and CRP Predict the Need for Mechanical Ventilation in COVID-19. *J. Allergy Clin. Immunol.* **2020**, *146*, 128–136.e4. [CrossRef] [PubMed]
8. Vélez-Paez, J.L.; Montalvo, M.P.; Jara, F.E.; Aguayo-Moscoso, S.; Tercero-Martínez, W.; Saltos, L.S.; Jiménez-Alulima, G.; Irigoyen-Mogro, E.; Castro-Reyes, E.; Mora-Coello, C.; et al. Predicting Mortality in Critically Ill Patients with COVID-19 in the ICU from a Secondary-Level Hospital in Ecuador. *Rev. Bionatura* **2022**, *7*, 1. [CrossRef]
9. Zhong, Q.; Peng, J. Mean Platelet Volume/Platelet Count Ratio Predicts Severe Pneumonia of COVID-19. *J. Clin. Lab. Anal.* **2021**, *35*, e23607. [CrossRef]
10. Sertbas, M.; Dağcı, S.; Kizilay, V.; Yazıcı, Z.; Elçi, E.; Özaydın, Ö.; Elarslan, S.; Şaylan, B.; Dayan, A.; Sertbas, Y.; et al. Mean Platelet Volume as an Early Predictor for The Complication of Coronavirus Disease 19. *Haydarpaşa Numune Med. J.* **2021**, *6*, 177–182.
11. Vélez-Páez, J.L.; Tercero-Martínez, W.; Jiménez-Alulima, G.; Navarrete-Domínguez, J.; Cornejo-Loor, L.; Castro-Bustamante, C.; Cabanillas-Lazo, M.; Barboza, J.J.; Rodriguez-Morales, A.J. Neutrophil-to-Lymphocyte Ratio and Mean Platelet Volume in the Diagnosis of Bacterial Infections in COVID-19 Patients. A Preliminary Analysis from Ecuador. *Infez. Med.* **2021**, *29*, 530–537. [CrossRef]
12. Liu, Y.; Du, X.; Chen, J.; Jin, Y.; Peng, L.; Wang, H.H.X.; Luo, M.; Chen, L.; Zhao, Y. Neutrophil-to-Lymphocyte Ratio as an Independent Risk Factor for Mortality in Hospitalized Patients with COVID-19. *J. Infect.* **2020**, *81*, e6–e12. [CrossRef] [PubMed]
13. Ma, A.; Cheng, J.; Yang, J.; Dong, M.; Liao, X.; Kang, Y. Neutrophil-to-Lymphocyte Ratio as a Predictive Biomarker for Moderate-Severe ARDS in Severe COVID-19 Patients. *Crit. Care* **2020**, *24*, 288. [CrossRef] [PubMed]
14. Basbus, L.; Lapidus, M.I.; Martingano, I.; Puga, M.C.; Pollán, J. Neutrophil to lymphocyte ratio as a prognostic marker in COVID-19. *Medicina* **2020**, *80* (Suppl. S3), 31–36.
15. Ramos-Peñafiel, C.O.; Santos-González, B.; Flores-López, E.N.; Galván-Flores, F.; Hernández-Vázquez, L.; Santoyo-Sánchez, A.; Montes de Oca-Yemha, B.; Bejarano-Rosales, M.; Rosas-González, É.; Olarte-Carrillo, I.; et al. Usefulness of the Neutrophil-to-Lymphocyte, Monocyte-to-Lymphocyte and Lymphocyte-to-Platelet Ratios for the Prognosis of COVID-19-Associated Complications. *Gac. Méd. Méx.* **2020**, *156*, 413–419. [CrossRef]
16. Liu, J.; Liu, Y.; Xiang, P.; Pu, L.; Xiong, H.; Li, C.; Zhang, M.; Tan, J.; Xu, Y.; Song, R.; et al. Neutrophil-to-Lymphocyte Ratio Predicts Critical Illness Patients with 2019 Coronavirus Disease in the Early Stage. *J. Transl. Med.* **2020**, *18*, 206. [CrossRef] [PubMed]
17. Mateu Campos, M.L.; Ferrándiz Sellés, A.; Gruartmoner de Vera, G.; Mesquida Febrer, J.; Sabatier Cloarec, C.; Poveda Hernández, Y.; García Nogales, X. Techniques available for hemodynamic monitoring. Advantages and limitations. *Med. Intensiv.* **2012**, *36*, 434–444. [CrossRef] [PubMed]
18. Abdelsalam, M.; Althaqafi, R.M.M.; Assiri, S.A.; Althagafi, T.M.; Althagafi, S.M.; Fouda, A.Y.; Ramadan, A.; Rabah, M.; Ahmed, R.M.; Ibrahim, Z.S.; et al. Clinical and Laboratory Findings of COVID-19 in High-Altitude Inhabitants of Saudi Arabia. *Front. Med.* **2021**, *8*, 670195. [CrossRef]
19. Ballaz, S.J.; Pulgar-Sánchez, M.; Chamorro, K.; Fernández-Moreira, E.; Ramírez, H.; Mora, F.X.; Fors, M. Common Laboratory Tests as Indicators of COVID-19 Severity on Admission at High Altitude: A Single-Center Retrospective Study in Quito (ECUADOR). *Clin. Chem. Lab. Med.* **2021**, *59*, e326–e329. [CrossRef]
20. Yuan, X.; Huang, W.; Ye, B.; Chen, C.; Huang, R.; Wu, F.; Wei, Q.; Zhang, W.; Hu, J. Changes of Hematological and Immunological Parameters in COVID-19 Patients. *Int. J. Hematol.* **2020**, *112*, 553–559. [CrossRef]
21. Hunter, C.A.; Jones, S.A. IL-6 as a Keystone Cytokine in Health and Disease. *Nat. Immunol.* **2015**, *16*, 448–457. [CrossRef] [PubMed]
22. Meduri, G.U.; Headley, S.; Kohler, G.; Stentz, F.; Tolley, E.; Umberger, R.; Leeper, K. Persistent Elevation of Inflammatory Cytokines Predicts a Poor Outcome in ARDS. Plasma IL-1 Beta and IL-6 Levels Are Consistent and Efficient Predictors of Outcome over Time. *Chest* **1995**, *107*, 1062–1073. [CrossRef] [PubMed]
23. Aziz, M.; Fatima, R.; Assaly, R. Elevated Interleukin-6 and Severe COVID-19: A Meta-Analysis. *J. Med. Virol.* **2020**, *92*, 2283–2285. [CrossRef]
24. RECOVERY Collaborative Group Tocilizumab in Patients Admitted to Hospital with COVID-19 (RECOVERY): A Randomised, Controlled, Open-Label, Platform Trial. *Lancet* **2021**, *397*, 1637–1645. [CrossRef] [PubMed]
25. Min, C.-K.; Cheon, S.; Ha, N.-Y.; Sohn, K.M.; Kim, Y.; Aigerim, A.; Shin, H.M.; Choi, J.-Y.; Inn, K.-S.; Kim, J.-H.; et al. Comparative and Kinetic Analysis of Viral Shedding and Immunological Responses in MERS Patients Representing a Broad Spectrum of Disease Severity. *Sci. Rep.* **2016**, *6*, 25359. [CrossRef] [PubMed]
26. Fajgenbaum, D.C.; June, C.H. Cytokine Storm. *N. Engl. J. Med.* **2020**, *383*, 2255–2273. [CrossRef] [PubMed]
27. Morgan, R.A.; Yang, J.C.; Kitano, M.; Dudley, M.E.; Laurencot, C.M.; Rosenberg, S.A. Case Report of a Serious Adverse Event Following the Administration of T Cells Transduced with a Chimeric Antigen Receptor Recognizing ERBB2. *Mol. Ther.* **2010**, *18*, 843–851. [CrossRef]

28. Çalışkan, S.; Sungur, M.; Kaba, S.; Özsoy, E.; Koca, O.; Öztürk, M.İ. Neutrophil-to-Lymphocyte Ratio in Renal Cell Carcinoma Patients. *Folia Med.* **2018**, *60*, 553–557. [CrossRef]
29. Ciccullo, A.; Borghetti, A.; Zileri Dal Verme, L.; Tosoni, A.; Lombardi, F.; Garcovich, M.; Biscetti, F.; Montalto, M.; Cauda, R.; Di Giambenedetto, S.; et al. Neutrophil-to-Lymphocyte Ratio and Clinical Outcome in COVID-19: A Report from the Italian Front Line. *Int. J. Antimicrob. Agents* **2020**, *56*, 106017. [CrossRef]
30. Yang, A.-P.; Liu, J.-P.; Tao, W.-Q.; Li, H.-M. The Diagnostic and Predictive Role of NLR, d-NLR and PLR in COVID-19 Patients. *Int. Immunopharmacol.* **2020**, *84*, 106504. [CrossRef]
31. Akilli, N.B.; Yortanlı, M.; Mutlu, H.; Günaydın, Y.K.; Koylu, R.; Akca, H.S.; Akinci, E.; Dundar, Z.D.; Cander, B. Prognostic Importance of Neutrophil-Lymphocyte Ratio in Critically Ill Patients: Short- and Long-Term Outcomes. *Am. J. Emerg. Med.* **2014**, *32*, 1476–1480. [CrossRef]
32. Ye, W.; Chen, G.; Li, X.; Lan, X.; Ji, C.; Hou, M.; Zhang, D.; Zeng, G.; Wang, Y.; Xu, C.; et al. Dynamic Changes of D-Dimer and Neutrophil-Lymphocyte Count Ratio as Prognostic Biomarkers in COVID-19. *Respir. Res.* **2020**, *21*, 169. [CrossRef]
33. Prozan, L.; Shusterman, E.; Ablin, J.; Mitelpunkt, A.; Weiss-Meilik, A.; Adler, A.; Choshen, G.; Kehat, O. Prognostic Value of Neutrophil-to-Lymphocyte Ratio in COVID-19 Compared with Influenza and Respiratory Syncytial Virus Infection. *Sci. Rep.* **2021**, *11*, 21519. [CrossRef]
34. Martínez, F.; Boisier, D.; Vergara, C.; Vidal, J. Neutrophil to lymphocyte ratio and inflammatory biomarkers as prognostic factors amongst patients with COVID-19: A prospective cohort study. *Rev. Chil. Anest.* **2022**, *51*, 80–87.
35. RECOVERY Collaborative Group; Horby, P.; Lim, W.S.; Emberson, J.R.; Mafham, M.; Bell, J.L.; Linsell, L.; Staplin, N.; Brightling, C.; Ustianowski, A.; et al. Dexamethasone in Hospitalized Patients with Covid-19. *N. Engl. J. Med.* **2021**, *384*, 693–704. [CrossRef]
36. Gong, J.; Ou, J.; Qiu, X.; Jie, Y.; Chen, Y.; Yuan, L.; Cao, L.; Tan, J.; Xu, M.; Zheng, W.; et al. Multicenter Development and Validation of a Novel Risk Nomogram for Early Prediction of Severe 2019-Novel Coronavirus Pneumonia. 2020. Available online: https://search.bvsalud.org/global-literature-on-novel-coronavirus-2019-ncov/resource/es/ppcovidwho-637 (accessed on 27 November 2022).
37. Ji, D.; Zhang, D.; Xu, J.; Chen, Z.; Yang, T.; Zhao, P.; Chen, G.; Cheng, G.; Wang, Y.; Bi, J.; et al. Prediction for Progression Risk in Patients with COVID-19 Pneumonia: The CALL Score. *Clin. Infect. Dis.* **2020**, *71*, 1393–1399. [CrossRef]
38. Grommes, J.; Alard, J.-E.; Drechsler, M.; Wantha, S.; Mörgelin, M.; Kuebler, W.M.; Jacobs, M.; von Hundelshausen, P.; Markart, P.; Wygrecka, M.; et al. Disruption of Platelet-Derived Chemokine Heteromers Prevents Neutrophil Extravasation in Acute Lung Injury. *Am. J. Respir. Crit. Care Med.* **2012**, *185*, 628–636. [CrossRef] [PubMed]
39. Fuchs, T.A.; Brill, A.; Duerschmied, D.; Schatzberg, D.; Monestier, M.; Myers, D.D.; Wrobleski, S.K.; Wakefield, T.W.; Hartwig, J.H.; Wagner, D.D. Extracellular DNA Traps Promote Thrombosis. *Proc. Natl. Acad. Sci. USA* **2010**, *107*, 15880–15885. [CrossRef]
40. Campos, A.; Scheveck, B.; Parikh, J.; Hernandez-Bojorge, S.; Terán, E.; Izurieta, R. Effect of Altitude on COVID-19 Mortality in Ecuador: An Ecological Study. *BMC Public Health* **2021**, *21*, 2079. [CrossRef] [PubMed]
41. Giamarellos-Bourboulis, E.J.; Poulakou, G.; de Nooijer, A.; Milionis, H.; Metallidis, S.; Ploumidis, M.; Grigoropoulou, P.; Rapti, A.; Segala, F.V.; Balis, E.; et al. Development and Validation of SCOPE Score: A Clinical Score to Predict COVID-19 Pneumonia Progression to Severe Respiratory Failure. *Cell Rep. Med.* **2022**, *3*, 100560. [CrossRef]

Disclaimer/Publisher's Note: The statements, opinions and data contained in all publications are solely those of the individual author(s) and contributor(s) and not of MDPI and/or the editor(s). MDPI and/or the editor(s) disclaim responsibility for any injury to people or property resulting from any ideas, methods, instructions or products referred to in the content.

MDPI AG
Grosspeteranlage 5
4052 Basel
Switzerland
Tel.: +41 61 683 77 34

MDPI Books Editorial Office
E-mail: books@mdpi.com
www.mdpi.com/books

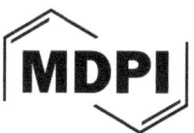

Disclaimer/Publisher's Note: The title and front matter of this reprint are at the discretion of the Topic Editors. The publisher is not responsible for their content or any associated concerns. The statements, opinions and data contained in all individual articles are solely those of the individual Editors and contributors and not of MDPI. MDPI disclaims responsibility for any injury to people or property resulting from any ideas, methods, instructions or products referred to in the content.

www.ingramcontent.com/pod-product-compliance
Lightning Source LLC
LaVergne TN
LVHW072357090526
838202LV00019B/2569